Autonomy and the Situated Self

Autonomy and the Situated Self

A Challenge to Bioethics

Rachel Haliburton

LEXINGTON BOOKS
Lanham • Boulder • New York • Toronto • Plymouth, UK

Published by Lexington Books
A wholly owned subsidiary of Rowman & Littlefield
4501 Forbes Boulevard, Suite 200, Lanham, Maryland 20706
www.rowman.com

10 Thornbury Road, Plymouth PL6 7PP, United Kingdom

British Library Cataloguing in Publication Information Available

Library of Congress Cataloging-in-Publication Data

Haliburton, Rachel Frances Christine, 1965-
Autonomy and the situated self : a challenge to bioethics / Rachel Haliburton.
pages cm.
Includes bibliographical references and index.
ISBN 978-0-7391-6871-4 (cloth : alk. paper) -- ISBN 978-0-7391-6872-1 (electronic)
1. Bioethics. I. Title.
QH332.H32 2014
174.2--dc23
2013032402

∞™ The paper used in this publication meets the minimum requirements of American
National Standard for Information Sciences Permanence of Paper for Printed Library
Materials, ANSI/NISO Z39.48-1992.

Printed in the United States of America

To my family

Contents

Acknowledgments

I would like to thank my friends and colleagues, Carol Collier, Mary Ann Corbiere, Susan Dodd, and Réal Fillion for their willingness to read drafts of this book. Your comments helped make the argument clearer and stronger, and your generosity in taking time from your own work to provide feedback on mine is very much appreciated.

Introduction

Bioethics tells a heroic story about its origins and purpose. The impetus for its contemporary development can be traced to concern about widespread paternalism in medicine, mistreatment of research subjects used in medical experimentation, and questions about the implication of technological developments in medical practice. Bioethics, then, began as a defender of the interests of patients and the rights of research participants, and understood itself to play an important role as a critic of powerful interests in medicine and in medical research. Bioethics has been phenomenally successful; since its modern incarnation (usually traced to the mid-1960s), it has spawned a multitude of academic journals, sponsored an innumerable number of conferences, found an important place for itself within universities and health care institutions, and given rise to the profession of "bioethicist." Bioethicists are considered qualified to make public pronouncements on issues of bioethical importance, to sit on Institutional Research Boards, and to guide others through the decision-making process when issues of bioethical concern arise. The bioethicist is seen by many—and often sees herself—to possess a particular kind of professional expertise, one that both legitimates the role she plays and makes her qualified to offer guidance and make judgments about issues of bioethical concern. The bioethicist, then, is a recognizable figure both within health care settings and outside of them: someone who occupies a respected place alongside physicians and hospital administrators, and who, like a lawyer or economist, can be called on by journalists to explain public events, or politicians, to help shape public policy. Both the attractiveness of bioethics as a field of study and research, and the respected place occupied by the bioethicist, are importantly predicated on the perception that bioethicists are willing to challenge medical practices if they conflict with the interests of patients, that they remain staunch defenders of the rights of research subjects, and that the purpose of bioethical argumentation, methodology, and education is, in large part, to protect the interests of the weak and vulnerable from mistreatment, exploitation, and harm.

This book offers a critique of contemporary bioethics, and of the way in which it has been co-opted by the very institutions it once sought (with good reason) to criticize and transform. In the process, it has become mainstream, moved from occupying the perspective of a critical outsider to enjoying the status of a respected insider, whose primary role is to defend both existing institutional arrangements and its own privileged position. It does this primarily through argumentation: by rigorously defending particular ways of thinking and acting, and by ruthlessly marginalizing or excluding alternative approaches. The mainstreaming of bioethics, then, has resulted in its domestication: it is at home in the institutions it would once have viewed with skepticism, and a central part of practices it would once have criticized. Consequently, I argue that, despite its very public successes, contemporary bioethics is largely failing to offer the ethical guidance it purports to be able to provide; that the move of the bioethicist from external critic of the medical system and critical observer of biomedical research to respected insider has encouraged many bioethicists to defend what they might once have criticized, and arguably still ought to; and that as the field has developed it has become increasing theoretically narrow, focused on procedural questions at the expense of substantive ethical analysis; self-congratulatory rather than self-aware or self-critical; and that mainstream bioethics and its practitioners serve as theoretical gatekeepers, who effectively exclude perspectives and claims that might challenge their assumptions and methods. The critique I offer considers the dominant theoretical claims, methods, activities, commitments, and assumptions of contemporary bioethics from a philosophical perspective.

The nature of this critique requires me to move between theory and practice, between abstract theoretical claims to first-person experiential accounts, and to take seriously ethical perspectives that mainstream bioethics marginalizes, dismisses, or towards which it is sometimes actively hostile. My claims, therefore, and the way in which they are made, are likely to be, at least initially, unfamiliar and perhaps unpersuasive to those who accept the parameters, methods, and assumptions of contemporary mainstream bioethics, so I want to set out, in this introduction, a brief account of the reasons for which I have engaged in this critique, describe the arc of the argument I present, and make some positive proposals for a richer and more complex model of bioethics than that which currently prevails.

I have taught courses in bioethics at the university level for nearly twenty years, have co-authored a bioethics textbook, and have participated on a number of ethics committees in various health care institutions, ranging from hospital, to hospice, to long-term care home. I began my work in bioethics with enthusiasm, seeing it as a discipline that had the power to provide important guidance to those tasked with making difficult ethical choices, as a necessary component of the education of any student planning to enter the medical field, and as a provider of the theoretical resources required to transform health care institutions into more ethical places. I became increasingly puzzled, however, by the difficulties many of my students were experiencing understanding the ethical framework provided by mainstream bioethics—by their inability to grasp the creative tension between Kantian commitments and utilitarian ones, or to understand how these commitments related to the important place currently occupied by autonomy. Moreover, I also became increasingly frustrated by my experiences on ethics committees: why were so many of the meetings I attended endless replays of the same issues? Why were staff members so reluctant to use the ethics tools we provided, and to bring ethical concerns forward? And why did these committees exist, anyway, since any attempt to make significant changes to institutional procedures was met with the response by administrators that the policies of the institution took precedence over any proposals made by the ethics committee?

I gradually came to the realization that, in practice, there was a significant gap between what bioethics purported to be able to do—namely, help individuals make better decisions when faced with ethical dilemmas in the context of health care, and make health care institutions into better, more ethically sound places—and what it actually seemed to be able to do. While mainstream bioethics did, indeed, provide frameworks through which ethical dilemmas could be filtered, articulated principles to be balanced in the course of making decisions, and offered a mechanism by which the resulting decision could be defended, it became increasingly unclear to me what made those decisions "ethical" ones, or what the bioethicist was offering that the thoughtful physician, caring nurse, responsible chaplain, or dedicated social worker would be unable to provide, at least given sufficient time and resources. Not that all physicians were thoughtful, or all nurses caring, of course, but this was a different issue from the question of what the bioethicist was offering, and, anyway, not an issue that needed the expertise of the bioethicist to be addressed: the real question was, how would the institution, its policies and practices, be any different if the bioethicist was not there, and if the ethics committee did not exist?

My practical experiences, then, led me to identify two sets of questions that were of philosophical significance. First, what is the precise nature of the professional expertise possessed by the bioethicist, and why is it thought to be needed in modern health care institutions? What distinguishes it from the ethical expertise possessed by others who can also be found there, such as personal support workers, addictions counselors, social workers, and chaplains, whose jobs all involve caring for patients in various ways, and require that their interests be protected and their concerns taken seriously?

Second, if such expertise actually exists, what did it mean that so many of the efforts of the various ethics committees in a variety of institutions of which I was a member were so unsuccessful, that there was such a gap between what we thought we were offering, and what was actually happening (very little) as a result of our efforts? Physicians tended to see the ethics committee, its policies and "tools" as superfluous to their professional activities, administrators needed to have an ethics committee as part of their risk management strategies and accreditation requirements, but didn't want to allocate much staff time to ethics education, and as for the staff themselves—well, they appeared to find our tools, no matter how many times we refined or simplified them, as both confusing and unhelpful. Moreover, this gap seemed to be endemic to most ethics committees, rather than afflicting only particular ones; colleagues reported similar experiences and frustrations as they worked with other committees and institutions, which suggested that the problem was systemic rather than discrete. Was the problem simply that bioethics, its commitments, methods, and principles, were not yet fully a part of the culture of these institutions? If so, then we just needed to work harder to ensure that they were fully integrated at all levels of the organization. As time passed, however, this simple answer seemed increasingly implausible: the institutions did give bioethics a central space, adopting Mission Statements, Codes Of Ethics, Patient Bills Of Rights, and so on, but these things seemed to make very little difference to the way that they actually ran.

At the same time as I was becoming aware that bioethics, in practice, seemed largely ineffective, despite its very public successes in being incorporated into the workings of health care organizations, I was growing increasingly dissatisfied, philosophically speaking, with the theoretical claims made by academic bioethicists, and the confidence and certainty with which sometimes astonishingly implausible conclusions were reached and the assertive form in which they were defended. Why, for example, were bioethicists so quick to welcome the encroachment of the market into every sphere of human activity, and to argue that the selling of organs by impoverished individuals in the third world should be understood as a free and equal win-win transaction for both buyer and seller? Why was bioethical discourse so comfortable with young women acting as paid surrogates, seeing this (again) simply as a freely chosen activity and one, moreover, that demonstrated female empowerment in action? How could bioethicists describe genetic enhancements of offspring in order to facilitate parental desires to have a particular kind of child not as a potentially disturbing extension of parental control over children, but as something that merely follows from respecting the right of parents to make autonomous choices?

Even when these larger issues were considered, the role played by the market in many areas of health care, reproductive choice, and pharmaceutical research went almost unchallenged. Why, when it came to matters of distributive justice, were so many bioethicists content to concentrate most of their attention on the question of what procedures should be used to distribute goods within a health care system, rather than on larger social, economic, and political questions, which consider who has easiest access to health care, and take seriously the fact that both health status and the outcomes of many medical treatments are correlated as much with socioeconomic status as they are to freely made lifestyle choices? The commitment to protect the weak and vulnerable, and to hold the powerful to account, that was so much a part of modern bioethics in its early years seemed largely to have disappeared.

These positions, moreover, had something of an air of orthodoxy about them: as long as they resulted from an application of the correct principles and were filtered through the appropriate procedures, to disagree with them was to render one something of a heretic, whose views did not need to be taken seriously. Mainstream bioethics, it was becoming clear, worked only within a very specific theoretical framework, and considered only a small number of perspectives to be legitimate participants in any debate.

Over nearly two decades, then, I experienced increasing dissatisfaction and even frustration with both bioethical theory and what I saw of bioethics in practice. I began to wonder whether there was not a connection: perhaps bioethics in practice didn't work well—or worked well only if one was willing to make, and to stick with, a number of implausible and difficult-to-justify working assumptions—because of its theoretical commitments. Moreover, I now believe that my increased dissatisfaction and frustration was generated, at least in large part, not only by my wider theoretical knowledge and extensive personal experience, but because over this period mainstream bioethics itself has been growing ever more procedural in method and ever more narrow in focus; indeed, some perspectives which were considered not only legitimate but important in the early years of bioethics have little or no place today, and the powerful critique of mainstream bioethics offered by feminist theorists has been largely ignored.

There is arguably a connection between the dramatic public success bioethics has enjoyed and its domestication. As it has narrowed its ethical focus and restricted the scope of what constitute legitimate theoretical perspectives and approaches, it has become more focused on procedural questions than on substantive ones. When bioethical issues are constructed in this way, they can be addressed through creating and applying the correct policies and procedures, instead of requiring that medical institutions and research practices be transformed or overhauled in any significant way. Bioethics has become so successful, that is to say, precisely because it no longer offers any kind of a threat; instead, it serves to provide a form of ethical legitimation to institutions and practices that does not require them to change in any substantial way.

Daniel Callahan, an important figure in the development of modern bioethics who has now become critical of its present form argues that bioethics has become strikingly ideological, functioning on the basis of a set of political and social commitments which serve "as a vital constellation of values" which reflect "the almost complete triumph of liberal individualism . . ."[1] While "liberal individualism does not function as a moral theory as philosophers have understood that concept, it is clearly present and pervasive as a litmus test of the acceptability of certain ideas and ways of framing issues."[2] As such, it shapes both what *can* be said, and *how* it can be said: "As a familiar constellation, it encompasses a high place for autonomy, for biomedical progress with few constraints, for procedural rather than substantive solutions to controverted ethical problems, and for a strong antipathy to comprehensive notions of the human good."[3]

Callahan observes that this form of bioethics marginalizes conservative and religious perspectives, treating them with "disdain and hostility."[4] I would add that it treats perspectives from the left (such as socialist or Marxist approaches), as well as those that don't fall neatly into the dichotomies of right-left, conservative-liberal, or religious-secular, such as feminism and virtue ethics, in much the same way: they, too, are marginalized and treated with disdain and hostility. And I would go further: any perspective which takes a substantive approach to questions of the human good (or even makes use of terms like "the human good"), which describes autonomy in relational rather than individualistic terms, which centers on virtues rather than principles, which makes issues of social and economic justice central rather than peripheral to its analysis, or which draws on theoretical resources which go beyond the bounds of an analytic and procedural method of conceptualizing the issues, is marginalized and dismissed.

This is a loss for bioethics, and it generates an impoverished version of what bioethics is, or might become. Philosophically speaking, some of the most interesting and compelling work in ethical theory is taking place within the contexts provided by feminist and narrative ethics, and some of the most challenging, radical, and potentially transformative ethical propositions are being put forward by those who draw on the resources provided by virtue ethics: to see these perspectives and approaches marginalized or dismissed by mainstream bioethics is understandable—it protects the privileged place bioethics now occupies within institutions whose practices these approaches would require it to critique—but it is theoretically problematic.

While Callahan, I believe, is correct to assert both that mainstream bioethics has become a form of ideology, with all the narrowness and limitations that that implies, and that underlying many standard bioethical positions and lines of argument is an (often unacknowledged) commitment to liberal individualism, the ideological assumptions of contemporary bioethics are more complex than his account suggests. Indeed, if this was all there was to mainstream bioethics, it would be both required to defend its liberal commitments more explicitly, coherently, and robustly than it currently does, and could be more easily dismissed as a partisan approach that can legitimately be challenged by those on the right and the left, and by those working within a feminist, narrative, virtue-based, or religious context. While mainstream bioethics works within a liberal framework, it both detaches that framework from the serious commitment to social and political justice that liberalism as a political theory requires, with all the trade-offs and economic disruption that such commitments might sometimes involve, and supplements it with a thoroughgoing acceptance of the market as an appropriate mechanism for regulating and facilitating autonomous choice; with ethical principles drawn largely from watered down versions of Kantian and utilitarian ethical theory, but which are claimed to encompass other values as well; and with a collection of decision-making procedures which purport to be rational in origin and universal in scope.

These supplementations allow bioethicists working within the mainstream to assert both that any insights that the virtue ethicist might offer are encompassed by the principled approach properly understood, and that virtue ethics is a subordinate and outdated approach that does not need to be taken seriously; to assure feminists that their concerns about gender can be dealt with when autonomy is adequately respected; to respond to those who work with narrative ethics that an analysis of stories is not a proper subject matter for philosophers, and that experiential accounts (which are neither rational nor universally applicable) should be treated with suspicion; and to tell those who explore bioethical questions from a religious perspective that they have nothing legitimate to say, unless and until they can translate their claims into terms which are rational, secular, and universal, and which demonstrate sufficient respect for individualism and autonomy.

Contemporary mainstream bioethics, then, has become ideological, but the form this ideology takes, while narrow, is multifaceted rather than one-dimensional. Because it is multifaceted, procedurally-based, committed to an individualistic understanding of autonomy, and organized around a relatively small set of principles, it is useful and effective in much the same way that utilitarianism can be useful and effective: as long as one is willing to work within the theoretical framework provided, apply the procedures which follow from it, and make the ethical commitments it requires, it can be an efficient way to make decisions. However, it is also often the case that the procedures produce results that seem unsatisfactory, or even beside the point: for example, if it is indeed the case that autonomous individuals ought to be left free to make their own choices in a medical context, unless those choices are harmful to others, then why engage in an ethical analysis at all rather than simply asking them what they want and determining whether what they want is affordable? The mainstreaming and domestication of bioethics, then, has so distorted the ethical commitments that inspired the creation of modern bioethics in the first place that much of the practical work that bioethicists do no longer makes sense. As a result, health care workers participating in "ethics education" workshops, or other members of ethics committees, often respond to the concepts presented by bioethicists, and to the decision-making frameworks they offer, with a mixture of bafflement and frustration: do we have to learn so much, do so much work, in order to discover that there are no right answers, and that we should respect the client's wishes, if possible?

Moreover, the assumptions needed to make the machinery of mainstream bioethics work (for instance, that it still makes sense to talk of free and autonomous choice in the context of serious illness and approaching death when the only options available are limited and unwanted, that the choice to have a child and the choice not to have a child are simply equivalent to one another, that clear and freely made autonomous choices should always be sought and respected, except when it's desirable to increase the number of organs available for transplant, in which case presumed consent is acceptable, and so on) seem as implausible and unconvincing as those required to get a fully fledged utilitarian or religious perspective off the ground.

Further, while the multifaceted nature of the constellation of ideas that compose mainstream bioethics combined with its ideological rigidity may help it defend itself from a variety of external criticisms, they also create internal tensions: they require bioethicists to alternate between Kantian assumptions and utilitarian ones, to accept liberal individualism but to detach it from its original home in political theory which provided individual choices with a context, and to argue that a commitment to autonomy doesn't require that the experiential accounts of patients ought to be taken seriously, as long as their right to make their own choices has been respected. In this book I argue that one source of these internal tensions lies in the fact that it makes use of incompatible conceptions of the self, incompatible understandings, that is to say, of what constitutes a moral agent, what it is that ought to move that agent to action, and what features distinguish an ethical choice from an unethical one. The way in which these diverse theoretical strands are drawn together in mainstream bioethics culminates in a conception of autonomy that revolves around the figure of the Choosing Self. It is this conception of autonomy that is largely assumed in contemporary bioethical discussions, and it is the desires of the Choosing Self that bioethics takes as givens, and the choices of the Choosing Self that bioethicists work to facilitate and defend.

While mainstream bioethics is multifaceted, all of its parts arguably fall within what Margaret Urban Walker calls a theoretical-juridical model of morality. This model is not itself a moral theory. Rather, "it is a kind of template for organizing moral inquiry into the pursuit of a certain kind of moral theory."[5] This model views morality "as a compact, propositionally codifiable, impersonally action-guiding code within an agent, or as a compact set of law-like propositions that 'explain' the moral behavior of a well-formed moral agent."[6] She contrasts the theoretical-juridical model of morality with a model she calls expressive-collaborative. Approaches which fall into the expressive-collaborative model focus as much on relationships as they do on individuals; take actual experiences as seriously as they do theoretical commitments; and, while not relativistic, see ethics as something that we create together, in particular times and places, rather than as something that results solely from the exercise of reason, which could emerge from one person's deliberations as long as that person is sufficiently rational and intelligent, and which purport to be universal in scope. Expressive-collaborative approaches usually lack the theoretical clarity and procedural certainties provided by theoretical-juridical approaches, but they also tend to be more open to competing perspectives, more creative, and more potentially transformative. Moreover, from the perspective of those working within the expressive-collaborative template, the clarity and certainty provided by their theoretical-juridical rivals is both illusory and costly. They are clear only because they ask us to leave out of our deliberations so much of what we might legitimately consider, certain only because they rigorously exclude competing perspectives, illusory because their advocates believe that their approach can satisfactorily cover all that needs to be said about the nature of ethics, and costly, because they ignore so many important elements of human experience. Two important perspectives that Walker identifies as falling within the scope of expressive-collaborative approaches are feminist ethics and virtue ethics; narrative ethics can be found on this side of the ledger as well.

The approach I defend in this book locates itself within the template provided by expressive-collaborative approaches, draws on theoretical sources that are already present in the bioethical literature but which have not been fully or extensively incorporated within standard discussions, and it is from this perspective that I critique what currently constitutes the theoretical commitments, methodology, and scope of mainstream bioethics. This critique, and the positive proposals which emerge from it, not only takes a theoretical position that self-consciously situates its analysis outside the theoretical-juridical template, but one that is committed to the belief that philosophical analysis can take different forms and employ multiple resources. It is only from a position outside the theoretical-juridical template that the assumptions of approaches that fall within it can be both adequately viewed and their methods and assumptions critiqued; any arguments that are made from within it necessarily must assume precisely what I want to question, and employ the methodology that I want to reject.

Consequently, the content, method, and tone of the critique I offer and of the positive proposals I present, as noted above, will be unfamiliar and may be unpersuasive to some; my argument may even be considered not to be *real* moral philosophy, if real moral philosophy is understood to follow the parameters set out by the theoretical-juridical template. But I believe that the subject matter considered by bioethics is important, and that it can do better; that it should be more philosophical and less ideological; that it should become more open to diverse perspectives and function less like a theoretical gatekeeper whose job it is to exclude them; and the arguments I present in this book and the way in which they are presented is meant to be a contribution to what I hope will be an ongoing conversation about what bioethics is and what it might become.

I propose that bioethics should make use of the resources provided by a contemporary version of virtue ethics, one that employs a conception of autonomy that is both relational and sees the self as situated within a rich moral universe in which experiential accounts and stories are considered to be sources of ethical knowledge, feminist concerns about gender, power, and exploitation are taken to be of fundamental, rather than peripheral, importance, and which locates the virtues in practices which are nurtured or hindered by particular institutional, social, economic, and political arrangements. Autonomy, like justice, is a concept that is rich enough to generate competing conceptions, and out of the theoretical resources provided by these various expressive-collaborative perspectives, I generate a conception of autonomy that stands as a counterweight to the version that currently dominates in mainstream bioethics. The model of the self that lies at the center of this expressive-collaborative conception of autonomy, and around which this conception revolves, I call the Situated Self. It is this Situated Self that I propose as a competitor to the Choosing Self. What I offer in this book, then, is both an analysis and critique of the conception of autonomy that is assumed in contemporary bioethics, the model of the self that results from this conception, and the consequences for bioethics of giving these things a central role. In addition, I propose an alternative conception of autonomy, one that is animated by a competing model of the self, and which can, I argue, better accommodate the ethical commitments that gave rise to the creation of bioethics in the first place.

Ironically, I believe that the very success that bioethics has enjoyed represents the most serious danger it faces: as it has grown to play an increasingly visible public role and to occupy an important place within the academy and within health care institutions, it has become both less self-reflective and less critical of powerful elements within society and within medicine than its origin story suggests it should be. Bioethicists have become protective of their status as respected insiders, and, as they have done so, they have become increasingly dismissive of ethical perspectives that might require them to criticize the activities that take place within the institutions that employ them. However, given that the original success of bioethics was predicated on its outsider status, on its willingness to criticize the status quo in order to protect the interests of patients and the rights of research subjects, its credibility depends on its commitment to challenge authority when necessary.

If mainstream bioethics doesn't change its ideological ways, refuses to risk its insider status by offending those with power and authority, or, indeed, becomes part of the power structures and institutional arrangements it once saw as its role to question, then it increasingly won't matter whether it exists at all. It will do little to ensure that health care institutions are ethical places, and will not be taken seriously by those who might require its help; instead, it will be viewed with suspicion, having become an integral part of the system it once challenged, and a defender of practices it would once have criticized. Either bioethics must overhaul itself from within, or another external approach is likely to appear to challenge it in turn, and, perhaps, eventually take its place. In the meantime, philosophical bioethics will be less effective than it should be in performing its central task: helping us to think clearly about issues of ethical importance in health care, protecting the interests of research subjects, and ensuring that the experiences patients have meet not only their medical needs, but that their suffering is acknowledged.

The argument falls into two parts and so does the book. The first part is an analysis of contemporary mainstream bioethics. This part of the argument sets out the framework of mainstream bioethics, and traces the theoretical sources that have led to the utter dominance of (a particular conception of) autonomy in bioethics today. This part of the argument follows lines of moral theorizing that fall into the theoretical-juridical model. Chapter 1 considers the "creation myth" offered by contemporary bioethics, and shows how elements of this myth are tied to the place currently occupied by principles in bioethical reasoning. Chapter 2 explores the tension between utilitarian considerations and Kantian ones, and the way in which this tension has shaped many aspects of discussions in bioethics, and why these tensions seem impossible to resolve. The fact that these important moral theories each seem to capture crucial insights that cannot be reconciled with one another has contributed to the place currently occupied by autonomy in bioethics: if we have no good way of choosing between Kantian intuitions and utilitarian ones, rather than making substantive moral claims, the default position becomes to simply ask people what they want. Consequently, within bioethics today, a lot of attention is paid to the concept of autonomy and what respect for it requires. Chapter 3 explores the conception of the self-employed within liberal political theory, and identifies ways in which this conception has been utilized within bioethics, since it is liberalism that provides the main theoretical foundation of bioethical claims about autonomy and clearly articulates why it is important that individuals be free to make their own choices.

Chapter 4, however, argues that this liberal self-employed within mainstream bioethics has now become almost entirely detached from liberal commitments, and therefore lacks the resources that liberalism provides to help shape individual choices, and to ask important questions about social and economic justice. Indeed, it is because it lacks these resources, perhaps, that it has largely allowed the market to determine which choices are available to individuals, and how these choices are facilitated. The dominance of this conception—and the figure of the Choosing Self that results from it—generates the paradox that bioethics conceived of in this way no longer needs bioethicists because it requires that bioethicists make no substantive ethical claims (except, of course, about the value of this conception of autonomy). This is the point at which bioethics becomes largely procedurally driven, and has very little of ethical importance to say. It is this form of bioethics that, I argue, is both self-defeating and ultimately unsustainable.

The second part of the argument (beginning with a discussion of feminist approaches to bioethics) considers some other approaches to bioethics that fall within the expressive-collaborative model. These feminist approaches are considered in chapter 5; they are important because, in addition to demonstrating what an approach that is expressive-collaborative in nature might look like, they both highlight important assumptions and omissions in contemporary mainstream bioethics, and illustrate the role played by mainstream bioethics (and bioethicists) in excluding competing perspectives from the discussion of bioethical issues. Feminist bioethicists are very clear that they only get to be considered "real" bioethicists if they give up their feminist commitments, and, as long as they refuse to do this, they are thought to have little of significance to say. Chapter 6 introduces virtue ethics, an approach to ethics that has been treated as subordinate to its competitors by many contemporary theorists, but which, I argue, provides important ethical insights that are difficult to find in other approaches. Virtue ethics also, in a contemporary form, can, I believe, encompass the insights of feminist approaches, and can also provide a foundation for a conception of autonomy that is not detached from questions of meaning and value, but which is firmly connected to substantive concerns about what might make some choices better than others. It is this conception of autonomy that is embodied in the figure of the Situated Self.

The next two chapters consider the role of narratives in bioethics, and the way that a literary consideration of case studies and first-person accounts of the experience of illness can provide important ethical insights that bioethicists should take seriously, and help us fill out in more detail what situated autonomy might look like. These chapters, then, articulate additional dimensions of the autonomy-based, neo-Aristotelian model of bioethics that I am proposing.

The final chapter squarely confronts the likelihood that the very success bioethics has enjoyed has become its greatest weakness: there is increasing evidence that, as bioethicists have become an important part of the medical and research systems they once challenged, they see their role not to be primarily concerned with the protection of patients and research subjects, but, rather, to protect their own professional positions by ensuring that the ethical analysis they provide lends support to the practices of that system, and protection to the medical practitioners and researchers within it. Unfortunately, the moral framework of mainstream bioethics—which ends up ensuring only that autonomy (understood simply as lying in choice) is protected, that questions of the good are explored in procedural rather than substantive ways, and that the market is allowed almost unfettered permission to shape health care and pharmaceutical research—not only lacks the moral resources required to evaluate itself, but, even more profoundly, embodies, in its moral framework and operating assumptions, much of what it should question. It is not only the case, that is to say, that mainstream bioethics largely *lacks* the resources required to evaluate itself; in addition, given what it actively endorses, it *can't* question certain practices which, from other perspectives, might be understood to be ethically problematic or even straightforwardly unethical.

Bioethics, I conclude, needs to question its own assumptions and current place, and, because the only way it can do this is by grounding itself differently, must reconstruct itself on a different basis. Alasdair MacIntyre's revolutionary Aristotelianism, supplemented by the feminist and narrative approaches considered in the second part of the book, provides a way to accomplish these goals. The final chapter, then, connects virtue-based ethical reflection within bioethics to larger questions of political, economic, and social justice. It also argues that bioethicists need to be constantly aware of the danger of co-option by the values of the institutions that employ them, and vigilant in their commitment to remaining self-critical and self-questioning.

In conclusion, then, the argument I offer is one that seeks to provide a basis upon which bioethics can better do justice to the ethical concerns and commitments that led to its creation and inspired its early practitioners. Mainstream bioethics, as currently constituted, has so depleted the theoretical resources upon which it draws that it is increasingly unable to make substantive ethical claims, and, as a result of the conception of autonomy it endorses, has found itself in a position in which it must defend what it would once have critiqued and can offer little guidance to those who must make difficult decisions in their own lives. In its present form, mainstream bioethics makes choices empty, procedures paramount, and questions of social and economic justice peripheral rather than central.

The alternative framework I propose is one that allows bioethicists to make substantive moral judgments and to engage in robust ethical debate without giving up a commitment to autonomy. Indeed, I argue that this conception of autonomy, and the framework for ethical thinking it requires, will better allow bioethics to achieve its goals of protecting the vulnerable and allowing individuals to make choices that are genuinely their own than it is currently able to, and will provide bioethicists with a basis on which to offer the kind of ethical guidance that justifies their claim to possess an important and unique kind of professional expertise.

NOTES

1. Daniel Callahan, "Individual Good and Common Good: A Communitarian Approach To Bioethics," *Perspectives in Biology and Medicine* 46, No. 4 (Autumn 2003): 496–507.

2. Callahan, "Individual Good and Common Good," 498.

3. Callahan, "Individual Good and Common Good," 498.

4. Callahan, "Individual Good and Common Good," 498.

5. Walker, Margaret Urban, *Moral Understandings: A Feminist Study In Ethics*, 2nd Ed. (Oxford: Oxford University Press, 2007), 7–8.

6. Walker, *Moral Understandings*, 8.

1

Contemporary Mainstream Bioethics

Chapter One

The Chimeric Self

Exploring the Landscape of Bioethics

INTRODUCTION: THE BIOETHICIST AND THE ETHICS COMMITTEE

The scene has now become familiar to me, and the parts the participants play predictable. I find myself sitting around a big table; my companions are people working in various aspects of health care: as physicians, as directors of long-term care facilities, as hospital administrators who determine how health care resources are distributed, or as chaplains in hospice or palliative care. We are all members of the institutional ethics committee. I am there as an ethicist, the person who in this role is supposed to help these people and the organizations they represent work through ethical issues, build "ethics capacity" in their institutions, create codes of ethics, and develop worksheets to guide the ethical decision making of employees. I am usually not the first ethicist to sit on a particular committee, and, sometimes, I exchange places with one of my colleagues so that the committee doesn't get stale, stuck in a rut. What is striking, however, is that nothing much ever seems to happen in the way of demonstrably advancing the role of ethics within the organization: we create new "ethics tools" (a refinement of our Ethics Guidelines, perhaps); we sponsor educational seminars for employees; we worry about how the "values statement" of the organization fits with professional Codes of Conduct, and with the actual practices of the institution; and we engage in variations on the same conversation: how can we ensure that employees behave ethically? How can we demonstrate that ethics are "lived" in the hospital (or hospice, or long-term care home)? Why can't we get staff to make use of the tools we provide? And why given that Ethics Committees are invariably created by administrators or boards do we find it so hard to persuade upper management that if they *really* want to run an institution that clearly functions in accordance with its stated ethical values, the institution must do more than simply cite a value when a workplace policy is created?

This is a book about contemporary bioethics; more particularly, it is a book about the gap between what bioethics purports to be able to do, namely, help people analyze, work through, and then make sound ethical decisions in the context of health care and what it actually does, which is generate both an extraordinarily extensive array of ethical "tools" and academic documents policies, frameworks, guidelines, principles, Codes, values statements, journals, and books, and an interminable discussion about what bioethics is, how it should be done, and its proper role in addressing practical ethical questions, without actually providing the ethical assistance upon which its existence is predicated.

After working in the field of bioethics for almost twenty years, what has become striking to me is how much the field of bioethics promises in the way of providing ethical clarity and practical guidance, and how little of either it actually seems able to provide. Many people have made successful careers as bioethicists; they provide media commentaries when stories with bioethical implications make headlines, they teach in universities and medical schools, and they provide policy advice to governments. Academic texts on bioethics and journals devoted to the subject abound; and bioethicists occupy an increasingly important role within many health care institutions. Moreover, bioethics plays a prominent social role in contemporary North American society. Despite all this activity, both theoretical and practical, bioethics has reached something of an impasse. While there is a general consensus on some theoretical positions—for example, in North America, paternalism within medicine has been largely replaced by the doctrine of informed consent—many of the issues with which bioethicists concern themselves remain intransigent. For example, the health care institutions I am familiar with are still at a loss to know what to do with "noncompliant" patients who won't do what seems to be clearly in their best interests, or when the family members of non-competent patients disagree about their treatment, which suggests that the theoretical move from paternalism to informed consent hasn't helped to resolve ethical issues around treatment decisions as much as might have been expected, given all the time and attention paid to the concept of informed consent, and the development of procedures meant to facilitate its exercise. Conversely, a number of the positions around which something of a consensus has been reached—such as the widespread acceptance that the sale of reproductive materials such as sperm, and the anonymity that usually accompanies that exchange, raise few, if any, ethical concerns—seem to justify practices that raise serious ethical questions. Given that decades worth of evidence from the practice of adoption clearly reveals that keeping secret information about biological parenthood has been damaging to many adoptees, why would so many bioethicists reach the conclusion that the experience of persons produced through sperm donation would be different? Indeed, why do so many bioethicists persist in calling a commercial transaction of this sort a "donation"?

When I began working in this field, I was able to articulate the ethical theories usually identified as the basis of bioethical reasoning with conviction. I was also able to present the principles, frameworks, and guidelines for ethical decision-making that arise from them with confidence because I believed that they could, indeed, help people "work through" ethical dilemmas so that they could make decisions that they could justify on ethical grounds. However, the gap between what bioethics purports to be able to do and its difficulty in actually performing those tasks points to a deep and philosophically interesting problem.

I now think that this impasse is generated by the fact that there is a fundamental incoherency at the heart of contemporary bioethics, one that results, at least in part, from the presence of competing and incompatible conceptions of the self. These conceptions tend to be implicit and therefore largely invisible, but they help shape what is seen to be morally significant: they tell us what is important and what is not, what a human being is and how creatures of this sort should behave, and how we should respond when we are threatened with infirmity, illness, and death. These conceptions, therefore, shape not only what are understood to be adequate responses to the ethical dilemmas that arise in medicine, but also, and even more fundamentally, how we identify and describe the dilemma in the first place, and the sort of reasoning we engage in as we consider it. An approach that is based on incompatible and competing conceptions of the self, given the central role that these conceptions play in our ethical thinking, is itself likely to be both theoretically incoherent and practically unhelpful. Moreover, because these conceptions are largely unseen, their role in generating conflicting moral rules and incompatible understandings of what is at stake in moral dilemmas goes largely unnoticed.

MORAL UNIVERSES AND CONCEPTIONS OF THE SELF

Sandel has observed that every political philosophy is predicated on a "philosophical anthropology"[1] which provides a conception of the person who is the central actor in that philosophy. Ethical theories, I argue, likewise presuppose an "ethical anthropology": a conception of the self which describes the most fundamental aspects of our humanity, and which sets out, on the basis of this description, instructions for the way in which each of us ought to treat other selves. Many moral philosophers use the term "person" in much the

same way I am using the term "self," namely, to encompass a list of fundamental human characteristics, and to designate those beings towards whom
we have moral obligations. Warren offers a simple test to distinguish persons
from non-persons (or to use my preferred terminology, selves from non-
selves): if a space traveler were to land on a strange planet occupied by
previously unencountered organisms, her first task would be "to determine
whether they are people and thus have full moral rights, or whether they are
things that she need not feel guilty about treating . . . as a source of food."[2]
There is no uncontroversial list of characteristics that constitute personhood
or selfhood, and there is no universal agreement on necessary or sufficient
criteria for self or personhood.[3] While the concepts of "self" and "person"
are indeed closely connected, they have slightly different connotations. I will
use the term "self" to indicate not only the externally observable presence of
certain criteria that allow us to recognize other beings as "persons" in the
sense that Warren employs, but also an internal awareness of one's own
mental states and personal identity which allow for the possibility of mutual
recognition between one self and another. This shifts the Warren test from
asking us to consider what other beings we would consider to be persons—as
entities towards whom we have moral obligations—to asking what beings
would have the capacity to recognize us in this way, as creatures towards
whom they have similar obligations. The distinction between "self" and "person" is rough, and any definition of either is likely to be incomplete and
contested; however, it does have important applications in bioethics because
it allows us to recognize (and to treat) the severely demented, infants, and
PVS patients as persons without expecting from them the full capacities of
responsiveness and engagement with others that we expect from *selves.*

Any ethical theory must provide some account of who *counts* as a being
towards whom moral obligations exist and who does not, whom we can
relate to as fellow citizens, who can relate to us in the same way, and what
we can eat for supper. These ethical anthropologies are crucially important,
often invisible or deeply hidden, and ultimately unavoidable. The particular
content of each anthropology is fundamental to the structure of the ethical
theory within which it is embedded: it is implicated in claims about what
constitutes rational choice, who counts as persons in the morally relevant
sense and why, and even what sorts of political arrangements and social
policies should be designed for this sort of self.[4] These ethical anthropologies
can remain hidden because they are usually presented as straightforward,
commonsense descriptions of what people actually are—at least if they
understand themselves correctly.[5]

Many contemporary theorists are suspicious of "all-encompassing models
of the self" because they see them as closely tied to overarching claims about
human nature, which ignore diversity and cultural differences.[6] However,
even to offer a *criticism* of such "all-encompassing" conceptions requires one

to have a different model against which the conception being criticized can be measured and found wanting. Conceptions of the self, then, are unavoidable and inescapable, whether they are presented in the form of particular carefully elaborated conceptual creations, or take less explicit and articulated forms, being embodied in practices, or revealed through the stories we tell and the ethical commitments we make. They are what ground our moral, social, and political assumptions; underpin our arguments about how we ought to live and what choices we ought to make; and account for many of our moral intuitions—the "gut-feelings" that we cannot always rationally defend and articulate but which can shape our perceptions of what is most fundamentally at stake in moral debates.

Ethical theories, in short, cannot function unless they provide, either implicitly or explicitly, a description of the sorts of creatures that count as persons, and as selves, in the relevant way. It is often easier to see the work that *someone else's* conception of the self is doing in his ethical thinking (particularly if we disagree with his assumptions and conclusions) than it is to see our own ethical anthropologies, even as they help us conceive and articulate our own values in the arguments we make and the conclusions we reach. Our opponents have flawed conceptions of the self; we are simply describing human beings as they really are.[7]

While conceptions of the self-play a crucially important role in shaping how we understand the world along its ethical dimensions (it makes an enormous difference, for example, whether we understand our selfhood to lie in our capacity to be autonomous choosers who can create our own systems of value, or see ourselves as embodied souls, whose primary purpose is to discover and respond to the demands of a divine creator) and in distinguishing those with whom we share moral space from objects that merely occupy physical space, what it is to be a self is difficult to pin down. Indeed, one might say that the complexity of the question of what it is to be a self is most clearly seen when we consider other questions that are connected to it. These questions include: Who are you? Who are we? And, who am I? What holds us together as one person over time? Where is "selfhood" located? In our capacity to reason? In our practices? In telling certain kinds of stories about ourselves, both to ourselves, and to others? In our embodiment? In our relationships with others, and in our capacity to enter into such relationships? Consider, for example, the way in which we might address the issue of abortion. The questions we ask, what values we believe to be most fundamentally at stake, and the conclusions we draw will all be shaped by the conception of the self we are (explicitly or implicitly) employing in our deliberations. If we believe that a fetus meets the requirements of selfhood as we understand them, we are unlikely to think that abortion can be justified, regardless of the particular circumstances in which someone might want to choose this option. If we see selfhood as residing in the capacity to be an autonomous chooser (a capacity that a fetus has clearly not yet achieved), then, not only are we unlikely to see the fetus as a self, but we will also be suspicious of any attempts to restrict individual choice when it comes to abortion. And, finally, if we conceive of the self as inescapably gendered and embodied, we will wonder why the protagonists in the abortion debate pay so little attention to the moral significance of the fact that only women can become pregnant.

However we answer these questions, as we have seen, there seems to be something reflexive about the notion of selfhood: we need other selves to recognize us as selves, just as we recognize them, and our selfhood seems to consist, at least in part, in this mutual recognition. As Todd May puts it, "The question of who we are . . . [is concerned with] who each of us is in our various groupings: who you are and who I am and who each of the other folks that we share the planet with is."[8] Christman argues, even more strongly, that selfhood is intimately tied up in the question of how others see us, and how we want them to see us: "Who should I say you are . . . ?"[9] It is because of this reflexivity, this mutual recognition required for attributions of selfhood, that questions of selfhood are so intimately tied up with questions of who *counts*, morally speaking: are (at least some) non-human animals selves in ways that we can recognize? If so, then it would follow that we have at least some moral obligations to them. And what sorts of human beings fall into (or out of) the category of selves: if embryos are not selves, where do we place them within moral space? When in our development do we move from persons towards whom moral obligations are owed, to selves, which can recognize the moral obligations that they have to others? What happens to selfhood as persons experience the progression of dementia?

In order to answer or, more precisely, begin to determine how we would answer any of these questions, we must presuppose, implicitly assume, or explicitly assert a particular ethical anthropology, and this assumption or assertion shapes how we understand our choices, our emotions, our selves, other people, and the world we share with one another. Consider three different accounts of selfhood and how each shapes the understanding of those who endorse it. First, if one believes that selfhood lies in the capacity to reason, and that the mind and body are distinct from one another, then it does not matter, in any significant way, in terms of maintaining our selfhood, whether we are encased in physical bodies or in machines. Schneider claims that "Many cognitive scientists suspect that the brain is a kind of computational system, and that relatedly, the person is fundamentally a sort of computational being."[10] On this view, if we could discover a way to do it, that computational system could be "uploaded" into a computer, which means that computers could house selves. Or, perhaps, computers could develop the characteristics that we associate with selfhood, including the capacity to recognize others in the appropriate way. If they did, they would arguably become persons towards whom we have moral obligations, and selves with whom we could develop relationships. In a world of potentially disembodied selves, our physical bodies are seen as accidental features, and the technology that might allow us to continue as selves after our bodies die becomes crucially important, for through it we might achieve a kind of immortality.

If, on the other hand, the most central elements of selfhood are seen to lie in our physical human embodiment, and in our capacity to develop relationships with others through and because of our bodies, then questions of gender and childrearing, as many feminists have argued, cannot be ignored, nor can the political and social policies that support and nurture or undermine and inhibit those relationships.

And consider a third possibility: that individuals cannot develop a full conception of who they are on their own, but only with, and through, interactions with others. Carrithers, for example, argues that what makes us human, despite the wonderfully diverse and strikingly different cultures that we can observe throughout history and around the world even today, is precisely the capacity to create cultures together. On his account, we all exist in an inescapable web which attaches us to others, and we cannot answer the question "Who am I?" without acknowledging that at least part of our answer will lie in how other people view us, in who *they* say *we* are. As Carrithers puts it, in a world in which we understand persons as active creators of culture, we must acknowledge that selves inhabit a world of understandings that are "mutual and reciprocal . . . in their nature interpersonal and intersubjective."[11]

Taylor goes even further and argues that any account of the self is incomplete unless we add that conceptions of selfhood are inextricably connected to beliefs about what is morally valuable. Selves exist, he believes, not only in physical space, but also in moral space. To answer the question of who we are as individuals is simultaneously and necessarily to ask where we stand with respect to our understanding of the good: "To know who I am is a species of knowing where I stand. My identity is defined by the commitments and identifications which provide the frame or horizon within which I can try to determine from case to case what is good, or valuable, or what ought to be done, or what I endorse or oppose."[12] We cannot understand who we are, he argues, until we orient ourselves within this moral space, "a space in which questions arise about what is good or bad, what is worth doing and what is not, what has meaning and importance . . . and what is trivial and secondary."[13]

Arguably, the converse of Taylor's thesis that we cannot give an adequate answer to the question of who we are without, in some way, saying something about what is important to us, what we think is valuable, and what we think is trivial, also holds: we cannot have an adequate moral theory which does not, explicitly or implicitly, provide some description of who we are.

An ethical theory provides what is essentially a description of moral space, a road map of the moral landscape, and this description requires a conception of the selves who act and move within this moral geography. Metaphorically-speaking, ethical theories are like travel guides which describe where the important cities are located and how they are linked to one another, what sorts of persons we can expect to encounter on our journey, how they might relate to us and how we ought to respond, and what dangers we should be aware of and how we might avoid them.

To present a conception of the self, then, is simultaneously to describe a world, indeed, a whole moral universe. Like science fiction writers, who create extraordinary worlds for their characters to inhabit and universes for them to explore, so, too, do the creators of ethical theories. Indeed, far from being straightforward descriptions of the "real world," ethical theories can be seen as imaginative utopian constructions: the worlds they describe are not ones that we *actually* live in, not ones that yet exist, but, rather, worlds that we ought to create together. We don't, for instance, live in Kant's rational world, or even Mill's utilitarian one, we don't live in a world composed of just societies inhabited by tolerant individuals as liberals describe them, nor in a world designed to inculcate and display the virtues. In much the same way that Anderson describes modern nation-states as "imagined communities" in which citizens "come to imagine themselves as though the whole nation were a face-to-face community,"[14] ethicists ask us to imagine that we meet with each other in an imagined ethical community. And just as the act of citizens imagining with one another a shared community "helps to create a real and effective sense of nationhood,"[15] so too, if we are willing to engage in the exercise of imagining a shared ethical community, we will come to understand ourselves and the persons we share this community with as participants in a mutual enterprise. Ethical theories, then, are both aspirational and hopeful: they give us something to work towards together, and they are confident that they can help us get there.

If we relate this aspect of ethical theorizing to bioethics, it follows that bioethics, too, has an important aspirational and hopeful dimension: that its purpose is to help human beings live better lives despite their physical frailty and in the face of their mortality, and that bioethicists are engaged in a mutual and collaborative effort, not simply to analyze what already exists, but, even more fundamentally, to transform, in light of this aspirational goal, the places and spaces within which they work and about which they think, write, and speak. My focus on conceptions of the self and the (often unnoticed and unacknowledged) work they do in shaping our ethical thinking is meant to be a contribution to this collaborative enterprise.

My aim in the first part of this book is to identify and describe the most important conceptions of the self that underpin contemporary North American bioethics. This is a form of bioethics that is sometimes called "mainstream" or "standard" bioethics because it provides the most common template for the exploration of bioethical issues, and the most influential basis for the justification of conclusions reached on bioethical questions. The presence of these conceptions of the self and the work they do in bioethics has gone largely unnoticed and uncommented upon in the bioethical literature, but, once they are noticed, the role they play in bioethical discussions is striking. These conceptions include the Kantian self, the utilitarian self, and the liberal self. The conceptions of the self assumed by these different theories are incompatible with one another; however, they structure debates in bioethics in ways that disguise this fact. Together, they compose a chimerical bioethical self: like the mythical Chimera, a creature composed out of the parts of a serpent, a lion, and a goat, this chimerical bioethical self is a creature that is pulled in different directions, shaped by competing and incompatible commitments, and, consequently, frequently at a loss to know what to think or do. What I will do in the first part of this book is detach this chimerical self into its component parts, explore each in turn, and demonstrate the way in which attempts to resolve the tensions between them lead to the development of the Choosing Self.

The Kantian and utilitarian selves will be considered together because they emerged at a similar period in history and are often played off against one another. It is now hard to think of utilitarianism simply and solely on its own terms, without simultaneously thinking of Kantian criticisms, and the converse is also true. Indeed, the conjunction of the two theories is so firmly formed that they can be said to come together to create what I will term the Troubled Self. The Troubled Self is a self that is torn between duty and happiness, between a completely rational world and one filled with pleasures and pains, between a world in which emotions like sympathy and benevolence form the basis of our recognition of our moral commitments to one another, and a world in which only reason can perform this task.

The liberal self, which will be considered in chapter 3, has become increasingly important in bioethics; while it is a modern self, which draws in part on certain features of both the Kantian and utilitarian selves (although not always explicitly) it is distinctive enough to be considered on its own terms. I shall call this self the Divided Self, and a central feature of this self is the place autonomy plays in its deliberations.

As noted, the self that emerges out of these various theoretical strands, and as a response to the tensions between them, is the Choosing Self, and it is this self that is increasingly dominant in mainstream bioethics. The Choosing Self is essentially the Divided Self utterly detached from its home within liberal political theory and organized around a conception of autonomy that, because it considers the freedom to make choices to be more important than questions about the value of the things chosen, would be largely unrecognizable to Kantians or utilitarians even though it sometimes makes use of the resources provided by their theoretical perspectives. The ascendancy of the Choosing Self in bioethics marks the point at which mainstream bioethics becomes almost entirely procedural in orientation, and largely uninterested in larger substantive questions about social and economic justice. Bioethics, understood in this way, has little to say, and it becomes unclear, as a result, what kind of expertise the bioethicist has to offer.

The theoretical perspectives out of which the framework of contemporary mainstream bioethics has been constructed all fall within the template provided by what Margaret Urban Walker calls a theoretical-juridical model of ethics; despite their differences, they all have a place within ethical approaches that see ethics as consisting in a set of law-like rules which are rationally determined, and assert that ethically defensible decisions are those that result from the correct application of these rules. Since the discussion of the first four chapters demonstrates that mainstream bioethics is running out of theoretical resources to address its own problems—the rise of the Choosing Self, that is to say, and the paradox of expertise that it generates, reveal a form of bioethics that is little more than a set of procedures encapsulated within a theoretical envelope that is itself a representation of a set of ideological commitments. The second part of the book, then, considers approaches that fall outside the theoretical-juridical framework, and which have been considered (when they are considered at all) largely peripheral to mainstream bioethics. I argue that these approaches can provide theoretical resources to bioethics that it is currently lacking and which it needs.

The second part of the argument begins with an exploration of feminine and feminist critiques of bioethics; the self that both approaches employ is a Gendered Self. This chapter provides an example of an expressive-collaborative approach to bioethics, and demonstrates the difficulties faced by anyone who wishes to challenge the assumptions of mainstream bioethics. The next chapter introduces the Virtuous Self and an older conception of ethics than those yet considered, namely, that proposed by virtue ethicists like Aristotle. It is in this ancient model suitably updated and supplemented by the insights provided by feminist and narrative ethics, I argue, that we can find the theoretical resources that are missing from competing perspectives. Like feminist approaches, virtue-based perspectives provide an outside standpoint on these other approaches because they are based on strikingly different foundational assumptions. I argue that virtue ethics can address many of the issues raised in the first part of the book, can provide the basis for a situated conception of autonomy, and can be enlarged to encompass feminist concerns about gender, power, and exploitation. The account of autonomy that emerges from this discussion is further filled out in the next two chapters, which consider case studies and illness narratives.

The final chapter puts the pieces of the Situated Self together, explores theoretical resources through which bioethics can evaluate itself, and demonstrates the connection between the sort of ethical guidance bioethics can provide and the need for bioethicists to make issues of social and economic concern central, rather than peripheral, to any analysis they provide. The Situated Self that emerges out of the conceptual strands considered in the second part of the book is designed to stand as a foil and a counterweight to the Choosing Self, and the conception of autonomy upon which this self and its activities are predicated is meant to provide an alternative to the version of autonomy that currently predominates in bioethics.

The approaches considered in the second half of the book might help to resolve the impasse that currently exists between what bioethics purports to be able to do, and its ability to actually follow through on this promise, because they provide ethical resources that will allow us to frame and discuss bioethical issues differently than mainstream approaches allow. Because I am interested in exploring the nature and dimensions of this impasse, and because its existence can only be observed when theoretical claims are connected to practice, I will move back and forth between my own observations (and the observations of others working in bioethics who have critically reflected on what it might mean to call oneself a "bioethicist") and theoretical considerations which, I will argue, shape our understanding of bioethics and bioethical issues in ways which are not always explicit or even clearly seen.

I want to make it clear, however, that my approach is meant to be not only critical of others, but self-critical as well: I want to explore the way in which "mainstream" bioethics has shaped my own activity when I occupy the role of an ethicist, and how this role might not only become more effective and helpful, but richer, more interesting, and, indeed, less bureaucratic and more philosophical. These reflections will, I hope, be helpful for others who are engaged in "doing bioethics" and who are also frustrated by certain accepted features of the field. Before exploring the Troubled, Divided, and Choosing selves, however, I will say more about the features of contemporary North American bioethics, and the central place currently held by principlism.

THE GRAND TOUR: PLACING BIOETHICS ON THE CULTURAL MAP

Bioethics occupies an important place in North American society. Bioethics is taught in religious studies, philosophy, and theology departments in many universities; bioethicists teach in medical schools and provide guidance in hospitals; and people working in the field help shape government policy with respect to how bioethical issues should be approached and how the possibilities opened up by medical and technological discoveries should be regulated. Bioethicists work on Institutional Research Boards that help determine what medical and pharmaceutical research is conducted, and they speak publicly when events with a bioethical dimension occur. When these events are reported in the media, individuals working in bioethics are often given the opportunity to offer their views which means, more fundamentally, that they are being given the opportunity to help shape public opinion on bioethical matters. For professional philosophers—those who make their living usually as faculty members in universities, speaking, teaching, and writing about philosophy—the opportunities provided by the significant cultural space occupied by bioethics in North America are both entrancing and unique. While much of what we have to say as philosophers seems to be of little interest to anyone outside of the academy, when we speak not as philosophers but as "bioethicists," our views are sought out, and our pronouncements are treated with respect. As philosophers, then, we have very little presence in the culture; as "bioethicists," in contrast, we are viewed as persons who possess an important kind of expertise.

In North American culture, then, bioethics currently occupies an important place in the public domain, and bioethicists, drawn from a variety of disciplinary backgrounds, play an important cultural role. As Fox and Swazey observe, contemporary North American bioethics is remarkable in the way in which it has moved beyond the "normal" social and cultural spheres in which it might be expected to operate: "Not only are bioethical questions, cases, and personages constantly, saliently, and often dramatically covered in the print and electronic media, but in addition, in a variety of ways, the executive, legislative, and judicial branches of government, at every level of the society, have been continually involved with them."[16]

Given the prominent cultural role played by bioethics and the public visibility of bioethicists, it is surprising to discover, when one examines bioethics more closely, that trying to define or describe what it is can be difficult. The field is amorphous and "ambiguous,"[17] and, because it draws on a large range of disciplinary sources (including ones that are legal, scientific, philosophical, medical, religious, anthropological, and sociological) it is profoundly multidisciplinary. Metaphorically speaking, bioethics is a tapestry that is woven out of many different intellectual, cultural, and social strands. As a result, any proposed description not only carries with it the challenge of describing the field accurately, but, simultaneously, tends to privilege a particular strand within the tapestry.

As a result, it is almost impossible to give a purely factual account of what bioethics is because any description includes a large component of normativity; that is to say, it tells us not only what bioethics *is*, but, more significantly, what the person providing that description thinks it *ought* to be. Is it a "field" or is it a "discipline"?[18] Should it strive for a universal ethics, or should it recognize pluralism and particularism? Should it be dominated by those with medical backgrounds, or by those with philosophical or legal ones? Should religious perspectives be considered when examining bioethical issues, or are they profoundly illegitimate in a pluralistic and secular society? The answers given to questions like these in any account of what bioethics is almost inevitably "make the case" for a particular conception of how bioethics ought to be understood.

Moreover, just as particular descriptions of what bioethics is both embody an argument for how the field ought to be characterized and what it ought to be, they also make the case for who can most convincingly (if they wish to do so) call themselves *bioethicists*. [19] As O'Neill puts it, those engaged in bioethical disputes and debates are "protagonists"[20]: they have an active interest in shaping the disputes and debates in particular ways, and, simultaneously, their participatory role helps determine the way in which bioethics itself is understood. Moreover, the positions the protagonists take are arguably sometimes driven as much by their (usually unacknowledged) emotional commitments as they are by their rational judgments. What strikes one immediately when one enters the domain of bioethics is both the tenacious nature of the debates with which bioethicists concern themselves[21] and the stridency with which the protagonists who take different sides on particular issues defend their views. [22]

This situation, perhaps, partially results from the fact that bioethics is a relatively new area of research, study, and application. While questions about the role of ethical judgment in medicine go back for hundreds of years (for example, the Hippocratic Oath is often understood to be an early form of medical ethics) the contemporary field is usually traced to medical, technological, political, and social developments in the United States that took place during the 1960s and 1970s. Even with this relatively short history, however, there are a number of myths of origin "about when, and the reasons for which, the modern field of bioethics took shape."[23]

Even the meaning of the term "bioethics" can be contentious. Reich identifies what he calls a "bifurcated birth" in 1970–71 for this term, with credit going to both VanRennselaer Potter at the University of Wisconsin and Andre Hellegers at Georgetown University.[24] Reich notes that, even at this early stage, there was some disagreement about the scope of the questions intended to be covered by this term, with Potter understanding the term to include not only medical concerns, but also broader issues such as the environment, while the scholars at Georgetown (though not, perhaps, Hellegers himself) understanding the term more narrowly, as covering an exploration of concrete medical issues concerned with: "(1) the rights and duties of patients and health professionals; (2) the rights and duties of research subjects and researchers; and (3) the formulation of public policy guidelines for clinical care and biomedical research."[25]

As a result of these considerations, the claim that any description of what bioethics is involves implicit normative commitments, and the observation that what is covered by the term was understood in different ways even by those who are credited with its invention and promulgation, I will, in the remainder of this section, make my own position clear.

I will begin the process of situating myself within the debate about the meaning and scope of bioethics by saying, first, that I shall use the term broadly, as encompassing not only "concrete medical questions," but also issues such as environmental concerns, concerns about the role technology may play in transforming not only how we live but also our bodies, and the political and social consequences of medical and technological developments, to name a few. Moreover, I shall consider the term "bioethics" to cover the areas of concern normally captured under the headings of "medical ethics" and "biomedical ethics." The reason that I have chosen to work with a broad understanding of what the term "bioethics" encompasses, rather than a narrow one, is that most of the questions with which bioethicists concern themselves have dimensions that go beyond medical settings and satisfactory responses to them are not simply synonymous with what is medically appropriate. Issues like euthanasia, abortion, or the appropriate use of genetic testing, for example, will never be reducible simply to medical decisions, but will always raise questions about the meaning and purpose of human life, the political and economic contexts within which medical choices are made, and the significance of particular choices in the lives of particular individuals.

Second, I will proceed by asserting the importance of images, metaphors, and narratives in bioethics. As Lakoff observes, "Language gets its power because it is defined relative to frames, prototypes, metaphors, narratives, images, and emotions. Part of its power comes from its unconscious aspects: we are not consciously aware of all that it evokes in us, but it is there, hidden, always at work."[26] Bioethicists often use metaphors, images, and thought experiments to advance their claims, and the field is characterized by an extensive use of case studies short narratives designed to make moral questions vivid and personal. Indeed, part of what makes bioethics a distinctive academic field is the reliance it places on these images, metaphors, thought experiments, and narratives. My own account will be no exception, although I will try to be self-conscious about my usage of these tools in a way that is largely absent in mainstream bioethical discourse.

I have already used the metaphor of bioethics being like a tapestry, composed of multiple strands. I now want to draw attention to the way in which the term "field" (which is often applied to bioethics) is not only a descriptive term which acknowledges the diverse sources which compose its subject matter, but can also be understood as a kind of geographic metaphor[27]: it suggests a *space* in which a wide range of issues can be presented and explored, and a number of positions on those issues staked out. If we think of bioethics as a *space*, then it becomes important for those working in the field to identify where they situate themselves within this space, and why. Although he does not use the word "field" in the way I am proposing, Chambers argues that this positioning is often engaged in by bioethicists through a process he calls "centering"; however, they usually do not explicitly acknowledge that this is what they are doing.

Chambers observes that many of those working in the field of bioethics give an account of how they got there, how they were invited into the "space" encompassed by that term. The story is often one of movement from the "outside" world of the "ivory tower" (to use another metaphor, whose very familiarity may make us forget what a striking image it presents[28]) which (also metaphorically speaking) stands on the edge of the field, outside the fence which forms the boundary between the domain of the philosopher and the sphere of the bioethicist, and into the world of the health care professional, who stands at the bedside of the patient. In this movement, we see "the remarkable journey that many scholars have taken in leaving their academic offices and entering into a hospital, medical clinic, or nursing home. Their roles were previously defined in a very different setting, one that in many ways is 'theirs,' and the journey into the hospital represents a movement into another's space."[29]

This movement into the field (to use the terminology I am developing), Chambers observes, not only literally describes a movement into a new physical setting, as individuals shift from the university to the hospital, long-term care home, or hospice, it also performs another function: it legitimizes their claim to be called "ethicists" or "bioethicists." "In moving to the bedside and into the world of the health care professional they have left the 'ivory tower' and thereby the abstract 'periphery' of academic moral philosophy. These metaphors portray ethicists as doing the real work, being inside, at the patient's bedside, as opposed to outside in a comfortable armchair."[30]

As individuals describe their move from their accustomed place "outside the fence" (from the comfortable classroom or office in the ivory tower) into the field of bioethics (through the corridors of the hospital or nursing home until they reach the bedside of the patient), they perform what Chambers calls an act of centering: "Centering provides order and coherence to our descriptions and arguments by producing a compelling metaphor or narrative that possesses what rhetoricians refer to as *energia*."[31] This "rhetorical energy" draws "on the reader's imagination in a manner that is distinct from how academic disciplines normally think their disputes proceed."[32] (It should be noted that I performed my own act of centering in the first section of this chapter).

There are three important and interrelated features generated by centering. First, by centering something "in the center of the field," something else is placed on the margins, or even pushed outside the fence: "The degree to which ethicists are able to center discussions of morality at the bedside [or on the ethics committee] marginalizes more traditional academic philosophers;

they are not 'where the moral action is.'"[33] Second, centering helps provide a meaningful and coherent order to the activities under discussion, and situates them in a specific location on the field: "In medical ethics, the traditional moral positions of philosophy come to be seen as relevant or irrelevant in relation to whether they help resolve the 'real' moral problems facing the clinical ethicist."[34]

Third, Chambers notes, centering is a powerful intellectual strategy because it forces those on the periphery to respond to it in terms which it sets out. For example, "traditional academic moral discourse" conducted by philosophers from their comfortable armchairs and in their safe classrooms, is challenged "by medical ethics through an appeal to the need for action outside of the academy."[35] If academic philosophers respond to this appeal (as many of us do, when we are invited inside the fence that separates the field of bioethics from the other parts of our discipline), we are forced to accept "the center as central."[36] Part of the reason we do this is defensive: academic philosophers tend to look down on applied ethics generally, and on bioethics in particular: one of my colleagues reports that she once heard bioethics referred to at a philosophy conference as "the phys-ed of philosophy"— certainly not a subject with which "serious" philosophers would concern themselves.[37] Centering allows those who have crossed the border between the domain of academic philosophy and entered the field of bioethics to, in turn, "marginalize the academic philosopher and . . . defend themselves . . . against the charge that they are no longer doing 'real' philosophy."[38]

Chambers observes that centering strategies in bioethics don't end once one has moved inside the fence; rather, bioethics is characterized by attempts to demonstrate why *this* particular part of the field is where the action *really* is. To further develop the field metaphor, it is as though a fair, with various booths and attractions, has been set up inside the fence, and their proprietors are competing to be the most popular. As Chambers puts it, "Centering is an activity that entails revealing why what one is doing is actually where the center is and thereby suggesting why one's rivals are working under an illusion that they are doing significant work."[39] Because bioethics is multi-disciplinary, each of the various disciplines which have set up booths feels compelled to make the case for their own privileged position on the field, and they need to make the case to their competitors using whatever persuasive tools they can find. Consequently, understanding the strategy of centering is, Chambers believes, important for understanding how arguments in bioethics are advanced and defended: "centering represents a crucial way in which debates proceed in bioethics and reveals that these debates proceed as much by metaphor and narrative as by logical argument."[40]

Centering, then, is nothing less than an attempt to determine not only *which* concepts shape debates in bioethics, but, even more fundamentally, *whose* concepts they are. Successful centering requires opponents to engage in arguments in terms that they have not chosen, and would not naturally choose. As Lakoff puts it, "If we hear the same language over and over, we will think more and more in terms of the frames and metaphors activated by that language. And it doesn't matter if you are negating words or questioning them, the same frames and metaphors will be activated and hence strengthened."[41] Even as we challenge a particular position, then, we simultaneously both acknowledge its importance and make it stronger.

I want now to depart slightly from Chambers' account. While I think that he is correct to draw attention to the role that centering strategies play in bioethics (and it is striking how many bioethicists, whatever their disciplinary background, tell "entrance tale[s]"[42] that both place them firmly in the center of the field and legitimize what they have to say, and, indeed, how seductively appealing this strategy is as I engage in it myself), it seems to me that many of those who use it are largely unaware that this is what they are doing. Fox and Swazey, for example, observe that a noticeable feature of contemporary American bioethics is the extent to which it explains, chronicles, and commemorates its beginnings, and the variety "of different narrative accounts about how, why, and where it began."[43] In addition, bioethics seems to feel the need to celebrate itself, in a way that is almost unique in the academic world; arguably, it is one of the few areas of relatively coherent intellectual and professional activity that spends almost as much time and energy observing itself and trying to define what it is, as it does on exploring the subject matter with which it is concerned.

At the same time, being self-referential and self-conscious does not always seem to translate into self-awareness: part of what is involved in these examples of centering, then, seems to be a desire to ignore the possibility that one's preferred account of what bioethics is and who gets to define it (which, as we have already seen, means also what one *wants* it to be) may, in fact, not be at the center at all. As Callahan points out, the ostensibly rational commitments bioethicists make to particular descriptions of what is at stake in bioethics, and how particular issues ought to be approached, analyzed, and resolved, sometimes mask unrecognized ideological commitments about which bioethicists can be self-deceived: "we can have trouble understanding our own deepest motivations, whether in judging our own commitments and predilections or appraising those of others . . . . [Many bioethicists] seem to know their own convictions far better than they know themselves."[44] This points to another important feature of the field metaphor: protagonists who have succeeded in making a place for themselves inside the fence often seem to feel the need to act as gatekeepers, whose job it is to exclude those who would like to introduce different perspectives, or challenge the positions of those who have already gained access to the theoretical space occupied by what is sometimes called mainstream bioethics. Their defense of their own positions, and of the central assumptions of mainstream bioethics, can be strikingly territorial: as some feminist scholars have observed, those who disagree with them are either not doing "real" bioethics, or have no right to call themselves "bioethicists."[45]

Given the diverse, multidisciplinary, and, therefore, contentious state of bioethics, centering is perhaps an unavoidable strategy. However, it seems to me important that it be engaged in self-consciously, rather than surreptitiously, or even obliviously. Consequently, I will make explicit claims about where I situate myself on the field: my focus will be primarily on American bioethics, and the discipline which I will draw on most extensively, and which provides not only the method for my explorations but also the framework within which they will occur, is philosophy. I will also, as I have already indicated, make reference to my own experiences when I have been placed in the role of "bioethicist." Bioethics is a field of inquiry that purports to be able to clarify, and sometimes even resolve, practical ethical questions and concerns, and my philosophical reflections are generated as much by my observations of bioethics in practice as they are by my theoretical judgments: if bioethics is able to do much less than it purports to be able to do, why is this the case, and what accounts for the important cultural space it currently occupies despite this failure? These experiences, then, are integral to my analysis because they provide insights into bioethics as it is currently practiced in health care settings.

There are three reasons why my focus will primarily be on the state of American bioethics. First, however we define the term "bioethics," and however narrowly or broadly we construe the issues, disciplines, and approaches that are covered by this term, the central contemporary understandings can be traced to, and are largely shaped by, intellectual, medical, social, and political developments that have occurred in the United States over the last forty years or so. Indeed, while bioethics may be starting to develop distinctive national forms in other parts of the world such as Europe and Asia, even in these places, bioethics remains partially shaped by the American form.[46] As a result, even challenges to the assumptions inherent in American bioethics recognize the central role it plays in defining the field.

Second, my observations are drawn from my own experiences working in a bioethical context shaped and framed by distinctly American or North American approaches to the subject. My experiences working on ethics committees in various health care organizations, for example, demonstrate the profound extent to which the theoretical ethical models we make use of have been framed by a particularly North American emphasis on freedom, and the resulting weight placed on individual autonomy and informed consent in health care.

Third, I accept the premise that the approaches to bioethics that I will be exploring, critiquing, and proposing throughout this book reflect a number of North American assumptions and commitments. This acknowledgement stands in contrast to the position taken by a number of advocates of some of these approaches, who make the claim that the values embedded in them are, in fact, *universal*, ones that everyone, everywhere, should be committed to. *If* they are right, then these explorations, critiques, and proposals would apply to a global bioethics. However, if other coherent approaches to bioethics exist elsewhere in the world, this will not in itself undermine my claims, since I do not purport to be making universal or global claims. I won't keep repeating "North American" or "American" bioethics. Unless otherwise indicated, this should now simply be assumed.

It is also important to say a little bit more about the role that the discipline of philosophy will play in my discussion. Philosophy provides one of the most important strands in the tapestry of contemporary bioethics; or to shift the metaphor, the booth occupied by philosophy in the field of bioethics is large, visible, and centrally located. To say this, however, is *not* to assert that philosophy occupies the *only* important site on the field, or that the voice of the philosopher should sound more loudly than the voices of, say, the physician, lawyer, and anthropologist, who also have booths to promote and protect. My examination will concern itself with exploring the various spaces and pieces of equipment within the philosophical booth, and will make some observations about where the booth is situated with respect to the other tents, booths, and attractions scattered around the field of bioethics. My project, moreover, will be one that moves back and forth between the ivory tower in which bioethics is taught, and its questions and concerns considered on an abstract level, and the more practical work that is done in medical settings: in ethics committees, on Institutional Research Boards, and at the bedside of the patient.

What does the booth set up by philosophy look like? What are its features? Which items are on display, and which are shoved to the back corners? While any attempt to describe the role played by philosophy will, like all acts of centering, place some aspects at the center and others at the periphery, the following features can be clearly observed.

First, contemporary theoretical ethics draws extensively on two main ethical theories, Kantianism and utilitarianism. The presence of these theories, moreover, can be discerned in many of the debates engaged in by bioethicists, and responses to bioethical issues frequently fall into recognizably utilitarian and Kantian camps. Second, another prominent theoretical source is rights-based; claims that certain actions are required or prohibited on the basis that they enhance or violate rights play a powerful role in modern ethical philosophy, and in contemporary bioethical debates. Frequently, rights-based claims are framed and justified by liberal individualism. Liberal individualism itself draws, in part, on elements present in the writings of Kant and Mill. Third, moral philosophers are increasingly drawing attention to the narrative features of the moral life, and they argue that important dimensions of our moral experience can best be illuminated—indeed, perhaps can only be illuminated—through stories. Some theorists working in bioethics have incorporated features of narrative ethics into their analyses; this approach, however, is not yet widely accepted, and many bioethicists ignore it completely. Fourth, another important dimension of bioethics is provided by feminist philosophy. Feminist philosophers often challenge utilitarian, Kantian, and liberal assumptions. While feminist perspectives have been employed by some of those working within bioethics, this perspective has not yet become a central part of the mainstream approach. Finally, an older ethical perspective usually called "virtue ethics" has some place in bioethics (particularly in considerations of the professional obligations of those working in health care), but its role tends to be diffused through (roughly speaking) communitarian and ethics of care approaches to moral reasoning. Consequently, even within the philosophical booth, only certain positions occupy a central place within the philosophical center: while principled, liberal, Kantian, and utilitarian approaches have been widely incorporated into the fabric of mainstream bioethics, perspectives based on feminist critiques, that understand narratives to be a source of moral insight, or which assert that the virtues ought to play a central role in any articulation of the moral life, are usually treated as peripheral. In the best case, they provide modest insights that can easily be incorporated by perspectives at the center; in the worst case, they are dismissed entirely. While the philosophical booth occupies an important place within the field of bioethics, that is to say, its contents are far more circumscribed than they arguably ought to be: moral philosophy encompasses much more than is conceived of in bioethics.

I want to examine some of the important sources that help compose the philosophical contributions to bioethics, their strengths and weaknesses, and the consequences of endorsing them. I will then propose a philosophical alternative that, while it will certainly not resolve all the issues that bioethics considers, may help us to discuss at least some of those issues differently, and see new possibilities for exploration as a result. However, as the points just made make clear, even within the philosophical booth, it is difficult to pin bioethics down; like other descriptions of the field, philosophical descriptions, too, often embody implicit normative commitments, and their proponents take their role as gatekeepers seriously. So the challenge becomes to find a way to maneuver through the field, identify the place of the philosophical booth, and then describe its most notable features in a way that allows for this exploration without predetermining too much how it ought to go.

I want to argue that, following Chambers' notion of centering, what we find at the heart of philosophical bioethics, at the center of the center, is principlism. Principlism is the idea that issues in bioethics can be analyzed, and even resolved, when we make use of ethical principles that allow us to articulate and balance competing moral intuitions and commitments. To say that principlism lies at the "center of the center" is not to say that everyone working in bioethics employs this approach, or even agrees with it (indeed, many bioethicists are highly critical of it); it is, however, to acknowledge that even those who disagree with it must be aware of it, and must make reference to it, even as they argue in favor of competing approaches. As Fox and Swazey note, the most widely-accepted form of principlism is the "four principles" approach developed by Tom Beauchamp and James Childress. The four principles they identify—respect for autonomy, nonmaleficence, beneficence, and justice—have become the "cornerstones of the chief conceptual framework of U.S. bioethics."[47] Moreover, as Callahan observes, principlism, despite its many critics, "has been one of the most widely used methodological tools for the resolution of ethical dilemmas . . . principlism has been particularly popular with clinicians and others who want a relatively clear and simple way of thinking through ethical problems."[48]

Principlism, in my experience, is widely used by ethics committees, and it is principlism that provides the primary ethical basis of the "tools" that persons working in health care settings are expected to use as they face ethical dilemmas. Indeed, for many members of the ethics committees I have participated on, "thinking ethically" simply *means* applying principles to the issues under discussion. Principlism, then, provides an important bridge between theoretical ethics and practical, or applied, ethics: when philosophers make the move from the ivory tower to the health care setting, they carry a knowledge of principlism with them, a knowledge which they are frequently required to disseminate to hospital, hospice, or nursing home staff. While it will not be all that they bring, nor perhaps even something they are happy to carry with them, it is a necessity, like a passport: you might not want to bring it with you when you travel, but you need to have it if you want to get anywhere.

I will argue that principlism is ultimately a flawed approach to bioethics, even on its own philosophical terms; however, the reasons for which it is problematic are revealing. Principlism provides a microcosm of philosophy's role within bioethics more generally, and it offers, therefore, a means of exploring and articulating the ways in which philosophers often consider bioethical questions. What I will argue is that, far from being the "mid-level" principles which do not require a commitment to particular ethical theories that their proponents purport them to be, underlying the four principles proposed by Beauchamp and Childress are the ethical theories of Kantianism, utilitarianism, and liberalism. Moreover, underlying *these* ethical theories lie hidden yet structurally important conceptions and descriptions of the nature of the moral universe. The conceptions of the self-assumed by these different theories are incompatible with one another; however, they structure debates within bioethics in ways that disguise this fact. More particularly, issues are presented as though they arise solely from the complexity of the subject matter, rather than, as I shall argue is often the case, from incoherencies in the way in which that subject matter is framed, organized, and discussed. An exploration of principlism, then, will provide a way to begin to reveal these hidden conceptions of the self and the unrecognized work they perform in bioethics more generally.

WHY ARE ISSUES IN BIOETHICS SO DIFFICULT TO RESOLVE SATISFACTORILY? THE INSTRUCTIVE CASE OF PRINCIPLISM AND APPEALS TO THE "COMMON MORALITY"

In this section, I will set out the main elements of principlism, as they are described and defended by Beauchamp and Childress in their well-known *Principles of Biomedical Ethics.* While theirs is not the only version of principlism that exists, and while some applications of their approach supplement the four principles they identify with others, their approach is both well known, and, as we have just seen, enormously influential. *Principles of Biomedical Ethics* stands as a central text in bioethics, and it is one that has helped shape both theoretical approaches to the issues with which bioethicists concern themselves, and as a model for the application of ethical reasoning to practical questions that need to be answered quickly and consistently within medical settings. *Principles of Biomedical Ethics*, over the course of a number of editions, provides a snapshot of the state of bioethics during various periods, because the theoretical approaches Beauchamp and Childress critique and employ reflect the most influential sources that existed when particular editions were written. (Casuistry, for example, is treated as an important type of ethical theory against which Beauchamp and Childress must make their case for principlism in the fourth edition, which was published in 1994. In the seventh edition that came out in 2013, however, casuistry is barely mentioned). I will use the term "principlism" to describe the version presented by Beauchamp and Childress, and my description of their theory will be based on what they say in the seventh, and most recent, edition.

I will proceed by explaining how their approach is designed to work. My contention in this section is that the elements that compose principlism are in tension with one another, and that analyzing these tensions illuminates larger problems within mainstream bioethics. In particular, identifying why this approach is unsatisfactory will help reveal the tension between the different conceptions of the self that underpin the different ethical theories its principles (I shall argue) are ultimately drawn from. Moreover, its claims to a particular kind of universalism reveal a striking and interesting lack of self-awareness, a trait that tends to afflict theoretical bioethics more generally: what are actually culturally and historically situated moral commitments are understood to be ones which apply to all people, everywhere. The way in which this claim to universalism is presented and defended, arguably, is both unpersuasive, and, ironically enough, unfairly minimizes the contributions made to western thought by great moral thinkers like Kant, Mill, and Aristotle.

The four principles that form the framework of principlism are, as we have seen, respect for autonomy, nonmaleficence, beneficence, and justice. Before examining what Beauchamp and Childress identify as the origin of these principles, it is important to have a clear sense of what they understand by each of these terms, given the central place occupied by these principles within mainstream bioethics.

They begin their presentation of the principles with a description of respect for autonomy. Autonomy encompasses the concept of self-rule, which requires both freedom from external control and an inner capacity to make adequate judgments about the choices available: "The autonomous individual acts freely in accordance with a self-chosen plan, analogous to the way an independent government manages its territories and sets its policies."[49] Autonomy, then, requires both "*liberty* (independence from controlling influences) and *agency* (capacity for independant action)."[50] Respect for autonomy, in their view, involves both negative and positive obligations. Understood as a negative obligation, autonomy "requires that autonomous action not be subjected to controlling constraints by others."[51] Understood as a positive obligation, it "requires both respectful treatment in disclosing information and actions that foster autonomous decision making,"[52] and they connect this obligation to the second formulation of the Categorical Imperative, which holds that rational beings must be treated as ends in themselves: "As some contemporary Kantians have argued, the demand that we treat others as ends requires that we assist them in achieving their ends and foster their capacities as agents, not merely that we avoid treating them solely as means to our ends."[53]

While they claim that the "order of our chapters [which places autonomy first] does not imply that this principle has moral priority over other principles"[54] because all four principles are meant to be balanced against one another, it is arguably the case that respect for autonomy will require that the other principles be applied in ways which support autonomy. It is respect for autonomy that many bioethicists understand as the central value they need to defend. Indeed, Callahan argues, in this principled approach, "autonomy turns out to be king: all the other principles lead back to it,"[55] and are interpreted in light of its requirements.

Nonmaleficence is a principle that requires us not to cause harm to others; while some philosophers assert that beneficence and nonmaleficence come together to form a single principle, Beauchamp and Childress think this to be a mistake: "In our view, conflating nonmaleficence and beneficence into a single principle obscures critical moral distinctions as well as different types of moral theory. Obligations not to harm others, such as those prohibiting theft, disablement, and killing, are distinct from obligations to help others, such as those prescribing the provision of benefits, protection of interests, and promotion of welfare."[56] Beneficence, then, is a principle that requires us to contribute to the welfare of others. Beauchamp and Childress note that the related values of beneficence and benevolence are central principles in utilitarian ethical thought. Beneficence is so central to utilitarian thinking, indeed, that many utilitarians "associate beneficence with the goal of morality itself."[57] While Beauchamp and Childress "concur that obligations to confer benefits, to prevent and remove harms, and to weigh an action's possible goods against its costs and possible harms are central to the moral life,"[58] they believe that beneficence must be balanced with the other principles they identify.

The final principle is justice. Beauchamp and Childress note that there is a formal principle of justice (which holds that "Equals must be treated equally, and unequals must be treated unequally"[59]), which is common to all theories of justice. What distinguishes one theory from another, then, is the way in which "equal" and "unequal" are spelled out. Material principles of justice, consequently, are needed to "specify the relevant characteristics for equal treatment . . . because they identify the substantive properties for distribution."[60] When Beauchamp and Childress fill out the formal principle of justice with material criteria, their account is suggestive, even though they arguably don't give a clear-cut and simple definition. They make several comments, however, that indicate that their preferred understanding of justice is both egalitarian and global, and supplemented by utilitarian considerations. Egalitarian theories of justice identify some basic goods that should be distributed equally. Beauchamp and Childress note that one of the most influential contemporary egalitarian theories is the theory developed by John Rawls. In addition, they acknowledge that their views on justice are shaped by cosmopolitan or global considerations: "This [global] approach . . . has deeply influenced the authors of this volume."[61] While global justice theorists take social inequalities as a focal point, and then extend their concerns beyond national borders, the version accepted by Beauchamp and Childress points to an acceptance of an essentially liberal theory of justice; indeed, they state that they often take a "perspective of egalitarian social justice [that] . . . orient[s] theory around the moral evaluation of social institutions and their responsibilities, legitimacy, and weaknesses,"[62] that is much like the theory presented by Rawls, but extended globally, rather than confined to a particular nation-state: "If the worst-off are the focal point of concern, as they are in Rawls's theory, then the situation of the worst-off—the global poor—should be addressed."[63] Since the way in which these issues are framed is shaped by liberal theory, their solutions will likewise fall within this framework as well;

a Marxist perspective on how these global inequalities might be addressed, for instance, would be a non-starter.

Beauchamp and Childress root the principles in something that they call "the common morality." The common morality is, in their view, universal: "All persons living a moral life know several rules that are usually binding: not to lie, not to steal others' property, to keep promises, to respect the rights of others, and not to kill or cause harm to others. . . . The common morality is applicable to all persons in all places and we rightly judge all human conduct by its standards."[64] The common morality has four central features. First, while the common morality is universal, it is not ahistorical or a priori; rather, it is rooted in human history and experience. Second, Beauchamp and Childress accept that *particular* moralities can differ from one another in ways that suggest that moral perspectives are plural, or even relative; however, they *reject* "moral pluralism (or relativism) in the *common* morality. No particular way of life qualifies as morally acceptable unless it conforms to the standards of the common morality."[65] Third, the common morality is composed of the moral beliefs that are held by all "morally committed persons,"[66] and, fourth, "explications of the common morality in books such as this one are historical products, and every *theory* of the common morality has a history of development by the author(s) of that theory."[67]

The four principles identified by Beauchamp and Childress are meant to capture the "general norms"[68] that are present in the common morality. However, while they provide general guidelines, they need further *specification* (a process of adding more specific content to the abstract norms represented by the principles) if they are to serve as action-guides. Beauchamp and Childress draw on Rawls's concept of *reflective equilibrium* to help specify and further refine the principles and define their appropriate application, and this process of revision and refinement can continue indefinitely: "The goal of reflective equilibrium is to match, prune, and adjust considered judgments and their specifications to render them coherent. We then test the resultant guides to action to see if they yield incoherent results. If so, we must further readjust the guides."[69]

Now that we have a clear sense of how principlism is supposed to work and where the principles are said to come from, two serious problems with this framework can be noted. First, the assertion that there is a common morality is unpersuasive, and the claim that all persons who are committed to morality share it is circular. Second, the principles identified by Beauchamp and Childress, even if they are widely shared by many North Americans (which they may or may not be), are, in fact, rooted in important ethical and political theories (most fundamentally, Kantianism, utilitarianism, and liberalism) that are central to Western ethical thought. (Indeed, is it primarily *because* these principles are rooted in these central theories that they have the force and weight that they do.) I will consider each objection in turn.

PROBLEMS WITH THE COMMON MORALITY

Beauchamp and Childress justify their claim that the common morality is universal by stating that it is the morality that is shared by all persons who are *committed* to morality. They go on to state that (of course!) not everyone that they might speak to (in the United States or elsewhere, presumably) will, in fact, be committed to these principles. Rather than acknowledging that this is a serious weakness in their account, they simply assert that their hypothesis "is that all persons committed to morality accept the standards of the common morality. It would be absurd to assert that all persons do, in fact, accept the norms of the common morality, because many amoral, immoral, or selectively moral persons do not care about or identify with moral demands"[70]; consequently, if empirical studies designed to test their hypothesis that the principles they articulate and the values that underpin them that they identify as being central to a universal common morality don't endorse them, all Beauchamp and Childress need to say is that they are obviously not persons who are committed to morality. While they acknowledge that some critics might assert that their argument is circular and their position self-justifying because they think "that we are defining the common morality in terms of a certain moral commitment and then allowing only those who accept the norms that we have identified to qualify as persons committed to morality,"[71] they confidently assert that "this risk is manageable through careful research design."[72]

This response is inadequate: it is, indeed, circular and self-justifying to define the "common morality" as one which is universally shared by all persons committed to morality, and then to assert that persons who do not share the values of the common morality are, therefore, simply persons whose perspective can be dismissed on the grounds that their disagreement with these values shows that they are, demonstrably, not committed to morality at all. Moreover, as Turner points out, there *are* people who have designed studies that explore cross-cultural moral commitments: they tend to be anthropologists and sociologists, rather than philosophers. What they have discovered undermines "the claim that there are cross-cultural norms supporting a 'universal' common morality."[73] Rather, what they find is that there are both areas of agreement and areas of conflict, and it is not sufficient, Turner argues, to simply say that those who express disagreement are either not committed to morality at all, or only selectively moral.

Turner makes two other important points. First, even if within a North American context we can find general agreement on the level of abstract moral principles, difficulties will appear when we try to apply them to specific cases: "Agreement at the level of general norms has no inherent practical significance since it is possible to desire markedly divergent policies and practices from the 'same' principle, maxim, or moral intuition."[74] For example, two individuals can each endorse the four principles presented by Beauchamp and Childress, but reach very different conclusions about such things as abortion or the legalization of physician-assisted suicide. Second, as noted above, there *are* scholars who have studied cross-cultural responses to moral questions, and have explored the extent to which moral views are shared even within an American context. As Turner observes, "if normative analysis is supposed to draw from moral views that are present in actual communities [as Beauchamp and Childress suggest], is it not reasonable to think that there needs to be a more concerted effort to connect American bioethics with the sociology, anthropology, and history of morality of America?"[75]

Following from the claim that there is no compelling evidence that a universal common morality exists, we can ask, however, whether the principles identified by Beauchamp and Childress might be widely agreed to (at least on an abstract level) in a particular cultural context, such as exists in the United States. In other words, to use their own terminology, is it possible that the "common morality" identified by Beauchamp and Childress is, in fact, a *particular* morality, rooted in time and place, and with an identifiable history? It is arguably the case that this is how we ought to understand their approach because, in many ways, the "common morality" described by Beauchamp and Childress is "an Anglo-American liberal morality that has little relationship to values in other settings around the world."[76] If this is a plausible assertion (which it appears to be), the principlism presented by Beauchamp and Childress occupies a strange place, somewhere between the universalism it aspires to and a true pluralism that the claim that the principles capture incompatible moral commitments that need to be balanced with one another might be seen to acknowledge.

Arguably, even if this intermediate position captured by principlism is *sustainable* (it does, it must be noted, provide us with a method for working through moral dilemmas and justifying our conclusions, and it has provided both bioethicists and persons working in health care in other capacities with a shared moral language, and this is a not inconsequential achievement),[77] it is *self-deceived*, or even *deceptive*. The arguments in support of a common universal morality are both circular and not supported by empirical evidence, *and* they fail to do justice to the contribution to ethical thinking in the western tradition made by philosophers. That is to say, justifying moral claims on the basis that they can be found in a common morality that is shared by all persons committed to morality *and* then asserting that anyone who does not share these views is obviously not a person with such a commitment so their views can legitimately be ignored, is unpersuasive, to say the least. Moreover, there is ample evidence that the perspective articulated in the principled approach is, indeed, one shaped by values that are most at home in Anglo-American thought *as a result* of the arguments presented by philosophers who worked within, and helped shape, this tradition. Respect for autonomy, for example, is not as strongly valued in less individualistic cultures as it is in North America.[78]

What is even more perplexing, given that Beauchamp or Childress present their claims in philosophical terms, is how little respect they pay to basic philosophical presuppositions, and how little credit they give to philosophers, particularly those who have presented the most powerful and philosophically satisfying ethical theories in the Western tradition for providing a justification for the principles they advance.

In terms of the first point, that this "common morality" approach is philosophically peculiar, one of the first things many philosophy professors tell their students in introductory classes is that the fact that "everyone agrees" with a particular viewpoint (even if that claim is factually true) tells us very little about whether or not that viewpoint is one that we ought to hold or accept. Indeed, the presence of almost universal agreement on something is just as likely to indicate the presence of a shared ideology as it is to signify the recognition of an objectively true understanding of reality that all rational and reasonable persons ought to recognize. As DeGrazia puts it, "there is nothing paradoxical in the Socratic thought that ninety, or even ninety-nine, percent of all people might share a moral belief, yet be wrong; experience reveals that moral judgment can be distorted in many ways."[79] Philosophically speaking, then, even if it were clearly and uncontroversially the case that the common morality as described by Beauchamp and Childress actually exists, is shared cross-culturally, is endorsed by a majority of individuals, and even if the principles they identify can be extracted from it, this tells us nothing (without much further investigation and analysis) about whether these principles are ones that we *ought* to accept as guidelines for moral reasoning and action. While a number of the philosophical arguments presented by Beauchamp and Childress in support of the principles they endorse appear to acknowledge this point, their assertion that it is their presence in the common morality that is their initial source and their ultimate justification undercuts the significance of this acknowledgment.

Even more perplexingly, while Beauchamp and Childress, in every edition of *Principles of Biomedical Ethics* give a significant amount of space to discussing prominent competing ethical theories, and even acknowledge (as we shall see more clearly in a moment) that the principles they generate have an important place in bioethics, they seem to have very little respect for the work these theories actually do in both articulating and justifying the principles they defend. There is a gap in their account between the discussions they provide of ethical theories and their acknowledgment of the importance of these theories (for example, in the 7th Edition of *Principles of Biomedical Ethics*, they provide an extensive discussion of utilitarianism, Kantianism, rights theory, and contemporary theories of justice), and their insistence that the principles they present are rooted, not in these theories, but, rather, in the "common morality." While they recognize that a "knowledge of these theories is indispensable for reflective study in biomedical ethics, because much of the field's literature presumes familiarity with them,"[80] and observe that each of the theories they consider "casts light on important aspects of moral thinking in biological sciences, medicine, and health care,"[81] they assert that it is to the common morality that we must look when we want to find a justification for the principles they present.

But this claim raises some significant questions. If the principles are drawn from the common morality, then why are ethical theories needed, let alone "indispensable" in bioethics? Conversely, if ethical theory is, indeed, indispensable, then what are we to make of the claim that the common morality is universal, and that from it we can derive principles of sufficient weight and complexity that they alone can provide the basis for an adequate analysis, and even resolution, of bioethical issues? Indeed, if the common morality is both so clear and so widely shared, why is moral theory (and specific applications of it, such as in the case of bioethics) needed at all? Surely, the common morality alone ought to provide all the guidance that is required, and we ought to be faced with fewer ethical issues than we currently are, and need fewer bioethicists to help us work through them.

Beauchamp and Childress try to bridge the gap between the principles they identify, and the ethical theory that they admit is indispensable, by asserting that, when we examine the theories closely, what we can see are large areas of agreement. "Agreement derives from an initial shared database, namely, the norms of the common morality."[82] Consequently, they assert, "We can say without exaggeration that the proponents of these theories all accept these principles of the common morality *before* they devise their theory."[83]

This claim is unconvincing for two distinct reasons. First, as we have already seen, we have good reason to think that there is no such thing as a universally shared common morality, and to the extent that the principles identified by Beauchamp and Childress can be found to be widely shared, it is in an Anglo-American, or even distinctly North American, context. This suggests that they have a particular history, and that they entered into North American culture largely as a result of the articulation of particular ideas by the philosophers who are credited with creating the theories that we now recognize to be indispensable to our moral thinking.

That is to say, Beauchamp and Childress arguably have the process backwards: even if we accept their assertion that these principles can be derived from the "common morality" (at least in North America), the reason they can be found both there and in major ethical theories in the western philosophical tradition is *not* because Kant and Mill (for example) simply articulated the ideas of the "common morality" when they devised their theories, but, rather, while they may have drawn on some culturally shared ideas, what they produced was significant because it described the nature of the moral life in new and uniquely powerful ways. As their ideas were read and discussed, their novel moral articulations entered into what Carrithers terms the "landscape of consciousness."[84] The landscape of consciousness is composed of the shared understandings of the world that are shaped by culture and history, and by powerful ideas presented by particular individuals that become widely accepted, in part, as a result of their novelty, their appeal, and their usefulness. In short, the reason we still read the works of thinkers like Kant, Mill, and Aristotle, and the reason why their theories remain indispensable, is *not* because they simply happened to provide good descriptions of ideas that we all share; rather, they are still read, and their ideas are still analyzed and applied, because they have something significant to say that no one else has managed to say as well, as insightfully, or as compellingly. If their ideas have a presence in our shared understandings, it is because they have helped shape those understandings, not because they are rooted in them.[85]

What is puzzling about the account given by Beauchamp and Childress is that they implicitly acknowledge the role played by ethical theories in their articulation of the principles, even as they explicitly deny their importance when they assert that the origin of these principles lies in the common morality itself. For example, as we saw above, they note that beneficence is a central value in utilitarian thought, and they present their preferred version of justice in egalitarian and global terms that are strikingly liberal, or even Rawlsian. (Even in an American context, in which the views of Rawls have had a prominent place in contemporary political and legal discourse, it is arguably unlikely that a survey of Americans would demonstrate that this is how most people understand justice, and it is utterly implausible to think that all those who do not understand it in this way are simply persons who are not committed to morality.)

Beauchamp and Childress, then, often seem to implicitly recognize what they explicitly deny: that the principles they propose are rooted in, and justified by, their presence in particular ethical theories; and that any adequate articulation of them requires appeal not to the common morality (their purported source) but to those ethical theories.

ETHICAL THEORIES AND CONCEPTIONS OF THE SELF

I will argue that, while ethical theories are indeed indispensable to bioethical reflection, the ethical theories we commonly draw on in contemporary bioethics (primarily Kantianism, utilitarianism, and liberalism[86]) are incompatible with one another; and their incompatibility exists, in large part, because each theory is organized around a distinct conception of the self. These conceptions of the self, moreover, are also incompatible with one another:

while the liberal conception, for example, draws on Kantian sources as well as Millian ones, it is incompatible with both, just as the Kantian self and the utilitarian self are incompatible with one another. However, as principlism demonstrates, contemporary bioethics tends to draw on each of these theories in ways that disguise this incompatibility.

It is important to recognize, then, that the tensions within principlism are a microcosm of the tensions within contemporary philosophical approaches to bioethics more generally. What bioethicists do, because we recognize that each major ethical theory contains undesirable elements, is try to use the bits of the theories that we like while leaving these undesirable elements out, but the trade-off is that we give up relatively coherent theories for incoherent hybrid approaches, and we have a difficult time analyzing and resolving ethical issues with any degree of consistency. If bioethics were able to do all that it purports to be able to do, after forty or more years of intense intellectual activity, we ought to have fewer issues to resolve and more satisfactory methods with which to approach them; however, many bioethical issues remain intractable, and even those about which something of a consensus has been reached (such as the central place occupied by respect for autonomy) often generate puzzles. Autonomy is best understood as a conception of human flourishing that requires the capacity to make choices, and circumstances within which these choices can be exercised: how well does this conception fit with the reality of serious illness, with all the constraints on free choice that result when someone is sick or dying? While choices ought usually to be respected, autonomy, in these circumstances, is an odd principle to refer to in order to justify them. As Brand-Ballard forcefully puts it, "Bioethicists would do well to take seriously the possibility that some considered convictions may be irreconcilable."[87]

The reason the "considered convictions" derived from important ethical theories are irreconcilable results not only from the fact that each theory has at its heart a particular conception of the self, which is to say, a particular understanding of what human beings are, but also that these conceptions are placed within an imaginary social, political, and moral universe which determines such things as what constitutes rationality, who (or what) counts as a being towards whom moral duties are owed, and what role society should play in shaping moral agents. These conceptions of the self, and the geography of the moral universes within which they are placed, are as incompatible with one another as a Darwinian universe is with a theocratic one, or an ideal Marxist world is with a world run on rigidly capitalist lines. The three ethical theories that I shall focus on, as already indicated, are Kantianism, utilitarianism, and liberalism. They are the theories most widely used in bioethics, and each of the principles identified by Beauchamp and Childress are arguably drawn from these theories (as they implicitly acknowledge when they explicate these principles by making reference to them). I will first explore the

"Troubled Self" that emerges when we try to balance Kantian commitments with utilitarian ones; in the following chapter, I will explore the liberal self that draws on elements present in the ethical theory of Kant and the political philosophy of J. S. Mill, but which is profoundly different from both.

NOTES

1. Michael J. Sandel, *Liberalism and the Limits of Justice* (Cambridge: Cambridge University Press, 1982), 50.

2. Mary Anne Warren, "On the Moral and Legal Status of Abortion," in *Contemporary Moral Problems* 8th Ed., ed. James E. White (Belmont, CA: Thomson-Wadsworth, 2006), 119.

3. M. Warnock observes, "Everyone who tries to come up with factual or scientific criteria for personhood gets into difficulties over what we are to say about infants or those who, though they once satisfied the criteria, are no longer able to do so, such as those in a coma, or suffering from dementia. But this is not just a little local difficulty. It is fundamental. For it is essentially for society to *decide* who . . . [Counts as a person]. There is no way of looking at facts about, say, a demented woman, and deducing whether she is a person." Mary Warnock, *An Intelligent Person's Guide To Ethics* (London: Duckworth, 1998), 85. Consequently, claims about who counts as a persons, just like claims about who counts as a self, are normative, not factual or descriptive.

4. Moral and political commitments often go together: once it is determined how people ought to behave, it must then be considered whether the political framework within which their actions must take place will encourage, allow, or prevent them from acting is this desired way.

5. Appeals to something like a "common morality," for example, are attempts to make the case that moral claims ought to be based on the views of "real" people and their judgments, not on a "model" conception of what people are. The ethical anthropology employed by Beauchamp and Childress, then, is dependent on the assertion that the persons who count as adequate moral agents are those who agree with the ethical values set out in their morality. It is, therefore, as much an artificial conception as are any of its rivals.

6. John Christman, *The Politics of Persons: Individual Autonomy and Socio-Political Selves* (Cambridge: Cambridge University Press, 2009), 1.

7. Consider the abortion debate, which can be seen as revolving around competing conceptions of the self: one side believes that fetuses are selves or potential selves in a way that is morally relevant, while the other side does not.

8. Todd May, *Our Practices, Our Selves: Or, What It Means To Be Human* (University Park, Pennsylvania: The Pennsylvania University Press, 2001), 1-2.

9. John Christman, *The Politics of Persons*, 1.

10. Susan Schneider, "Introduction," in *Science Fiction and Philosophy: From Time Travel to Superintelligence*, ed. Susan Schneider (Oxford: Wiley-Blackwell, 2009), 6.

11. Michael Carrithers, *Why Humans Have Cultures: Exploring Anthropology and Social Diversity* (Oxford: Oxford University Press, 1992), 90.

12. Charles Taylor, *Sources of the Self: The Making of the Modern Identity* (Cambridge, Massachusetts: Harvard University Press, 1989), 27.

13. Charles Taylor, *Sources of the Self*, 28.

14. Described by Michael Carrithers in *Why Humans Have Cultures*, 141.

15. Michael Carrithers, *Why Humans Have Cultures*, 141.

16. 16 Renee C. Fox and Judith P. Swazey, *Observing Bioethics* (New York: Oxford University Press, 2008), 7.

17. Fox and Swazey, *Observing*, 146.

18. Onora O'Neill, for example, states that "Bioethics is not a discipline, nor even a new discipline; I doubt whether it will ever be a discipline. It has become a meeting ground for a number of disciplines, discourses, and organizations concerned with the ethical, legal, and social questions raised by advances in medicine, science, and biotechnology." Onora O'Neill, *Autonomy and Trust in Bioethics* (Cambridge: Cambridge University Press, 2002), 1.

19. Many philosophers are uncomfortable calling themselves bioethicists, because this title suggests both too much and too little. First, it suggests a kind of expertise in practical ethics that is incompatible with the open-ended exploration of issues that many philosophers take as a hallmark of their discipline. Second, the constraints imposed by mainstream bioethics have become ideological, and are not, therefore, amenable to philosophical challenge. Conversely, however, many of those working in the field wear the label of "bioethicist" with pride. What it means to be a bioethicist—what sort of training is required, whether one needs to be certified in some way—is also a subject of some controversy. I will use the term "bioethicist" loosely, to mean anyone who claims to be doing ethical work in a health care related context, whether his or her background is in philosophy, law, medicine, or some other appropriate discipline.

20. O'Neill, *Autonomy and Trust*, 1.

21. Consider, for example, the case of abortion, which seems no closer to a satisfactory resolution now than it did forty years ago, or physician-assisted suicide, about which different political and legal jurisdictions have simply reached different, and incompatible, conclusions.

22. These claims are similar to the ones that Alasdair MacIntyre makes in his analysis of contemporary moral discourse in *After Virtue* (Notre Dame, Indiana: University of Notre Dame Press, 1981); in a sense, bioethics can be understood as a microcosm of issues which beset moral philosophy more generally, although the distinctive features of bioethics (in particular, its multidisciplinary origins, its prominent cultural role, and its very practical concerns) require a similarly distinctive analysis.

23. Fox and Swazey, 29.

24. Warren Thomas Reich, "The Word 'Bioethics': The Struggle Over Its Earliest Meanings," *Kennedy Institute of Ethics Journal* 5, no. 1 (1995): 19—34.

25. Reich, "Bioethics," 20.

26. George Lakoff, *The Political Mind* (New York: Viking Penguin, 2008), 15.

27. Notice, for instance, what a different mental image is created if bioethics is called a "field" rather than a "discipline": "discipline" is much narrower, more focused and stringent, than the open and unpredictable image generated by the term "field."

28. "Professor X" amusingly (but with serious intent) plays with this image in his book *In The Basement Of The Ivory Tower* (New York: Viking Penguin, 2011).

29. Todd Chambers, "Centering Bioethics," *Hastings Center Report* 30, no. 1 (Jan. Feb. 2000): 22 29.

30. Chambers, "Centering," 23.

31. Chambers, "Centering," 23.

32. Chambers, "Centering," 23.

33. Chambers, "Centering," 23.

34. Chambers, "Centering," 23.

35. Chambers, "Centering," 23.

36. Chambers, "Centering," 23.

37. I owe this story to my colleague, Dr. Carol Collier.

38. Chambers, "Centering," 23.

39. Chambers, "Centering," 23.

40. Chambers, "Centering," 23.

41. Lakoff, *Political*, 15.

42. Chambers, "Centering," 23.

43. Fox and Swazey, *Observing*, 123.

44. Daniel Callahan, "Bioethics and Ideology," *Hastings Center Report* 36, no. 1 (Jan. Feb. 2006): 3.

45. As Helen Bequaert Holmes puts it, "Those who wish to get tenure, and to have papers published—that is, to get paid for 'doing' ethics—can write and speak only within accepted paradigms. We can't rock boats." Helen Bequaert Holmes, "Closing The Gap: An Imperative For Feminist Bioethicists," *Embodying Bioethics: Recent Feminist Advances*, ed. Anne Donchin and Laura M. Purdy (Lanham: Rowman & Littlefield Publishers, 1999), 57.

46. As Fox and Swazey observe, "U. S. bioethics and bioethicists have played a leading role in erecting the conceptual and organizational scaffolding for what is termed international or global bioethics in establishing its agenda, and in conveying its analytic perspective and sub-

stantive foci. American bioethicists have been primary architects of the international bioethics organizations that have been created, and among the most active and influential participants in them. Furthermore, they have been recurrently called upon by international organizations concerned with health to assume ethics-relevant offices within them, and to provide expert ethical counsel and instructions." Fox and Swazey, *Observing*, 225.

47. Fox and Swazey, *Observing*, 334.

48. Daniel Callahan, "Individual Good and Common Good: A Communitarian Approach To Bioethics," *Perspectives in Biology and Medicine* 46, no. 4 (Autumn 2003): 496—507.

49. Tom L. Beauchamp and James F. Childress, *Principles of Biomedical Ethics*, 7th Ed. (New York: Oxford University Press, 2013), 101.

50. Beauchamp and Childress, *Principles*, 102.

51. Beauchamp and Childress, *Principles*, 107.

52. Beauchamp and Childress, *Principles*, 107.

53. Beauchamp and Childress, *Principles*, 107.

54. Beauchamp and Childress, *Principles*, 101.

55. Callahan, "Individual Good," 505.

56. Beauchamp and Childress, *Principles*, 151.

57. Beauchamp and Childress, *Principles*, 203.

58. Beauchamp and Childress, *Principles*, 203.

59. Beauchamp and Childress, *Principles*, 250.

60. Beauchamp and Childress, *Principles*, 251.

61. Beauchamp and Childress, *Principles*, 277.

62. Beauchamp and Childress, *Principles*, 278.

63. Beauchamp and Childress, *Principles*, 278.

64. Beauchamp and Childress, *Principles*, 3.

65. Beauchamp and Childress, *Principles*, 4.

66. Beauchamp and Childress, *Principles*, 4.

67. Beauchamp and Childress, *Principles*, 4.

68. Beauchamp and Childress, *Principles*, 13.

69. Beauchamp and Childress, *Principles*, 405.

70. Beauchamp and Childress, *Principles*, 5.

71. Beauchamp and Childress, *Principles*, 417.

72. Beauchamp and Childress, *Principles*, 417.

73. Leigh Turner, "Zones of Consensus and Zones of Conflict: Questioning the 'Common Morality' Presumption in Bioethics," *Kennedy Institute of Ethics Journal* 13, no. 3 (Sept. 2003): 193—218.

74. Turner, "Zones of Consensus," 196.

75. Turner, "Zones of Consensus," 213.

76. Turner, "Zones of Consensus," 202.

77. Although, as Turner succinctly puts it, "If this approach was as successful as its proponents claim, most of the major issues in bioethics ought to be well on their way to resolution." "Zones of Consensus," 208.

78. Fox and Swazey argue that the strong emphasis placed on the value of autonomy in American bioethics has had a profound effect on the kinds of analyses that bioethicists engage in: "Perhaps the greatest deterrent to the incorporation of social and cultural analysis into the matrix of bioethics has been the primacy that the field has accorded to a conception of individualism and individual rights that emphasizes the values of autonomy and self-determination what has come to be known in the terminology of bioethics as the principle of 'respect for persons,' as well as 'respect for autonomy.' This accentuated individualism has its origins in what Andrew Delbanco (1999) identifies as one of the prominent ideas 'around which American society and culture have been organized since the beginning of the country's history a distinctively American conception of the self that has roots in the Protestant Christianity of the seventeenth-and eighteenth-century New England Puritans.'" *Observing Bioethics*, 153 154.

79. David DeGrazia, "Common Morality, Coherence, and the Principles of Biomedical Ethics," in *Kennedy Institute of Ethics Journal* 13, no. 3 (Sept. 2003): 219 230.

80. Beauchamp and Childress, *Principles*, 351.
81. Beauchamp and Childress, *Principles*, 351.
82. Beauchamp and Childress, *Principles*, 384.
83. Beauchamp and Childress, *Principles*, 384.
84. Michael Carrithers, *Why Humans Have Cultures: Explaining Anthropology and Social Diversity* (Oxford: Oxford University Press, 1992), 86.
85. Charles Taylor exhaustively documents the interplay between the expression of ideas by particular individuals, and the way in which those ideas, in turn, shaped both culture and individual self-understandings, in *Sources of the Self: The Making of the Modern Identity* (Cambridge, Massachusetts: Harvard University Press, 1989). Another example of this process is provided by Robert B. Talisse, who traces the influence of John Rawls and the way in which his thinking has helped shape contemporary understandings of liberalism, liberal conceptions of the self, and conceptions of justice, and how these understandings have subsequently moved into the larger American culture. While Talisse places Rawls within the context of the history of liberal thought, he notes that Rawls's achievements extend well beyond both a re-statement of already existing ideas and the world of professional philosophers: "Rawls is among the few contemporary philosophers whose work has exerted considerable influence over academic disciplines other than philosophy. Rawls's works are studied in departments of economics, political science, sociology, and in law schools throughout the world, and his ideas have helped to shape and develop these areas of inquiry. Even more remarkable is the fact that Rawls has gained the esteem of persons outside the academy." Robert B. Talisse, *On Rawls: A Liberal Theory of Justice and Justification* (Belmont, CA: Wadsworth-Thomson, 2001), 5. Some of those influenced outside the academy, Talisse notes, have been politicians, who have translated his views into public policies. These policies, in turn, have helped shape the views of members of the general public.
86. While liberalism is usually understood to be a political theory, in bioethics it is used as a moral theory as well, particularly when questions of distributive justice are being discussed. Also, as we shall see in Chapter 3, the most prevalent conception of the self in contemporary bioethics is essentially the liberal self.
87. Jeffrey Brand-Ballard, "Consistency, Common Morality, and Reflective Equilibrium," *Kennedy Institute of Ethics Journal* 13, no. 3 (Sept. 2003): 231—258.

Chapter Two

The Troubled Self of Bioethics

The Unhappy Offspring of Immanuel Kant and J. S. Mill

INTRODUCTION: THE TROUBLED SELF OF BIOETHICS

In the spring of 2011, the Ontario Minister of Health was the subject of a number of critical news reports, negative editorials, and hostile commentary on radio and television. Her transgression was to follow the recommendation of experts in evidence-based medicine to fund the $40,000 a year per patient cost of Herceptin, a drug used to treat breast tumors, only when the tumors reached a certain size. One patient, who was denied government funding of the drug because her tumors were deemed to be too small, mounted a successful campaign through social media; after the Minister made the mistake of publicly stating that "We cannot have a health system where the stories that land on the front page of the paper determine our health-care policy,"[1] she was so savagely criticized that she had to back down and agree to fund the costs of the drug for this particular patient. While there were a few dissenting voices (Andre Picard summed up the opposing side when he asked, "Are the angry, unabashed supporters of [this patient] seriously suggesting that an insurance program be it public or private has to pay for every single treatment no matter how marginal the benefit, how high the cost and how grave the risks?"[2]), most people seemed satisfied with this outcome.

This case, and the issues it raises, was discussed in a hospital ethics committee that I sit on; the discussion revealed the fault lines (as many of our discussions do) between utilitarian principles and Kantian ones, and the almost insurmountable difficulty of accommodating both of them in a satisfactory way, and the equal impossibility of choosing one over the other. While members of the committee (which includes hospital administrators, who have to make difficult decisions about how to spend money every day, and usually use utilitarian-type reasoning, weighing costs versus benefits, when they do so) acknowledged that tough choices always have to be made, that evidence-based cost-benefit decisions are probably the best that we can hope for, and that the entire health care system will collapse unless costs are controlled, they still find themselves torn. Reflecting Kantian-type considerations[3], members noted that it does seem deeply unfair, and even unjust, that some people, often for reasons beyond their control, are fortunate enough to come out on the "winning side" when cost-benefit decisions are made, while others, through no fault of their own, find themselves on the "losing side." The discussion was inconclusive, and no one seemed entirely comfortable making a whole-hearted case in support of the initial stance of the Minister of Health, or for the now-famous patient.

ORIGINS OF THE TROUBLED SELF

The three ethical theories that have traditionally had the strongest presence in bioethics are Kantianism, utilitarianism, and liberalism.[4] Sometimes this role is explicit, and demonstrated when bioethicists frame their claims and ground their arguments in one or another of these theories.[5] Sometimes, in contrast, their presence is implicit; it reveals itself not in specific theoretical appeals, but, rather, in the shape of the arguments presented, in the assumptions that underpin them and which are not themselves defended, and in the terminology which is used.[6]

The conceptions of the self that animate these three central moral theories are incompatible with one another, and their presence has contributed to the intractable nature of many bioethical debates. However, since the primary insights of these theories are widely accepted by bioethicists, the fact that they are incompatible with one another is usually seen to indicate not the presence of competing conceptions of the self and distinctive understandings of the nature of the moral life that accompany such conceptions, but, rather, as revealing irresolvable and unavoidable complexities that are inherent in the issues themselves.

However, when we start *noticing* the presence of these conceptions of the self, and that they don't arrive unencumbered but carry worlds with them, we can begin to play these conceptions off against one another, explore how they shape our moral assumptions, influence our deliberations, and even help structure what we understand to be a genuine moral dilemma. We can, in short, act as ethical anthropologists, who understand that there can be "different representations of some subject, representations which may compete but which may also be just alternatives, each offering some advantages in manipulating the matter at hand."[7]

If we do this, we might avoid falling into one of the common traps of contemporary bioethics, which is to get caught up in the travails of the Troubled Self, the self that is torn between Kantian commitments and utilitarian intuitions (or vice versa). Many of the enduring issues in bioethics have the Troubled Self at their heart, as we can see when we consider the following issues: the morality of legalizing physician-assisted suicide for the competent and euthanasia for the incompetent; using prenatal testing and selective abortion to limit the birth of infants with disabilities or to respond to parental desires to have a certain kind of child; and the ethics of medical research using human subjects.

In all of these cases, as we shall see, the method of reasoning employed by Kantians and utilitarians is so fundamentally different that there is no clear way of reconciling their approaches. At the same time, we cannot simply assert that one approach is clearly superior to the other, since both appear to offer ethical insights that we not only ought not to ignore, but, more importantly, ought to take seriously in our own deliberations. To say that the approaches taken by these theories are fundamentally different does not mean that they will always reach conflicting conclusions about what ought to be done in any particular set of circumstances (although they will frequently do so), but it does mean that features of the moral landscape that they draw our attention to will be incompatible with one another, as will the justifications they offer for that conclusion. Moreover, in bioethics, our delineation of what is at issue, and what plausible positions might be taken in any debate, often naturally fall into Kantian and utilitarian oppositions.

First, consider the question of whether the legalization of physician-assisted suicide for competent individuals who desire to end their lives, or the euthanasia of those who are incompetent but who are clearly suffering, would be a good thing, or a bad one, for those individuals, for those who love them, and for society. If one addresses this question through the framework provided by utilitarianism, one is able to argue that, if the legalization of physician-assisted suicide and euthanasia would reduce suffering, then such legalization is perhaps not only morally permissible, but even morally required.

As Vaughn notes, in classical utilitarianism, the good is defined as happiness, and all issues are judged on the basis of how much happiness the various possible actions open to us might produce for everyone who is affected by them: "From this perspective, euthanasia or assisted suicide for someone suffering horrible, inescapable pain might be permissible because ending life would bring about the most net happiness."[8] In addition, he notes, appeals to the utilitarian principle of beneficence would suggest that, "If we are in a position to relieve the severe suffering of another without excess cost to ourselves, we have a duty to do so. To refuse would be cruel, inhumane, and wrong."[9] And we can note that the same kind of reasoning that makes this conclusion appropriate in the case of the competent can be extended to the suffering incompetent as well: if we can justify helping the competent to end their lives because doing so will end their suffering, the same principle suggests that we should end the lives of those who are suffering even if they cannot make this request for themselves. What is most important, that is to say, is the fact of suffering, not determinations of competency or incompetency.

Further, utilitarians who take seriously the injunction that we should work to produce the greatest amount of happiness for the greatest number of people might also argue that physician-assisted suicide and euthanasia should be legalized because it would reduce health care costs, which would be beneficial for society as a whole. As Battin puts it, those making a case for legalization assume "that the projected cost savings from euthanasia and assisted suicide are an additional reason favoring legalization. . . . This is a view compatible with the utilitarian background of these arguments: Even though some losses might be borne by a few, the imposition of these losses would produce the greater good for the greater number."[10]

Where utilitarians would focus their discussions of this question, then, would not be on the moral permissibility or impermissibility of killing or of helping someone to die. Rather, they would focus their attention on the question of whether, *in fact*, particular legislative proposals would reduce suffering and costs, or whether such legislation would increase suffering because it would make people fearful of seeking medical attention in case they are euthanized against their will, and whether costs would increase because of additional safeguards that would need to be built into the health care system in order for such legislation to receive sufficient public support.

For the Kantian, however, the most important questions raised by this issue are very different, and he would find the question of whether or not physician-assisted suicide should be legalized very easy to answer, at least in the case of those who are competent: killing someone without their consent is clearly ruled out, but so is committing suicide (whatever our reasons), or asking someone else to help us end our lives. In the first case, we would be failing to recognize the duties we have to others, in the second, the duties we have to ourselves, and, in the third, the physician would be failing to act as a moral agent should, were he to agree to our request. As Vaughn straightforwardly puts it, "What is clear in Kant's theory is that suicide is prohibited because it treats persons as mere things and obliterates personhood. . . . It is also clear on Kant's view that competent persons must not be killed or permitted to die."[11]

In addition, for the Kantian, unlike the utilitarian (whose primary concern with respect to the legalization question is suffering, not competency), Vaughn argues that it is the incompetent who raise the most significant and difficult questions as a result of the connection Kant draws between personhood and rationality: "it is not obvious what Kant's opinion would be of individuals no longer regarded as persons because they have lapsed into a persistent vegetative state. Would respect for persons demand that they be kept alive at all costs—or that we perform non-voluntary euthanasia to allow them to die with dignity?"[12] In short, then, the sides taken by utilitarians and Kantians with respect to the ethical implications of legalizing assisted suicide and euthanasia fall into what appears to be a natural and even inevitable division: the moral imperative to reduce suffering whenever possible, versus the requirement that we treat persons in accordance with principles of respect and dignity, and preserve life as much as we can.

Second, consider the issues raised by prenatal testing, selective abortion, and eugenics. Do potential parents who undergo prenatal testing to determine whether the fetus has a condition that will cause the potential child to be born with a disability have the right to choose to selectively abort on the basis of that test result? Indeed, might they even have an obligation to undergo such testing, and should they be encouraged to choose selective abortion if the fetus tests positive for a condition that will cause a disability? Finally, do parents have the right, not only to choose to avoid the birth of a child who will suffer from a disability, but also to choose to have a child with particular traits that they believe to be valuable? Again, the fault lines around these questions tend to be drawn along explicitly Kantian and utilitarian lines.

As Munson notes, a case for negative eugenics, which seeks to reduce the frequency of undesirable traits in a population through the creation of social policies designed to achieve this goal, can easily be justified through an application of the principle of utility: "the aim here need not be the remote one of improving the human population but the more immediate one of preventing an increase in sorrows and pain that would be caused by an impaired child."[13] Indeed, from a utilitarian perspective, it might even make sense to come up with a list of conditions which ought to be tested for prenatally, and, if a fetus is discovered to have any of them, abortion might be not simply permissible but actively encouraged.

Further, on utilitarian grounds, it might be considered beneficial, not only to discourage individuals from giving birth to children with undesirable traits, but to encourage them to reproduce children with desirable ones; as Munson notes, only utilitarianism, of the major ethical theories available to bioethicists, is likely to provide support for "a program of positive eugenics" in which the goal "of increasing the frequency of desirable traits in the human species might, in terms of the principle of utility, justify placing restrictions on reproduction."[14] In an essay that picks up on this theme, Savulescu argues that, according to a (utilitarian-type) principle of "Procreative Beneficence," parents have an obligation to produce the "best children possible," and that the means for doing so include prenatal testing and selective abortion."[15]

Someone who views these issues through a Kantian lens, in contrast, will reason very differently, and will draw very different conclusions about the purposes of prenatal testing, and the permissibility of selective abortion. Even if she is not entirely certain that a fetus meets the requirements of personhood as a Kantian would understand them, she would be hesitant to make judgments about whose lives are worth living and whose lives are not, and concerned about the degree of parental control over offspring expressed in these utilitarian proposals. As Savulescu states, the following objections are usually made to proposals like his, and we should note that they are either explicitly Kantian, or inspired by Kantian ethical considerations: "One common objection to genetic selection . . . is that it results in harm to the child. There are various versions of this objection, which include the harm which arises from excessive and overbearing parental expectations, using the child as a means, and not treating it as an end, and closing off possible future options."[16] In a claim that supports Savulescu's contention of the sorts of objections that are offered in response to proposals like the one he is making, in her argument about a child's "right to an open future," Davis states, "Deliberately creating a child who will be forced irreversibly into the parent's notion of a 'good life' violates the Kantian principle of treating each person as an end in herself and never as a means only."[17] Again, the battle lines seem inevitable and natural: increasing happiness and reducing suffering, versus respect for persons, which requires us to treat all persons as ends in themselves, regardless of their particular abilities or disabilities.

Finally, consider the issue of research and experimentation using human subjects. While such research produces benefits, it also involves unavoidable risks to participants, no matter how carefully designed the research protocol, and how scrupulous the investigator. Despite these risks, utilitarians must view such research positively. As Vaughn observes, it meets all the requirements set out in the utilitarian moral system: "Through medical research, the causes of disease are unmasked, disease preventions are devised, treatments are developed, and the true worth of common but untested therapies is determined. Thus, human well-being is advanced."[18] Indeed, given their ethical framework, utilitarians might sometimes endorse experimentation that imposes great costs (pain, suffering, and even death) on a small number of subjects, as long as the results that come out of the research benefit a sufficiently large number of people. Munson observes that a utilitarian perspective on research using human subjects does not even require that they give informed consent, and he further notes that "the principle of utility suggests that the best research subjects would be 'less valuable' members of the society, such as the mentally retarded, the habitual criminal, or the dying."[19]

Kantians, in contrast, will be inclined to view research on human subjects with a great deal of suspicion, given the requirement that persons need to be treated as ends in themselves, and never only as a means to benefit others—a requirement that all research, with the possible exception of research on treatments that may offer a benefit to the chosen participants, given their own health situation, risks violating. Consequently, many of the strongest arguments against particular experiments are made by those working within a Kantian framework, and most of the safeguards now built in to such research (particularly the requirements around informed consent) are Kantian in origin. As Vaughn notes, the Kantian approach to research is distinctive and powerful: "Its means-ends requirement—the prohibition against using persons as though they were things—was implicit in the strong condemnations of the Nazi medical experiments, the Cold War Radiation research, the Tuskeegee Study, and many others. It proscribes the coercing of research subjects, deceiving them, and diminishing or destroying their autonomy."[20] Indeed, not only does a Kantian perspective place limits on what we may do to others, it also places limits on the risks we may agree to take: while we can, as autonomous individuals, choose to volunteer as research subjects, the experimental procedures we agree to participate in must be ones that are responsive to the duties we have to ourselves. Once again, both perspectives seem to capture something fundamentally correct—medical research has conferred enormous benefits on human beings in general, and yet a number of particular individuals have suffered and even died in pursuit of this goal. In this case, utilitarianism seems to go too far, and Kantianism—at least if we take the means-ends formulation seriously—seems to allow too little.

In short, for the utilitarian, the ends will always justify the means, as long as the ends are important enough and benefit enough people, and the means an effective way to achieve them. For the Kantian, in contrast, the ends can never justify the means, however good our intentions, and however efficient our methods. And most of us are caught somewhere in the middle. We can experience situations, or imagine scenarios, in which physician-assisted suicide seems the most ethical response to someone's suffering, conditions for which selective abortion seems the most humane choice, and articulate benefits achieved for all of us through research on human subjects. On the other hand, few of us are entirely comfortable fully embracing utilitarian reasoning, or the moral commitments that follow from it: we would not want assisted suicide or euthanasia to be a regular part of end of life treatment, to have selective abortion encouraged through widespread social policies, and we believe that experimentation on human subjects can only be ethically performed when rigorous safeguards are in place, safeguards that must be found someplace other than in utilitarian theory.

The point here is not that it is difficult to *balance* these perspectives with one another. It is, far more fundamentally, that these approaches to moral decision making and reasoning are so different from one another that their commitments and outlook can hardly even be compared, just as, while they are both varieties of fruit, apples are difficult to compare to oranges. What happens, in particular cases, is that we must choose to privilege one account over the other. Sometimes, we will come down on the utilitarian side, and will justify our choice by an appeal to consequences, happiness, and utility; sometimes, we will come down on the Kantian side, and will justify our decision by an appeal to intentions, rights, and the means-ends formulation of the Categorical Imperative. Many of the debates in bioethics are driven precisely because different people will choose differently, with respect to particular cases or issues, which side of the divide is most compelling or most defensible, and, even if we have chosen differently, it will be hard to make the case that our opponent's choice is clearly wrong, and our own favored position clearly right. Indeed, if we are being fair, we will have to acknowledge that we, too, could have chosen differently, and for good reasons. Both theories employ conceptions of the self that are compelling, and both descriptions of the moral universe through which their self moves and acts contain elements that appear insightful, appealing, and even correct; consequently, while they cannot be reconciled with one another, we cannot easily claim that one is clearly better than the other. In short, neither approach is entirely satisfactory, but neither can be easily dismissed, so we are stuck with both and often pulled between them.

The presence of these competing conceptions of the self, moreover, contribute to what are arguably larger inconsistencies within the field of bioethics itself, in which arguments and lines of thinking that are widely accepted with respect to one issue are rejected in the case of another. For example, the right of individuals to freely choose for themselves on the basis of reasons which seem valid to them (a right which is supported by both Kantian and liberal conceptions of the self) is widely accepted as the basis of the requirement that patients give informed consent to medical procedures, and as a justification for the free use of reproductive technologies which sever the genetic, gestational, and social aspects of parenthood. Likewise, most bioethicists accept that it would be a good thing if the supply of organs available for transplantation were increased, even if this means moving towards a system of presumed consent and shifting away from whole-brain definitions of death to cardiac-based criteria, a position that relies heavily on (not always explicit) utilitarian considerations.

The Troubled Self is troubled precisely because it feels pulled in different directions, for reasons that are simultaneously compelling and contrary to one another. It wants to do justice to both intentions and consequences, feels that, on occasion, we ought to weigh costs and benefits, and that, in other situations, to approach ethical decisions in this way would be to distort what is most fundamentally at issue, we want to promote the common welfare, and we want to treat people as ends in themselves. Its presence, ironically enough, is revealed not only in explicit references to Kantian or utilitarian moral theory, or through the application of concepts that draw on these theories, but is also in the principled approach we considered earlier. Two of the principles—beneficence and non-maleficence—are usually thought to reflect the consequentialist orientation towards ethical reasoning which is most persuasively and influentially articulated by utilitarians, while autonomy and justice are frequently understood to derive, by both direct and indirect means, from Kantian commitments (often, in bioethics, supplemented by a liberal gloss). So, far from avoiding the conflict between ethical theories that this principled approach was designed to do, it actually embodies it.

Moreover, when these principles are applied in "real life" situations, when we discuss particular cases in ethics committees, or try to come up with ethically sound policies for health care institutions which also meet organizational constraints, the conflicting sides tend to fall along Kantian and utilitarian lines, and unless we are willing to commit ourselves wholeheartedly to one theory or the other (which few are willing to do, since both appear to capture fundamental ethical insights and to exclude other features that an adequate moral account would include), we find ourselves stuck: we have no reason to choose one side over the other, and we frequently end up experiencing a lack of confidence in the decision that is eventually made. A feeling of moral distress—a sense of unease—generated by the fact that we feel that we are unable to do what we know we have good reason to do, or because we recognize that we remain torn between conflicting reasons, can result. In addition, as we shall see, the central place occupied by autonomy, and the increasing detachment of the value of autonomy from other ethical and political commitments reflects, at least in part, a recognition that, given that we cannot easily choose between utilitarian and Kantian commitments, we need to find some alternative to both, one which does not, itself, require us to make substantive moral claims which might appeal to one or the other of these theories.

It is now time to flesh out the utilitarian and Kantian conceptions of the self, and to describe the moral space within which these selves choose, act, and think. While it is common to present the conflict between Kantian and utilitarian moral thinking as lying primarily in whether it is our intentions which are most important or the consequences of our actions, if we shift our thinking towards asking what conceptions of the self lie at the heart of each theory, other, less frequently remarked upon but arguably even more significant differences reveal themselves. We can see that the emphasis on intentions, in one case, and on consequences, in the other, *result* from these fundamental distinctions, rather than being the *cause* of them. Neither Kantian deontology nor utilitarian consequentialism can tell us who is to count as a self, in the sense that is necessary for the attribution of moral agency and personhood; they only tell us how those who count as selves ought to think and act, and towards whom they have moral obligations.[21] I will consider three aspects of these competing conceptions of the self: the model of enquiry which tells us how to arrive at ethical knowledge, and what form that knowledge should take; the place of emotion in the life of the moral agent; and the space that non-human animals occupy in the moral universe articulated by the theory.

My account of Kantianism and utilitarianism will be selective, not comprehensive;[22] what I want to identify are the central features of each theory which most clearly distinguish it from its rival, and which reveal the conception of the self which lies beneath these features. The aspects I will explore, moreover, are important to the role these theories play in bioethics, where they come together to form an identifiable self, but one that is pulled in different and incompatible directions. I should also note that the selves I describe are the ideal selves which meet the requirements of moral agency, as these requirements are set out by Kant, and by the utilitarians: they are not precisely "us"; they are, rather, what these theories tell us we ought to be, and can be, if we only try hard enough and in the right way.

It is important to note that the selves that underpin Kantianism and utilitarianism are both eminently rational: their moral decisions rely upon a rational analysis of what they ought to do in any given situation, given the principles that they believe a commitment to moral behavior imposes upon them. However, because the selves described in each theory are strikingly different from one another, and because the moral landscapes within which they are placed are mapped so differently, the answers they give to moral questions, and the reasons for which they arrive at these responses, can diverge enormously. Metaphorically speaking, it is as though (to adapt a phrase borrowed from Nina Rosenstand) they inhabit different "moral universes":[23] ones containing worlds with very different histories, customs, religious beliefs, political arrangements, and even different requirements for moral citizenship. In order to map these universes and identify their inhabitants, we must act like anthropological explorers. I will describe the Kantian self and the moral world it inhabits first, and then do the same for the utilitarian self.

THE ECCENTRICITIES OF THE KANTIAN SELF

The central role that Kantian theory has played in Western ethical thought has made many of Kant's claims about the nature of duty, the importance of autonomy, and the requirement that moral actions be universalizeable so familiar to us that we tend not to notice how distinctly odd is the self that animates his account, and how decidedly strange is his description of the moral landscape within which that self is placed. So this is where I want to begin: with noticing how odd the Kantian self is, and how many of its features could have just as easily been created by a writer of science fiction as by a philosopher.

The most obvious characteristic of this self is its supreme rationality; the Kantian self recognizes, through the exercise of reason, that he has a duty to treat rational creatures as ends in themselves, not merely as tools for his own purposes.[24] Consequently, emotions, even positive ones like love, affection, and sympathy, must be recognized by the Kantian self as things which can distract him from his duty, so he must ignore them in his moral deliberations: he ascertains what he must do through the application of the Categorical Imperative, an entirely logical test which allows him to distinguish morally required actions from those which are morally indifferent or morally wrong. The Kantian self, moreover, must be detached from his own immediate desires and ends when he recognizes that he must not make an exception of himself when determining how he ought to act. For the Kantian self, autonomy lies in the rational capacity to determine what the moral law is, and to follow it for its own sake: as Kant puts it, "A rational being belongs to the realm of ends as a member when he gives universal laws in it while also himself subject to these laws. He belongs to it as a sovereign when he, as legislating, is subject to the will of no other."[25] In Kant's account of autonomy, unlike the liberal account that we will explore in the next chapter, autonomy consists in discovering and obeying moral laws that are ascertained through the exercise of logical reasoning. What is important for the Kantian self, then, are his intentions: as long as they arise from a Good Will—a Will that uses reason to identify the moral laws, and acts according to these laws for the sake of duty—the consequences of his actions are utterly irrelevant: "The moral worth of an action does not lie in the effect which is expected from it or in any principle of action which has to borrow its motive from this expected effect. For all these effects . . . could be brought about through other causes and would not require the will of a rational being, while the highest and unconditioned good can be found only in such a will."[26] Conversely, of course, it follows that two nearly identical actions performed in nearly identical circumstances, and producing nearly identical results, can actually carry very different moral weights: if one is performed for the sake of duty while the other is not, only one will meet the requirements of Kantian morality, while the other will only appear to do so.

We can now explore the moral space through which Kantian selves move, and it's important, once more, to notice what a uniquely odd landscape this is. It's one that is, again, so profoundly strange (appealing and even sublime, perhaps, as an ideal towards which we should aim, but strikingly different from that assumed within other ethical approaches, and from that inhabited by any actually existing persons) that it could have been presented as a fictional creation, rather than a philosophical account of how we should understand morality. Consider, in particular, the following features. First, this is a world in which only rational beings have value: as Kant puts it, "Beings whose existence does not depend on our will but on nature, if they are not rational beings, have only a relative worth as means and are therefore called 'things'; on the other hand, rational beings are designated 'persons' because their nature indicates that they are ends in themselves, i.e., things which may not be used merely as means."[27]

This means that nonhuman animals are essentially *things*; they carry no direct moral weight, and they are not fellow citizens of the moral universe occupied by human beings. While Kant believes that we ought not to be gratuitously cruel to them, the reason for this is not because we have any moral duty towards the animals that are affected by our actions, but because "he who is cruel to animals becomes hard also in his dealings with men."[28] Moreover, Kant's assertion that we have moral obligations only to rational beings raises questions about where we should place human beings who lack rationality: are newborn babies creatures toward whom we have moral obligations? Are people with advanced Alzheimer's citizens of the moral universe, or 'things' like animals?

On the other hand, Kant's views suggest that we might extend moral citizenship to beings as yet undiscovered or uncreated. Rosenstand asks, "Would Kant respect a thinking android or computer, or a rational alien. . . ? If these beings are *rational*, they qualify as full members of our moral universe, and humans have no right to use them as tools."[29] Paradoxically, the Kantian conception of the self appears broad enough in one way to encompass extraterrestrials, androids, and computers (as long as they are sufficiently rational), but too narrow in another way to easily include a grandmother suffering from advanced dementia, a newborn child, or someone in a persistent vegetative state.[30]

A second surprising feature of Kant's moral universe is that moral reality and moral appearance are so different that many of our instinctive ways of thinking about the moral life are turned upside down. Consider two examples. Imagine two people who live next door to one another for many, many years, and whose lives have been very similar: they each raise families, hold down jobs, attend religious services, and make important contributions to the community through their volunteer work and charitable contributions. One, however, did these things because she felt that she had a duty to contribute to her family and her community, and she acted as she did because of this recognition. The other, in contrast, did these things because he loved his wife and children, enjoyed socializing with those with whom he did volunteer work, and felt good about his charitable commitments. Only the first person, in Kant's mapping of the moral universe actually acted as a proper moral agent should; the actions of the second, in contrast, have no moral weight. As Kant observes, "there are . . . many persons so sympathetically constituted that without any motive of vanity or selfishness they find an inner satisfaction in spreading joy and rejoice in the contentment of others which they have made possible."[31] However, he bluntly continues, "I say that, however dutiful and amiable it may be, that kind of action has no true moral worth. . . . For the maxim [on which they acted] lacks the moral import of an action done not from inclination but from duty."[32] Even in her treatment of family and friends, then, the Kantian self ought to act primarily for the sake of duty: she has only indirect and subordinate reasons to demonstrate love or affection to particular people.

Second, consider two people, one of whom, for reasons beyond her control, never manages to achieve anything significant in her life; she has few resources, material or social, and so is unable to contribute to the well-being of others. She lives, let us imagine, on a small pension, earned after years of quiet office work, and her only companion is her cat. However, she has a Good Will, acts for the sake of duty, and always follows the moral rules that she rationally identifies through the application of the Categorical Imperative. The second woman, in contrast, was highly successful in business, made enormous amounts of money, and took an early retirement in order to set up a charitable foundation to vaccinate children in the third world. As a result of her actions, many lives are saved. However, she does these things not for the sake of duty, but because they make her feel better about herself, and she also enjoys the attention she gets from the media as a result of her work. In this moral universe, only the first woman demonstrates the characteristics of the ideal Kantian self; the second, for all her achievements, is a moral failure. As Kant poetically puts it, when it comes to the Good Will, even if it achieves nothing, "it would sparkle like a jewel in its own right, as something that had its full worth in itself. . . . Usefulness or fruitlessness can neither diminish nor augment this moral worth."[33]

Third, as these two examples make clear, in Kant's delineation of the moral universe consequences are not merely *less* important than intentions, they are actually morally *meaningless*. Consequently, an action that has bad consequences can actually be morally good (if it was done for the right reasons, as Kant defines them), while an action that has good consequences (but was performed for the wrong reasons) has no moral worth.

The final distinctive feature of the Kantian moral universe is that, in it, moral rules are *discovered*, not *made*: they exist independently of time, place, circumstance, and human wants, needs, beliefs, and desires. Moral reasoning, for the Kantian self, reveals objective moral truths that are external to each moral agent. In this picture, moral reasoning involves "the same kind of logical reasoning that establishes such indisputable truths in mathematics and logic as 2+2=4, No circles are squares, and All triangles are three-sided."[34] Consequently, all Kantian selves, if they reason correctly, will arrive at the same moral truths, and these truths will be absolute: in just the same way that it would be a logical impossibility for some squares or triangles to be circles, so too, it must always be wrong to lie, break promises, or waste our talents because these actions are logically inconsistent with the moral rules that reason reveals to us.

The Kantian self, in short, is rational and logical; moved to act by duty, not inclination or emotion; and capable of radically separating the intention which leads to an action from the consequences that follow from it. The world the Kantian self inhabits is one in which moral reality and moral appearance are profoundly different from one another, and saints and sinners not always easy to tell apart. It is a world, finally, in which computers might one day meet the requirements for personhood, while sentient creatures, and even some human beings, fail to do so.

THE PLEASURES AND PAINS OF THE UTILITARIAN SELF

The utilitarian self is a distorted mirror image of the Kantian self, and the moral universe described by utilitarians into which this self is placed is almost precisely the reverse of the Kantian one. For the utilitarian self, the goal of morality is to increase the overall amount of happiness and decrease the overall amount of pain; in the first instance, for those he encounters in his own life, and, in the second, for all sentient beings. As a result, *consequences*, whatever achieves this goal are important, and intentions are essentially meaningless. Mill makes this point in memorable terms when he states that "He who saves a fellow creature from drowning does what is morally right, whether his motive be duty, or the hope of being paid for his trouble; he who betrays the friend that trusts him, is guilty of a crime, even if his object is to serve another friend to whom he is under greater obligations."[35] Moreover, in the utilitarian view, considerations of the goodness or badness of the person performing an action "are relevant, not to the estimation of actions, but of persons"[36]; bad people, therefore, can do good things, and good people bad ones: it all depends on what the consequences of their actions turn out to be, not the reasons for which those actions were performed.

In the utilitarian moral universe, then, rather than looking for timeless and objective moral rules that we can apply in the same way to any situation in which we find ourselves, the utilitarian self will adjust her actions precisely to the particular set of circumstances in which a decision is required. For the Kantian self, the particular circumstances in which moral choices are made are almost as irrelevant as the consequences of that choice (if it's always wrong to lie, then the circumstances in which we might be tempted to lie are unimportant); for the utilitarian self, in contrast, the particular details of the situation in which a moral choice is being made are crucially significant: depending on these details, a lie might be wrong; but it might, in other circumstances, prevent hurt feelings, protect an important secret, or even save a life.

The utilitarian self, moreover, must rely on a particular species of feeling in order to be motivated to act morally. It is often observed that there is a significant gap in the utilitarian account between what it is rational for each person to do, and what morality requires of him. Mill asserts that the way in which utilitarians determine that humans desire pleasure and seek to avoid pain—a belief that provides the foundation of the utilitarian moral system— is not through an abstract logical analysis of the nature and duties of rational beings, but, rather, through observation and experience. The merits of the utilitarian principle "can only be determined by practiced self-consciousness and self-observation, assisted by observation of others."[37] However, while it might be rational for each individual to seek to maximize her own happiness and minimize her own pains, and to use reason to determine what to do to achieve this goal, it is quite another to say (as utilitarians do) that each of us is obligated, according to the same rational principle, to increase the *overall* levels of happiness for the largest number of people, even, perhaps, at a high cost to ourselves.

This gap can only be bridged, many commentators believe, by a feeling of benevolence or sympathy. Sidgwick, for example, considers that the "gap between desire for one's own happiness and desire for the general happiness can only be filled by an 'intuition' albeit a *philosophical* rather than a commonsense intuition of Rational Benevolence, to the effect that each individual is morally bound to regard the good of every other individual as much as his own."[38] Mill himself believes that it can be bridged through appropriate social and educational policies: "education and opinion, which have so vast a power over human character, should so use that power as to establish in the mind of every individual an indissoluble association between his own happiness and the good of the whole."[39] And this brings us to another feature of the utilitarian self that distinguishes it from its Kantian cousin: rather than looking to reason to discover objective, independent, and timeless truths, the utilitarian self sees moral goals as ones that can be achieved incrementally, as we understand the world more clearly, design our societies in increasingly better ways, and determine what social and political policies work best to increase happiness and decrease suffering. As the above quote suggests, the utilitarian self places a high degree of importance on education: it is education that will train people to care as much for the well-being of others as for their own well-being. Indeed, Mill has such a high degree of confidence in the power of education that he believes that this feeling of benevolence or sympathy can be extended not only to all human beings, "but, so far as the nature of things admits, to the whole sentient creation."[40]

This last claim that utilitarian principles apply not only to human beings but also to all sentient creatures sets the utilitarian moral universe apart not only from the world of the Kantian, but from most other ethical theories as well. Bentham, a prominent utilitarian, famously said that what distinguishes fellow citizens of the moral universe apart from objects toward whom no moral obligations exist is the capacity to feel pain: "The question is not, can they reason? Nor, can they talk? But, can they suffer?"[41] Peter Singer, a contemporary utilitarian, suggests that utilitarianism revolves around a principle of equality which holds that each is to count for one, and count equally, and that this principle applies both to humans and to (sentient) nonhuman animals. What this principle requires in practice is not identical *treatment*, but, rather, *equal consideration*. Equal consideration for different beings will result in different practical choices, depending on the characteristics of the creature that will be affected by our actions: "concern for the well-being of a child growing up in America would require that we teach him to read; concern for the well-being of a pig may require no more than that we leave him alone with other pigs in a place where there is adequate food and room to run freely."[42]

The utilitarian self, and the world in which this self is placed, look, on the surface, much more like us, and the "real" world we actually inhabit, than the self and the moral terrain described by Kant. On closer examination, however, this world reveals itself to be a strange construction as well. Not only is it difficult for us to actually care about the pleasures and pains of others as much as we care about our own pleasures and pains—as Blackburn puts it, the world described by the utilitarians "would be a world of indiscriminate sympathy: a nice world, but not quite the world we live in"[43]—but it is also a world in which the potential candidates for what I have been calling "moral citizenship" increase exponentially. If Kant's criteria seem to limit moral citizenship in ways that are difficult to justify (by, for instance, potentially excluding newborn infants), the candidates for entry into the utilitarian ranks of beings who count morally raise intellectual and practical questions. Where, for example, do we draw the line? Do we include dolphins but exclude fish? Do we include cats and dogs but exclude insects? If we follow Warren's proposal that moral personhood provides the dividing line between creatures we can eat and creatures we can't, must the utilitarian self (at least in its human incarnation) be a vegetarian? Moreover, being a consistent utilitarian may force us to count some nonhuman animals more heavily in our calculations than some human beings; as Singer puts it, while it is usually the case "that if we have to choose between the life of a human being and the life of another animal we would choose to save the human, but there may be cases in which the reverse holds true, because the human being in question does not have the capacities of a normal human being."[44]

This last point brings us to another distinguishing characteristic of the utilitarian moral universe. This is that we must assume that we can, at least roughly, *quantify* or *weigh* the options open to us, so that we can determine which of the choices we make will, in fact, increase the overall amount of pleasure or happiness with the least amount of pain. The utilitarian self, then, inhabits a world in which pleasures and pains are *quantifiable*. Bentham tells us that, when trying to determine what we should do, we should "sum up all the values of all the *pleasures* on one side, and those of the pains on the other. . . . Take the balance, which on the side of *pleasure*, will give the general *good tendency* of the act, with respect to the total number or community of individuals concerned; if on the side of pain, the general *evil tendency*, with respect to the same community."[45] These kinds of analyses of trade-offs are ones that the utilitarian self must make all the time: it is, in fact, this sort of assessment which constitutes the practical guidance that utilitarianism offers to us, and it is a way of looking at the world which has been incorporated into contemporary cost-benefit analysis (an approach to decision-making which plays an important role in many areas of applied ethics, including bioethics). We are now, perhaps, so accustomed to this way of thinking that we don't notice how odd it is to believe that happiness and unhappiness (or benefits and costs) are things that actually can be weighed and measured. As James Rachels observes, while the idea that we should strive to increase happiness now sounds like a "mild truism," it's actually a profoundly "radical idea,"[46] and one with, as Singer's views on animals demonstrate, potentially radical consequences. It follows from this idea, for instance, that no action is inherently forbidden, even murder; and that almost any action we engage in, whether we see it as involving a moral choice or not, potentially has morally relevant consequences.

The utilitarian self, in short, is moved by benevolence and sympathy to count the well-being of others as being as significant as her own; must be deeply engaged in the political, social, and educational dimensions of her society in order to ensure that utilitarian values are inculcated in all citizens; and is willing to extend this benevolent concern for the overall well-being or happiness to all sentient creatures, but must also be willing to ruthlessly sacrifice the well-being of some (or even her own well-being, or that of someone she loves) if that is what is necessary to increase the overall amount of happiness or to decrease the overall amount of pain. The ideal utilitarian self, then, must take on the role of a benevolent, rational, and disinterested spectator, one who is more concerned to increase the overall level of happiness than to enhance her own.

CONCLUSION: THE TURN TO AUTONOMY

Thinking simultaneously in both Kantian and utilitarian terms has become an inescapable part of our mindset in bioethics, which is why it can be said that the two selves have been combined to form one conception, namely, the

Troubled Self. These theories are like conjoined twins: it's hard to think about, or apply one, without simultaneously thinking about the other as foil, as critic, and as competitor. As a result, Kantianism is often used to demonstrate flaws in the approach taken by utilitarians, and vice versa, and it is hard to place ourselves wholeheartedly in either of the distinct moral worlds each theory creates. Like the concept of a mountain requiring a valley, or a hero needing a villain, these theories have become inextricably linked to one another.

Consequently, we often approach the ethical questions that arise in bioethics in terms of binary oppositions: we think that both *consequences* and *intentions* are important, and we often don't know which should take priority in our moral deliberations when they seem to conflict; we believe that ethical judgments should be responsive to situations *and* that there should be absolute moral rules that cannot be broken regardless of circumstance; we think that emotions such as sympathy and empathy are important in shaping our treatment of others, particularly in the case of what are sometimes called the "caring" professions (such as nursing and medicine), *and* that emotions should not distract us from our moral obligations, which should not be influenced by how we feel; and, finally, we are willing to engage in a cost-benefit analysis in many cases, even as we recognize (and feel uncomfortable about) the fact that such an analysis may violate the rights of at least some of the individuals who are affected by the choices made as a result of this analysis.[47]

Kantianism and utilitarianism underpin other concepts that are widely employed in bioethics, such as measuring, in quantifiable terms, the outcomes of health care policies, respect for the dignity of patients, and the doctrine of informed consent. Consequently, utilitarianism and Kantianism form a significant part of the very warp and woof of the tapestry that is bioethics, and their interlocking strands are difficult to disentangle. Indeed, many of the discussions in bioethics are structured so that they implicitly depend on the interplay between these two theories, even as the tensions between them make the issues difficult to resolve.

While it is unarguably the case that our ethical thinking generally, and bioethics often demonstrates this, is profoundly and unavoidably shaped by these two theories, it would be a mistake to think that this demonstrates that Kant and the utilitarians simply discovered and articulated aspects of the moral life which are simply *true*. As Rachels observes, "Philosophers like to think that their ideas can change society. Often it is a vain hope: philosophers write books that are read, perhaps, by a few like-minded thinkers, while the rest of the world goes on unaffected. On occasion, however, a philosophical theory can profoundly alter the way people think."[48] Utilitarianism and Kantianism fall into this category. They have shaped our thinking in ways that would have been utterly unthinkable to moral philosophers in the ancient and medieval worlds: these theories make no reference to virtue in the classical sense; no reference to God as the source of moral commands; and at the heart of each theory lies a very modern commitment to individuality and equality—which partially accounts for the ease with which they can be compared to one another—but each theory fills these concepts out in very different ways—which partially accounts for their overall incompatibility. In Kantian terms, this commitment is reflected in the claim that each rational being has a worth and dignity equal to the worth and dignity of every other moral agent, and so it can never be legitimately overridden; in utilitarian terms, each is to count for one, and no one for more than one, and this means, in practice, that individual interests can be outweighed by the good of the many. These ideas, which seem so natural to us now, emerged from particularly powerful works of the imagination that have shaped how we understand not only what morality is, but even what we, as human beings, most fundamentally are. The fact that the conceptions of the self assumed by these theories, and their mapping of the moral space inhabited by these selves are radically different from one another, coupled with our acceptance of them, results in the birth of the Troubled Self of bioethics. The presence of this Troubled Self influences the way in which issues are framed, shapes the ways in which they are analyzed, and contributes to the difficulty we have resolving them. It frequently (and apparently naturally) forces us to think in familiar but oppositional terms, and to think of these oppositions as being rooted in the difficult nature of the issues bioethics considers, rather than in the presence of the Troubled Self that animates our examination of them.

Because we are torn between the worlds of the utilitarian and Kantian selves, and have no good way to choose one over the other, bioethicists have increasingly turned towards the idea of autonomy as a way to avoid the moral impasses generated by the Troubled Self. Autonomy, in simple terms, is a conception of human flourishing which holds that we live better lives when the choices we make are our own, rather than things which have been decided for us by others. As an idea, autonomy owes some of its elements to Kant; however, Kant's view of autonomy connects this concept to our rational capacity to recognize the moral law, and to act on it for the sake of duty. Kantian autonomy, then, is tied to the idea that autonomous beings are responding to criteria that exist independently of them, and that it is in accordance with these criteria that particular choices can be evaluated as corresponding or not corresponding to what is morally required. In contemporary mainstream bioethics, however, autonomy is given a distinctly liberal gloss, in which the ideal of what it is to flourish as an autonomous being is tied to our capacity to determine, for ourselves, what gives meaning and value to our own lives. On this account, there is no requirement that others share our beliefs about value, and nothing outside of ourselves (with, as we shall see, the notable exception of the Harm Principle) against which our choices can be measured and evaluated.

Before turning to this conception of autonomy, and showing the way in which it culminates, in bioethics, in the figure of the Choosing Self, I want briefly to demonstrate the way in which appeals to autonomy understood in the second way can help provide an escape from the difficulties experienced by the Troubled Self. I will return to the three issues we looked at in some detail above, namely, assisted suicide and euthanasia, selective abortion and eugenics, and research using human subjects.

First, as we saw, the question of whether or not it would be a good idea to legalize assisted suicide and euthanasia, when considered in utilitarian and Kantian terms, results in the unsatisfactory conclusion that these practices ought to be both encouraged and discouraged. The easiest way out of this impasse is to turn to the person in question in any particular case in which assisted suicide is contemplated and ask what she wants (something that can only be easily done, of course, in a context in which assisted suicide is legal). The strongest arguments in support of the legalization of assisted suicide and euthanasia in bioethics today, as a consequence, are autonomy based, and make appeal to the principle of self-determination. As Brock puts it, "self-determination as it bears on euthanasia . . . [requires us to recognize] people's interest in making important decisions about their lives for themselves according to their own values or conceptions of the good life, and in being left free to act on these decisions."[49] Moreover, the same line of thinking can be extended, in at least some cases, towards those who were formally but no longer competent. If, for instance, they made an advanced directive, or clearly articulated their wishes while competent, then we are respecting them as (formerly) autonomous and self-determining persons if we make decisions on the basis of these wishes. If we take the concept of autonomy to be the appropriate lens through which to examine the question of legalization, bioethicists do not have to reach any conclusions about the rightness or wrongness of euthanasia and assisted suicide in some clear and uncontroversial way; they simply have to ensure that autonomous choice is respected, and leave the determination of the morality or immorality of the choice to end a life in this way up to the individual in question. Moreover, an autonomy-based approach to this issue suggests that one person's determination that assisted suicide is morally wrong means only that he should not choose it for himself; it does not follow from this determination that he has the right to impose his beliefs upon anyone else, whose conception of what constitutes the good life may be different.

Second, the framework provided by autonomy also provides a way out of the selective abortion and eugenics debate. As the President's Commission Report on Screening and Counseling For Genetic Conditions put it, "Nowhere is the need for freedom to pursue divergent conceptions of the good more deeply felt than in decisions concerning reproduction. It would be a cruel irony, therefore, if technological advances undertaken in the name of providing information to expand the range of individual choices resulted in . . . social pressures to pursue a particular course of action."[50] Consequently, the authors argue, genetic counseling should be presented in a way that respects the autonomy of the prospective parents, who can determine for themselves whether they wish to bring a child into the world that will suffer from a disability. Whether or not they choose to selectively abort as a result of a genetic test is, and should be, entirely their own decision. This same principle supports the right of parents to choose desirable traits, in accordance with their own beliefs about value, as well.

Davis asks whether, given this approach, we can make an argument against the autonomous right of Deaf parents to ensure, through the use of genetic technologies, that their children are also Deaf. Despite her willingness to argue against this use of technology on the basis of a Kantian claim that children ought to be treated as ends in themselves, which, she believes, rules out deliberately creating Deaf children, Davis ultimately suggests that the only thing that can stand up to an autonomy-based argument is another autonomy-based argument: "A decision, made before a child is even born, that confines her forever to a narrow group of people and a limited choice of careers so violates the child's right to an open future that no genetic counseling team should acquiesce in it. The very value of autonomy that grounds the ethics of genetic counseling should preclude assisting parents in a project that so dramatically narrows the autonomy of the child to be."[51]

Finally, the easiest way out of the debate about using human beings in medical research is also to turn to autonomy, which is expressed through the requirements of informed consent. These include the requirements that potential subjects be fully informed, that they be competent, and that their consent be freely given. While vestiges of the Troubled Self remain—such research recognizes the utilitarian commitment to improve the level of happiness experienced by human beings in general, and the idea of giving consent partially responds to the Kantian obligation that research subjects be treated as ends in themselves—in contemporary bioethics, it is informed consent itself, and the procedures for obtaining and ensuring it, that have become fundamentally important. What makes a research proposal ethically acceptable, and the conduct of researchers ethically sound, is now tied at least as much to the procedures used to obtain consent as it is to judgments about the merits of the research, or to measures meant to ensure the safety of participants.[52] As Brannigan and Boss describe it, according to the doctrine of informed consent, "Prospective subjects should be adequately informed of the nature and risks of the experiment as well as alternatives in the case of therapeutic experimentation so they can make an autonomous decision about whether or not to participate."[53]

While it is clearly the case that the concept of informed consent serves as a crucial safeguard for research subjects and arguably must be a central part of any ethically sound research protocol, what is most important about the role it now plays for the purposes of our discussion is that it moves us away, once more, from the tribulations of the Troubled Self. Bioethicists can focus their attention on the requirements for achieving genuine informed consent, and on policies that ensure that these requirements have been met, rather than determining whether the potential benefits for the general public of particular research proposals outweigh the risks experienced by the participants: reaching the answer to this question can be largely left in the hands of prospective research subjects, who can decide for themselves whether or not they want to participate in the research, and the choice to participate becomes both an expression of their autonomy, and something for which they are ultimately responsible.

NOTES

1. Deb Matthews, quoted in Christie Blatchford, "Chemo Begins, Public Campaign Continues," *Globe and Mail*, March 15, 2011, 7(A).
2. Andre Picard, "Denying Herceptin Was A Necessary Evil," *Globe and Mail*, March 17, 2011, 1(A).
3. I say "Kantian-type" rather than simply "Kantian," because, while their concerns were expressed in the form of recognizably Kantian principles, speakers did not necessarily use Kantian terminology to do so.
4. While liberalism is most often understood as being primarily a political theory, in bioethics it serves as an ethical theory as well.
5. The following quotations are representative of this sort of explicit reference. First, in an examination of whether persons have the right to die at a time of their own choosing, Kamm references a Kantian argument: "The idea that there are limits on what we may do to ourselves as persons derives from Immanuel Kant. In his moral writings, Kant said that rational humanity, as embodied in ourselves and others is and should be treated as *an end in itself, and not a mere means* to happiness or other goals." (F.M. Kamm, "A Right To Choose Death?," in *Contemporary Issues In Bioethics*, ed. Tom L. Beauchamp and LeRoy Walters, 6th Edition (Belmont, CA: Thomson-Wadsworth, 2003), 189). Likewise, in an exploration of whether or not it is morally acceptable to use children as research subjects, Ross points out that arguments against using children in this way tend to draw on Kantian principles, while arguments that support using children as research subjects are usually utilitarian: "The moral justification for the child's participation in such research is utilitarian; it permits the enrolment of a child as a research subject if the costs (harms and risks) to the child are significantly outweighed by the potential benefit to society at large." Lainie Friedman Ross, "The Child as Research Subject," in *Contemporary Readings In Biomedical Ethics*, ed. Walter Glannon (Orlando, FL: Harcourt College Publishers, 2002), 158.
6. For example, Boetkes and Waluchow observe that "Mill's utilitarianism is an ancestor of modern theories of cost-benefit analysis, which are assuming an ever-increasing role in controversies surrounding the allocation of money in various forms of health care." (Elisabeth Boetkes and Wilfrid J. Waluchow, *Readings in Healthcare Ethics* (Peterborough, Ontario: Broadview Press, 2000), 11. They go on to observe that, "Between them Kant and Mill zero in on the roles played respectively by intention and consequences in shaping our moral responses. One cannot get very far in discussions of ethics without paying deference to the Kantian notions of autonomy and universalizeability, or the injunction to treat human beings as ends in

themselves and not merely as means. Similarly one cannot ignore Mill's emphasis on protecting and promoting human happiness or well-being." (Boetkes and Waluchow, *Readings in Healthcare Ethics,* 11). Likewise, Brannigan and Boss observe, "Basing moral decisions on a cost/benefit calculation of social worth is an example of the application of *utilitarianism.* (Michael C. Brannigan and Judith A. Boss, *Healthcare Ethics In A Diverse Society* (Mountain View, CA: Mayfield Publishing Company, 2001), 25). Finally, Glannon states "despite the difference in the ethical theories they defend, Kant's principle of respect for persons and Mill's principle of liberty together form the basis of autonomy and informed consent in biomedical ethics." Walter Glannon, *Contemporary Readings In Biomedical Ethics* (Orlando, FL: Harcourt College Publishers, 2002), 14.

7. Michael Carrithers, *Why Humans Have Cultures,* 154.

8. Lewis Vaughn, *Bioethics: Principles, Issues, and Cases* (New York: Oxford University Press, 2010), 534.

9. Lewis Vaughn, *Bioethics,* 531.

10. Margaret Pabst Battin, "Physician-Assisted Suicide," in *Healthcare Ethics In a Diverse Society,* ed. Michael C. Brannigan and Judith A. Boss (Mountain View, CA: Mayfield Publishing Company, 2001), 528.

11. Lewis Vaughn, *Bioethics,* 536.

12. Lewis Vaughn, *Bioethics,* 536.

13. Ronald Munson, *Intervention and Reflection: Basic Issues In Medical Ethics* 8th Ed., ed. Ronald Munson (Belmont, CA: Thomson-Wadsworth, 2008), 291.

14. Ronald Munson, *Intervention and Reflection,* 291.

15. Julian Savulescu, "Procreative Beneficence: Why We Should Have The Best Children," in *Intervention and Reflection: Basic Issues In Medical Ethics* 8th Ed., ed. Ronald Munson (Belmont, CA: Thomson-Wadsworth, 2008), 321.

16. Julian Savulescu, "Procreative Beneficence," 324.

17. Dena S. Davis, "Genetic Dilemmas and the Child's Right To An Open Future," in *Intervention and Reflection: Basic Issues In Medical Ethics* 8th Ed., ed. Ronald Munson (Belmont, CA: Thomson-Wadsworth, 2008), 343.

18. Lewis Vaughn, *Bioethics,* 205.

19. Ronald Munson, *Intervention and Reflection,* 27.

20. Lewis Vaughn, *Bioethics,* 205.

21. As Warnock notes, in a discussion of whether or not it is morally acceptable to use human embryos in research, "no purely utilitarian argument could serve to settle the question of who *should* count. The central question, what status should be accorded to the early embryo… [has] to be settled by different means…" Mary Warnock, *An Intelligent Person's Guide To Ethics* (London: Duckworth Overlook, 1998), 75. And the same is true of Kantianism: it is only *after* we determine who (or what) counts as a rational being in the morally relevant sense that we can apply Kantian reasoning to them.

22. I will not, for instance, explore the differences between Mill's version of utilitarianism, and Bentham's, or between act and rule utilitarianism; nor will I consider the question of whether the various articulations of the Categorical Imperative presented by Kant add up to one principle or several.

23. Nina Rosenstand, *The Moral of the Story,* 5th Edition (New York: McGraw-Hill, 2006), 280.

24. As Kant famously tells us, we must "Act so that you treat humanity, whether in your own person, or in that of any other, always as an end and never as a means only." Immanuel Kant, *Foundations of the Metaphysics of Morals,* ed. Robert Paul Wolff (Indianapolis: Bobbs-Merrill Educational Publishing, 1969), 54.

25. Immanuel Kant, *Metaphysics of Morals,* 59.

26. Immanuel Kant, *Metaphysics of Morals,* 20.

27. Immanuel Kant, *Metaphysics of Morals,* 53.

28. Immanuel Kant, "Our Duties To Animals," in *Contemporary Moral Problems,* 8th Edition, ed. James E. White (Belmont, CA: Thomson-Wadsworth, 2006), 378.

29. Nina Rosenstand, *Moral of the Story,* 280.

30. As Munson notes, Kant's emphasis on the importance of rationality as the hallmark of beings towards whom we have moral obligations ends up making his theory unhelpful for some of the most difficult bioethical issues. Is a fetus, for example, a person in the relevant sense? And how ought we to care for an infant with serious birth defects? Munson observes that cases of this sort make it clear "that the notion of a person as an autonomous and rational being is both too restrictive and too arbitrary. It begs important moral questions." Ronald Munson, *Intervention and Reflection*, 754.

31. Immanuel Kant, *Metaphysics of Morals*, 17.

32. Immanuel Kant, *Metaphysics of Morals*, 17.

33. Immanuel Kant, *Metaphysics of Morals*, 13.

34. Jacques Thiroux, *Ethics: Theory and Practice*, 5th Edition (Englewood Cliffs, New Jersey: Prentice-Hall, 1995), 68.

35. J.S. Mill, "Utilitarianism," in *Utilitarianism, On Liberty, and Considerations on Representative Government*, ed. H.B. Acton (London: Dent, 1972), 19.

36. J.S. Mill, "Utilitarianism," 21.

37. J.S. Mill, "Utilitarianism," 40.

38. H.B. Acton, "Introduction," in J.S. Mill, *Utilitarianism, On Liberty, and Considerations on Representative Government*, ed. H.B. Acton (London: Dent, 1972), xix.

39. J.S. Mill, "Utilitarianism," 18.

40. J.S. Mill, "Utilitarianism," 12.

41. Jeremy Bentham, quoted in Peter Singer, "All Animals Are Created Equal," in *Contemporary Moral Problems*, 8th Edition, ed. James E. White (Belmont, CA: Thomson-Wadsworth, 2006), 382.

42. Peter Singer, "All Animals," 381.

43. Simon Blackburn, *Being Good* (New York: Oxford University Press, 2001), 88

44. Peter Singer, "All Animals," 387.

45. Jeremy Bentham, quoted in Nina Rosenstand, *Moral of the Story*, 216.

46. James Rachels, *The Elements of Moral Philosophy* 2nd Edition (New York: McGraw-Hill, 1993), 92.

47. And, of course, this is the case in other branches of ethics as well. As Held notes, a similar pattern exists in business ethics. "Debates in business ethics often follow a certain formula. You identify a problem, like affirmative action, employment at will, or sexual harassment and then choose an ethical theory to apply to the problem. So, for example, you might decide to focus on your particular issue from a *deontological* perspective and emphasize respect and duty. On the other hand, someone else might address the same issue from a *utilitarian* perspective and thus stress results and the greater good. In such a case there will inevitably be an insuperable impasse when the demands of respect don't produce the best results or when the greater good can't be attained because respect is getting in the way. For example, one may argue against employment at will and for due process on the basis that insofar as employees are human beings and demand respect they can't be fired without good reason. Likewise, a utilitarian could argue that employment at will functions best, allowing an employer flexibility in hiring and firing that will lead to greater efficiency and productivity." Jacob M. Held, "'The Rules of Acquisition Can't Help You Now': What Can The Ferengi Teach Us About Business ethics?," in *Star Trek and Philosophy: The Wrath of Kant*, eds. Jason T. Ebel and Kevin S. Decker (Chicago: Open Court, 2008), 119—120.

48. James Rachels, *The Elements of Moral Philosophy* 2nd Ed. (New York: McGraw-Hill, 1993), 90.

49. Dan W. Brock, "Voluntary Active Euthanasia," in *Biomedical Ethics* 4th Ed., ed. Thomas A. Mappes and David DeGrazia (New York: McGraw-Hill Inc., 1996), 391.

50. Quoted in Gena S. Davis, "Genetic Dilemmas," 339.

51. Gena S. Davis, "Genetic Dilemmas," 345.

52. This issue will be explored more fully in Chapter Nine.

53. Michael C. Brannigan and Judith A. Boss, *Healthcare Ethics*, 345.

Chapter Three

The Divided Self

Liberal Politics and the Rise of Autonomy in Bioethics

INTRODUCTION: ETHICS COMMITTEES AND THE NON-COMPLIANT CLIENT

At a recent ethics committee meeting, we discussed a fictionalized case which asked us to determine how a resident of a long-term care facility who suffered from pica, a disease that causes cravings to eat non-food items, should be treated. According to the case study, the resident had managed to eat a pair of rubber gloves, which perforated his stomach, which led to a trip to emergency, surgery, and an extensive stay in the intensive care unit. Upon his return to the long-term care home, he was belted into a wheelchair when he couldn't be directly supervised, in order to minimize the chance that he would ingest something harmful or even fatal. The ethics committee was asked to consider whether such constraints were acceptable, and what the home might do to ensure both the resident's safety and respect for his autonomy. After heated discussion, which focused primarily on why this case was even considered to pose an ethical issue at all (of course such restraints were morally wrong!) committee members concluded that the only thing that needed to be ascertained was the man's competency: if he was competent, then he should be allowed to wander freely and ingest whatever he wished. I suspect that if this conclusion were to be shared with people who were unfamiliar with the central assumptions that currently prevail in bioethics, they would find this to be a surprising, perhaps even disturbing, result.

The cases we examine in ethics committees tend to coalesce around a small number of issues. The facts of each case will vary, but the central underlying ethical concern, often, will not be particularly unique. If bioethics cases were literary works, we would say that they fall into particular genres (mysteries, science fiction, romance); if they were songs, we would place them into musical categories (jazz, rock, classical). Many bioethics cases, as the last chapter indicates, revolve around the figure of the Troubled Self, and the pull between consequentialism and deontology; as members of the ethics committee, we often try to resolve this pull by employing the resources of principlism. However, a larger (and ever-increasing) number of cases falls into what might be called the autonomy genre, which means that they are primarily concerned with issues of competency, harm, and choice. The central figures in this genre are the Divided Self and the Choosing Self, and ethical dilemmas in this category center either on the clash between the choices made by these selves and (what are often understood to be) relatively objective standards of medical practice and relatively clear concerns about the possibility of harm, or around questions of competency. Moreover, since (a liberal conception of) autonomy occupies such an important place within principlism, principlism itself both contributes to the development of the Divided Self and the ultimate triumph of the Choosing Self, and makes it difficult for this self to be constrained by competing ethical principles. This chapter will consider the Divided Self, whose legitimate exercise of autonomous choice is placed within the context of liberal political theory, and so limited by the requirements of liberal justice; the next will describe the Choosing Self, whose autonomous choices are constrained only by the Harm Principle, and facilitated by the market.

One particularly common form that the autonomy genre takes is what can be called "the case of the non-compliant client." I should note that, in our discussions, the term "client" is usually used, rather than the term "patient": this reflects the move away from the assumption that sick people have shared goals that are shaped by objectively valid medical criteria, to the assumption that each individual will have his or her own unique set of desires, commitments, and conceptions of the good, and that the role of health care institutions is to facilitate the choices that result from these factors as much as possible. Consequently, I will use the term "client" in this chapter, to indicate that a number of the ideas that are connected to the Divided Self are in play when this term is used.

The non-compliant client is often a resident of a long-term care institution, or someone who is being supported in her own home by a health care team, and she comes in many forms: the hungry diabetic, who can't seem to stay away from the junk food dispensing vending machine; the nursing home resident who has friends smuggle in alcohol; or the person with a tendency to choke, who refuses to eat mashed-up food or to drink thickened liquids.

In keeping with the underlying themes that accompany such cases, and the standard bioethical approach that currently frames them, the first question we discuss is whether the client is competent. If competency is questionable, then we postpone further discussion until a formal assessment can be made. If, however, competency is not at issue, my job, as an "ethicist," is to remind the other committee members of the importance of autonomy, of allowing individuals to make their own choices, even when those choices may be harmful to them, and ones we don't approve of. This reminder is hardly needed: we must be careful, we all agree, not to make judgments about what people want, as long as those choices affect only themselves, and we must, at all costs, avoid imposing our own values on our clients.

Health care ethics committees, Thomas May argues, serve three primary functions: education, case consultation, and policy development.[1] In my experience, education consists primarily of designing "ethics tools" which are based on the four principles of biomedical ethics (sometimes supplemented by other principles and values), and then explaining to the staff, who are expected to use them that, as long as those they are dealing with are competent, autonomy takes precedence, and their primary role is to support client choice as much as possible; policy is problematic precisely because respect for client choice often conflicts with resource constraints, which means that not all choices can be respected; and case consultations are primarily concerned with ascertaining competency, and then either respecting client choice if the person is competent, or identifying the appropriate substitute decision maker, whose choices then are the ones we need to respect.

These observations reflect the fact that contemporary bioethics revolves around the principle of (respect for) autonomy. As Wolpe puts it, "For better or worse . . . autonomy has emerged as the most powerful principle in American bioethics, as the basis of much theory and much regulation, and has become the 'default' principle. . . . Indisputably . . . patient autonomy has become the most powerful principle in ethical decision making in American medicine."[2] This means that, while the Troubled Self still has a role to play, the dominant conception of the self in contemporary bioethics, both theoretically and practically, is now the Divided Self, or its close relative, which will be explored in the next chapter, the Choosing Self: conceptions of the self that are constructed around the idea that human flourishing is constituted by the attainment of (a certain kind of) autonomy, and demonstrated through the choices that individuals make.

The Divided Self, moreover, exists within a particular political and social framework, and cannot, ultimately, be adequately characterized or described apart from this context. An exploration of the world of the Divided Self, then, necessitates an excursion into currently dominant forms of political and social philosophy that exist outside the medical domain. It is these dominant political and social forms that largely shape issues in bioethics today, not only in the way they are discussed and resolved, but also, and even more importantly, how they are framed and identified *as being* ethical issues in the first place. To say that various versions of the Case of the Non-compliant

Client constitute an important element in the autonomy genre of the bioethics case is to say not only that the issues raised by such cases occur frequently and manifest a similar pattern; it is also to say that they occur as often as they do, and take this familiar form *because* the current framework of bioethics tends to construct the moral universe in such a way that ethical dilemmas often mean nothing more nor less than the clash between what an individual wants and what, because of limited resources, concerns of potential harm to that individual, or for reasons of policy, might be thought good for them, for others, or for society.[3]

The Divided Self that is generated by this account is divided in two ways, internally and externally. First, it can stand apart from its own commitments, even its deepest ones because they always remain, in principle, revisable; second, all of us have an obligation to treat our own values as private things, not ones that others necessarily share with us. In public in our roles as citizens, as members of ethics committees, as bioethicists, we have a moral obligation to respect the choices that other people make, and to tolerate even or especially those we deeply disapprove of, in order to help ensure that our shared public spaces allow the maximum amount of freedom for all to pursue their own particular conceptions of the good. The Divided Self, furthermore, is not split only into public and private parts, but its private part is also further divided: into the part that has the capacity to choose what it values and which stands apart from the values chosen, and the part which acts on the basis of the values that are currently held. In what follows, I shall explore both kinds of division more extensively.

AUTONOMY, BIOETHICS, AND LIBERALISM

Liberalism is often simply identified with political freedom. However, what underlies liberal claims about the importance of freedom is a commitment to individual autonomy. Autonomy, in simple terms, captures the idea that each of us lives a better life when we discern our own conceptions of the good, articulate goals for ourselves in light of those conceptions, and make choices that are designed to help us achieve those goals. Autonomy, then, requires that individuals possess certain rational capacities (small children, for example, are not considered to be autonomous, nor are persons suffering from advanced dementia) and that they live in a social and political environment that actually allows them to develop their own conceptions of the good and gives them the freedom to make choices in light of those conceptions. We cannot exercise our autonomy, that is to say, whatever our rational capacities, if we are engaged in a daily struggle to survive; nor can we exercise our autonomy if we live in a community or state which imposes a particular conception of the good upon us. Persons living in a theocracy, for example, which requires them to live their lives in accordance with the religious values endorsed by the state, are not able to fully exercise their autonomy (although autonomous individuals can choose to submit to religious authorities, if this is what their conception of the good requires).

Many theorists, then, believe that autonomy can only be fully exercised within a genuinely democratic political system that values freedom and which provides opportunities for people to experiment with different ways of living, and to make choices that others don't approve of. Autonomy, in this account, is closely tied to what might be called the virtues of citizenship[4]: the conceptions of the good that individuals identify with and act upon must not violate the Harm Principle, the idea that we can do what we like, as long as our choices are not harmful to others (or, at least, not harmful to them in ways that they have not consented to)[5]; and each of us, as fellow citizens, must be tolerant of one another, *particularly* when our conceptions of the good conflict.

There are several reasons why a conception of the autonomous self, which has its origins in political philosophy, in considerations of the appropriate relationship between individuals and the state, has found a home in bioethics, and why the Divided Self has come to play such an important role.

First, there has been a justifiable move away from *paternalism* in medicine to a focus on *informed consent*, and on the right of patients to make choices for themselves, for reasons which are significant to them, in matters which are as profoundly personal as their own health and what is done to their bodies.

Second, the rise of autonomy in bioethics, arguably, can be traced (in part) to the failures of the Troubled Self. If the two dominant ethical theories of modern Western thought, utilitarianism, and Kantianism, often clash with one another, and, consequently, offer us little clear moral guidance, and if we have no overarching and always compelling reason to choose one theory rather than the other, then we need something else to guide us. What an emphasis on autonomy allows us to do, at least when it is the choices of competent persons that are in question, is defer to the clients. As Gawande observes, doctors are fallible, and medical treatments are full of uncertainties: if we often don't know what the "correct" medical choice is, the "correct" ethical choice is also unclear. However, decisions must still be made: "if both doctors and patients are fallible, who should decide? We want a rule. And so we've decided that patients should be the ultimate arbiter."[6] An emphasis on autonomy in medicine and in bioethics, then, can simplify ethical dilemmas: the client is both free to choose, and ultimately responsible for the consequences of that choice.

Third, autonomy, as used in bioethics, attaches what is often presented as a simple ethical principle to a particularly powerful and influential political theory, namely, liberalism. Once this connection is made, the scope of the principle extends far beyond the medical context, and allows bioethicists to address questions of policy, questions of distributive justice, and questions about the role that health care should play in a just society. While the principles of justice and autonomy, as we saw in the last chapter, can be traced, in part, to Kant, once they are attached to this political framework, they take on a distinctively liberal gloss which departs from their Kantian origins and in which, indeed, the views Mill expresses in *On Liberty* also have a significant role to play.[7]

Liberalism is built around the idea that individuals will have different and often incompatible or even incommensurable conceptions of the good. Consequently, for liberals, the just state, which treats its citizens as equals, will be a state which allows the maximum amount of freedom possible for citizens to explore, choose, and enact, different ways of life, compatible with a similar amount of freedom for everyone. The role of the government, then, is not to impose a particular conception of the good upon its citizens; rather, it is to provide a framework within which individuals are free to pursue their own conceptions of the good life, and to protect their right to live in ways which others may not approve of (again, as long as those conceptions are not harmful to others).

Liberalism, Macedo argues, holds "an ideal of persons as self-determining and unpredictably self-transforming creatures,"[8] who make choices about how they want to live, and, often, examine and revise these plans and projects. Liberal politics brings liberal justice and liberal autonomy together by imposing "the rule of impersonal law and individual rights" which protects "the liberty to explore various ways of realizing the good life, and . . . exercise self-critical, self-transforming reflective capacities."[9] What is most important, in this account, is not that we make the *right* choices, in some objective sense, but that the choices we make are *our own*.

The just liberal state, moreover, will go beyond merely providing a framework within which citizens can choose freely, and provide protections for the choices they make, it will also have a distributive role: it must distribute goods and opportunities in such a way that each citizen will have a similar chance to fulfill his own vision of what his life should be like. As Dworkin puts it, for the liberal, equality requires that "resources and opportunities should be distributed, as far as possible, equally so that roughly the same share of whatever is available is devoted to satisfying the ambitions of each."[10]

Much of North American political and social culture is influenced, both constitutionally and in the self-understandings of citizens, by liberalism. Medicine, as a social practice, is shaped by the larger cultural milieu in which it operates, and so is bioethics. Consequently, May argues, "the role that moral beliefs play in bioethics will be limited, in a social context, by the political rights of individuals."[11] Liberalism is a particularly powerful political theory for a number of reasons. First, it is centered on an appealing account of who we are, and of the importance of respecting the choices we make. It tells us that we are individually important, and, consequently, so are our particular conceptions of the good. It uses the language of rights, as they provide important protections for our freedom to choose. Moreover, this conception of the self as free, as self-directed, as capable of forming its own life plans, has become an integral part of the self-understandings of most North Americans: even people whose political views differ sharply will share this conception of the self, and their political disagreements will be focused on which government policies can best ensure necessary freedoms, not on whether freedom itself is important.

In addition, liberal thinkers have provided a sophisticated, intricate, and comprehensive political and moral account of the nature of the just state and of who we are, which is (arguably) currently unrivalled. As Buchanan, Brock, Daniels, and Wikler (who unapologetically and influentially explore bioethical questions within an explicitly liberal framework) ask, "What justifies our reliance on a liberal framework for our ethical inquiry?"[12] They answer "that a liberal approach to moral and political philosophy is to date the most carefully worked out and defended approach available. In our opinion, there simply are no antiliberal or nonliberal (e.g. communitarian) moral-political theories that come close to the degree of systematic argumentation and power that we find in the writings of liberal thinkers. . ."[13] Whether or not they are correct to believe that there are no worthy competitors to the liberal framework, they are correct to state that liberalism has vanquished most of its rivals, at least in contemporary bioethics: most bioethical debates, now, occur *within* the liberal framework, rather than *between* advocates of liberalism and proponents of alternative approaches. Indeed, as we shall see in the next chapter, this framework has become so much a part of mainstream bioethics that its correctness is assumed to such an extent that its usage no longer needs to be defended.

I want to draw attention to the hyphenated phrase "moral-political" that is used in the above quote to describe the role that liberal theory plays in bioethics. As the discussion so far suggests, this linking is absolutely correct. There is an inherent connection between the *moral* claims made by bioethicists working within the liberal tradition, and the *political* framework within which individual choices are described and facilitated. I will argue, further, that if we tease out the various threads which compose the Divided Self along multiple dimensions, we will see that there is a three-way correlation between the Divided Self, the moral landscape within which this self considers and makes choices and designs plans of life, and the political framework which both helps determine which choices are compatible with the demands of citizenship and which provides the political space within which individuals have freedom to move in response to their own judgments about what gives meaning and value to life. We can, therefore, describe this theoretical approach using a three-way hyphen: liberalism, we might say, is a self-moral-political theory. Each of these aspects simultaneously relies upon, and supports, the other two.

We can see this combination of self-moral-political in Thomas May's account of the role that ought to be played by bioethicists in a liberal society. May argues that the dominance of autonomy in bioethics both naturally follows from the commitments made by a liberal society, and that these commitments have implications for ethics committees and for the bioethicists who sit on them. First, May argues that there is no such thing as a purely *factual* medical judgment. Consequently, there is no objectively correct choice that a patient *should* make. Rather, medical judgments about what treatments are "appropriate" are themselves normative judgments: "Whether a given treatment is appropriate depends on whether the potential benefits of that treatment outweigh the burdens it imposes on the patient. This judgment requires that we consider the patient's perspective in assessing the benefits and burdens of treatment."[14] From this perspective, there is no such thing as a "non-compliant client" (at least if the individual in question is competent); rather, what such cases represent is that the persons who brought the case forward do not properly understand their role, which is simply to respect the choices that clients make, whatever they happen to be.

This claim has implications for ethics committees as well. The role of the bioethicist on such committees is twofold: first, to ensure that the correct procedures are followed, and that the process is legitimate and fair; and, second, to protect the autonomy of those implicated in the case under discussion.[15] In May's view, given the importance of autonomy, "ethical expertise" does not (and should not) be taken to mean that the bioethicist has any privileged expertise *in ethics*. Indeed, the bioethicist must prevent fellow committee members from imposing their own values, and she must be scrupulous in ensuring that they don't express any substantive (as opposed to procedural) moral views of their own. Most fundamentally, he believes, the role of the bioethicist is nothing less (and nothing more) than "to protect patient autonomy. There is no 'power' claimed, no special knowledge about the 'morally right' answer. The ethicist merely offers assistance in recognizing how judgments of appropriate treatment are affected by presuppositions of value, and helps to identify and analyze values relevant to a particular decision. The ethicist does not impose a decision."[16]

While there is an intricate and superficially appealing connection between self-moral-political in this theoretical perspective, I want to argue that this conjunction of elements is unhelpful when inserted into the context of bioethics. In bioethics, we need to see clearly what the conception of the self that anchors this account looks like, and how it fits within the context of medicine. We also need to distinguish *moral* questions from *political* ones, in a way that is difficult to do if we simply accept the moral-political conjunction in a strong form. The dominance of this perspective in bioethics means that moral questions and concerns are often conflated with political questions and concerns, and the result is frequently jarring and sometimes misleading. Moreover, it almost inevitably compels us to frame bioethical questions in particular ways that blind us to the possibility that there may be other (potentially more fruitful) ways of exploring them. However, at the same time, if we detach the conception of the self that underpins liberalism from a robust attachment to its political commitments, the resulting conception of the autonomous self is even less satisfactory. Defenders of the dominant role played by a liberal conception of autonomy in bioethics, I argue, find themselves on the horns of a dilemma: if the conjunction of the self-moral-political dimensions of the Divided Self is tightly asserted, the result is a political conception of the self that fits poorly with the moral issues with which bioethicists concern themselves; on the other hand, if the moral dimensions of this self are abstracted from a robust commitment to liberal political values, what results is the Choosing Self whose presence undermines any claim that bioethicists might make to possess the specialized expertise that legitimates the public and professional roles they occupy. This chapter will consider the first horn of the dilemma; the next, the second.

My critique of the liberal account, and of the Divided Self which animates it, I must make clear, applies primarily to the role it plays in bioethics, and is not intended to be a fully developed critique of liberalism more generally. Indeed, I shall argue that, when it comes to explicitly political questions even within bioethics—for example, questions about the distribution of health care goods—liberalism can be, indeed, a helpful and even illuminating approach to employ. What I want to assert, however, is that we distort our moral thinking in subtle ways when we view moral questions through the lens provided by what is essentially a political theory, and that the Divided Self fits awkwardly with many of the issues that are encountered in medicine.

JOHN RAWLS AND THE CREATION OF THE DIVIDED SELF

I have been using the term "autonomy" as though it is a clear and uncontroversial concept. However, despite the dominant role it plays in contemporary political and moral philosophy, there is no clear consensus about what autonomy is, or about how its implications—personal, moral, social, and political—ought to be understood. Consequently, it is helpful to locate our discussion in a particular account, and then explore some of the ways in which this account fits with, or supports, the use made of this concept in bioethics. While there are a number of philosophical strands that contribute to the creation of the Divided Self, arguably the most influential contemporary articulation of them, and the one which is most clearly implicated in bioethics, is the account provided by John Rawls.

Many, if not most, of the liberal assumptions which implicitly underlie the Divided Self, and the claims which justify central conclusions about the domain of personal choice in a health care context and the limitations on government interference that follow from these claims, either explicitly reference Rawls, flow from his account, or are elaborations on ideas that he initially proposed. It is striking how often Rawls is used to underpin particular lines of argument in bioethics, and how often, indeed, his position is cited to justify the conclusions reached. As Talisse observes, "The number of books and articles building upon, and influenced by the ideas of John Rawls persistently increases and it is almost impossible now to find a recent book on political theory which does not contain multiple references to Rawls's work."[17] And the same is true in bioethics: Rawls's views are often present, either explicitly or as part of the background against which issues are framed and analyzed. Even critics of his approach and of liberal presumptions more generally acknowledge the importance of these views even as they reject them.

I should note, of course, that Rawls's account draws on a number of historical trends and concepts in liberal theory, including a concern with the social contract, the role of the Harm Principle, the interplay of Kantian and utilitarian ethical thinking, the pluralistic nature of the good, and the place of the market in modern democracies; however, what Rawls does with these strands is tie them together in an innovative and powerful way, and give them a new influence in theoretical and practical moral and political discourse.

The fact that liberalism has become an inescapable self-moral-political theory in bioethics is, arguably, largely because of the power and attractiveness of the Rawlsian account, and the Divided Self of bioethics owes most of its features to the conception of the self that Rawls articulates in *A Theory of Justice* and elaborates more fully in *Political Liberalism.* Consequently, in order to see the features of the Divided Self more clearly, we need to explore Rawls's claims about the nature of the just state, as well as how he presents and supports these claims. This Rawlsian account performs three important functions in bioethics.

First, it introduces us to a particular understanding of who we are which is predicated on a particular kind of self: one that is fundamentally individualistic (it is as individuals that we meet in the original position); rational (capable of articulating and pursuing plans of life); and reasonable (willing to reach agreements with other selves on matters of mutual importance). It's important to note, however, that the individualism of this self does not preclude, as some critics assume, making communal commitments. The point is that such commitments, if made by autonomous persons, must be *chosen*, not *given* by their families or communities, or *imposed* on them by the state.

Second, this self is placed in an explicitly *political* context. Its existence is predicated on the claim that goods are plural, that we will never be able to reach agreement on a shared conception of the good, or on the features of a genuinely good life; consequently, given that liberalism connects its conception of the self to its claims about the nature of the just state, the primary purpose of political arrangements, at least if they are just, is to allow the maximum amount of freedom for all to pursue their own conceptions of the good, compatible with the Harm Principle. Consequently, the Divided Self must be willing to separate his personal values and moral commitments from his public obligations to tolerate, or even respect, the choices made by others, particularly when he disagrees with those choices.

Third, the Rawlsian account (or variations upon it) profoundly shapes the most widely accepted account of distributive justice used in bioethics today. (As we saw in the last chapter, utilitarian thinking, in the form of a cost-benefit analysis, is also used to distribute goods and services; however, this method of distribution is usually understood to respond to the idea that these things should be distributed *efficiently*, rather than *justly*. Indeed, cost-benefit distributions can be—and, indeed, often are—criticized on justice-based grounds).

Before exploring these strands in more detail and depth, I want to examine the Rawlsian account of liberal justice, the particularly compelling moral claim that underlies it, and the strikingly imaginative approach to contract theory that Rawls takes through the presentation of what is essentially a thought experiment constructed around the complementary ideas of the veil of ignorance and the original position. My discussion will focus primarily on the claims Rawls makes in *A Theory of Justice*, with one important addition drawn from *Political Liberalism*, and will be selective, not exhaustive.

Rawls's claims in *A Theory of Justice* arise from one central idea: that differences in natural abilities and social background are, morally speaking, completely arbitrary. This claim leads to the expression of two other central assertions. First, that the social structure of society is unjust if it (inappropriately) takes these arbitrary differences into account. For example, a society is unjust if a child born into an impoverished family will have little opportunity over her lifetime to better her lot, or if women are excluded from entering the workforce because of their gender. Second, Rawls argues that the government of a just society should be neutral between competing conceptions of the good life: it should not, for example, privilege atheists over those who are religious, or people who derive meaning and pleasure in their lives from camping in wilderness parks over those who enjoy collecting stamps. These two claims are connected to the moral insight that animates Rawls's discussion because, on Rawls's view, our talents and abilities and, of course, our family background, often influence what it is that we find valuable in life.

Since none of us deserves our starting place in society, neither do we deserve our greater (or lesser) capacities, the "fundamental problem of justice," Rawls says, is to regulate those inequalities that arise from the fact that the basic structure of society "favors some starting places over others in the division of the benefits of social cooperation."[18] We should notice that, on this account of justice and injustice, the world that we actually live in is profoundly unjust, since undeserved starting places and natural abilities have a profound effect on how our lives are likely to go: for example, a child born into a wealthy family will have access to good schools, skiing trips, orthodontic treatments, and, if some of the proponents of genetic enhancements turn out to be correct, may one day be even further privileged by the insertion of genes which confer additional advantages; a child born into a poor family, in contrast, might not enjoy any of these benefits. Rawls must tell us, then, what follows if we take seriously the claim that such morally arbitrary differences are responsible for determining so much about how people's lives are likely to go, want to design a society in which these differences between persons are justly compensated for, and how we might arrive at principles of justice that are adequate to address this problem.

Rawls's complementary ideas of the original position and the veil of ignorance provide a mechanism to determine what a just society would look like, and how the principles that govern it can be reached. We are asked to imagine that the original position is a kind of giant meeting in which individuals get together to choose the principles of justice that will govern their society. In these circumstances, it is reasonable to suppose that principles that benefit certain persons more than others as a result of arbitrary fortune and circumstance would not be chosen; likewise, the principles adopted should not reflect the views and aspirations of particular individuals. It also seems reasonable "to suppose that the parties in the original position are equals,"[19] with equal rights when it comes to proposing and choosing principles.

Rawls, then, wants the original position to be designed in such a way that the agreements reached within it will be fair, whatever they happen to be. Arbitrary distinctions between individuals must not influence the outcome, and all must be equally represented as moral persons. The aim of the original position, he says, "is to rule out those principles that it would be rational to propose for acceptance, however little chance of success, only if one knew certain things that are irrelevant from the standpoint of justice."[20] Rawls ensures that the parties in the original position will also rule these things out of their deliberations by proposing that we imagine them meeting behind the veil of ignorance. This means that the parties do not know many facts about themselves: "no one knows his place in society, his class position or special status, nor does anyone know his fortune in the distribution of natural assets and abilities, his intelligence, strength, and the like."[21] They do not even know what conceptions of the good they hold.

Consequently, Rawls argues, those meeting behind the veil will choose the two principles of justice: the first states that everyone has an "equal right to the most extensive total system of equal basic liberties compatible with a similar system of liberty for all"[22]; the second asserts that social and economic inequalities "are to be arranged so that they are both: (a) to the greatest benefit of the least advantaged . . . and (b) attached to offices and positions open to all under conditions of fair equality of opportunity."[23]

Through this exercise, Rawls manages to make it plausible that principles that are quite radically egalitarian if taken seriously and applied consistently would be chosen out of self-interest. Those individuals who meet in the original position agree to these principles because, if they do not, they may find themselves seriously disadvantaged when the veil of ignorance is lifted, and they find out who they are and where they are placed in society. Conceptions of the good, then, are restricted right from the start: all reasonable conceptions must be in accordance with what the principles of justice require. As Rawls puts it, in a now-famous phrase, "in justice as fairness the concept of the right is prior to that of the good."[24] In short, the two principles chosen in the original position (but only because the parties are meeting behind the veil of ignorance) are acceptable to those choosing because they are "those a person would choose for the design of a society in which his enemy is to assign him his place."[25] An additional feature of Rawls's account is that he claims that a just society will provide its citizens with primary goods, those things—social, economic, and political—that are necessary for the successful execution of any life plan.

Rawls's theory is, of course, familiar to many; indeed, in liberal circles, his claims have provided the foundation for the arguments presented by other theorists, who work out detailed applications of how these claims might be applied to situations and institutions that Rawls himself did not consider. As we have already seen, contemporary bioethics is a field in which this account occupies an important place; indeed, many of the features of mainstream bioethics are drawn from, or rely upon, Rawls's theory of justice, and the conception of the self that lies beneath his claims. There are four aspects of this conception that have become important hallmarks of the Divided Self (and its less political offspring, the Choosing Self) that currently dominate bioethics.

First, this self is rational, self-interested, and individualistic. It is, Rawls says, capable of understanding basic social, political, and economic concepts; while it is also capable of accepting the necessity of principles of justice to govern its actions, it does so for self-interested reasons; and it is as individuals that we meet behind the veil, and as individuals that we emerge from behind it. Consequently, while the principles of justice that govern the space we share with others, it is primarily our individuality that they protect.

Second, the most important characteristic of this self is its autonomy, its capacity to choose: this is far more important, on this account, than the things chosen. Consider one of the few concrete examples Rawls provides. He asks us to imagine a man of normal intelligence and psychology, "whose only pleasure is to count blades of grass in various geometrically shaped areas such as park squares and well-trimmed lawns."[26] For this person, the most rational long-term plan is to arrange matters so that he will have as much time as possible to pursue his favored activity, since it is this activity that constitutes his conception of the good: "It will be for him the end that regulates the schedule of his actions, and this establishes what it is that is good for him."[27] Importantly, it follows from this that, even if we might believe a life oriented around this activity to be wasted, we must recognize both that we have no objective basis on which to make this judgment, and no right to interfere with his choice to live his life in accordance with this particular conception of the good.

Third, the self that is left when we strip away the features that are hidden behind the veil (an imaginative exercise each of us ought to be able to engage in) is more of a ghostly substrate than an identifiable person. Try to do this thought experiment: imagine who *you* would be behind the veil of ignorance. It will become clear that the questions that were identified earlier as helping to articulate what it means to be a self—who am I? who are you? who do you say I am? and who should I say you are?—are almost unanswerable. At most, we can say that we are rational and self-interested fellow citizens, who share a commitment to particular principles of justice, but these questions seem impossible to answer in any more meaningful and substantive ways.[28] Once we strip away the things we don't know about ourselves, and are left with only a ghostly remnant of who we actually are, make the assumption that we choose the principles of justice we do because we are self-interested, and that we possess some knowledge of political and economic principles, it's not clear what distinction between persons remains in Rawls's account, either. Anyone, in this set of circumstances, would make the same choices and for the same reasons, so it doesn't really matter who we *actually* are. Our distinct characteristics (ironically enough, given the emphasis on autonomy and the requirement that we be free to choose our own plans of life) are entirely irrelevant.

The final characteristic of the self as articulated in this account that I want to draw attention to is a feature that is implicit in *A Theory of Justice* and which becomes explicit in *Political Liberalism*. In *Political Liberalism*, Rawls acknowledges that one of the problems facing liberal democracies is stability: if they are inhabited by autonomous citizens pursuing divergent and even incompatible conceptions of the good (some of which, indeed, may be incompatible with liberal principles), how can we ensure that they will retain a sufficient commitment to the liberal ideals necessary to maintain the liberal state? Rawls argues that the liberal self must be willing to split herself into two sharply distinct parts, the public part, which accepts that it must abide by liberal political arrangements, and the private part, which can pursue conceptions of the good as it sees fit (as long as they are willing to defer to the public conception if it and the private one come into conflict). As he puts it, "I assume that for the purposes of public life, Saul of Tarsus and St. Paul the Apostle are irrelevant to our public, or institutional, identity."[29] (Or, as Rorty even more dramatically puts it in his endorsement of this split, an autonomous liberal self "can divide herself into a private self-creator and a public liberal . . . the same person [can] be, in alternate moments, Nietzsche and J. S. Mill"[30]). Consequently, on Rawls's account, free and equal citizens have two moral powers: they have a sense of justice, and they can devise (and revise) their own conceptions of the good.

RAWLS'S THOUGHT EXPERIMENT AND THE IMAGINATIVE CONSTRUCTION OF A MORAL UNIVERSE

Before turning to a consideration of the impact Rawls has had on bioethics, I would like to draw attention to some additional features of his account. While the *rationality* that is demonstrated in his theory is often commented upon, I want to point to a less-noticed feature of his discussion. This is the way in which Rawls's principles of justice, his conception of the self, and the features of the moral universe through which this self moves, are based on what is essentially a work of the imagination.

First, Rawls's account centers on a thought experiment. The concepts of the original position and the veil of ignorance not only make vivid Rawls's contention that the distribution of many social goods and individual talents are morally arbitrary and, hence, something which needs to be addressed in a just society, they also provide support for the principles of justice which come out of this thought experiment and for Rawls's claim that "the right is prior to the good," as well as for his assertion that, if we follow the correct procedures, what results from them will be morally acceptable. Without the thought experiment, the same claims could have been made, but they would be both less appealing and less convincing. This thought experiment, moreover, sets out the parameters of the Divided Self; and this conception of the self would be far less attractive and plausible without the thought experiment that introduces it to us.

This is worth mentioning because many of those who make use of the Rawlsian account in bioethics fail to note the *significance* of the fact that it is a thought experiment that underpins Rawls's account in multiple ways. Instead, they treat Rawls's conclusions as though they are somehow simply *true*, as things which fundamentally capture the essential attributes of justice, and which describes human beings as we *really* are. To point out that these conclusions are largely justified by a thought experiment that clearly sets out in advance limits for our thinking about justice and selfhood is not to say that this account doesn't capture something insightful about the nature of justice or tell us something illuminating about who we are; that would be an argument which goes beyond the scope of this discussion. But it is to say that this account is *not* simply true, nor a straightforward, commonsense description of reality, either, although it is often treated as such, particularly when used as a rejoinder to someone who is either critical of the liberal framework, or critical of the conclusions reached on bioethical issues by theorists who view them through the liberal lens.

Second, this thought experiment (as is the case with all thought experiments) is hypothetical, as much as work of the imagination as of the intellect. Consequently, the conception of the self that it presumes and reinforces is no more a straightforward conception of "who we are" than competing accounts, be they utilitarian, Kantian, communitarian, Marxist, or anything else. As Sandel observes, "Rawls's hypothetical social contract is even more imaginary than most. Not only did his contract never happen; it is imagined to take place among the sorts of beings who never really existed, that is, beings stuck with the kind of complicated amnesia necessary to the veil of ignorance."[31] Consequently, Sandel goes on to say, "Rawls's theory is doubly hypothetical. It imagines an event that never really happened, involving the sorts of beings who never really existed."[32]

Third, this account of the self, imaginary or not, true or not, is tremendously appealing: if we accept it, it allows us to be both self-interested (it is only because the parties in the original position do not know certain facts about themselves that they agree to the principles of justice that they do), and yet be committed to justice, tolerance, and other democratic values. And it allows us to see ourselves as persons who can design, live out, and experiment with different ways of living. (Just as its supporters seldom remark on how imaginary this conception of the self is, its critics don't always seem to notice just how attractive both it and the just and democratic world it inhabits really are.) Moreover, as noted above, most North Americans have been shaped to some extent, culturally speaking, by elements of this self. In some sense, for many of us, this self or parts of it *are* "who we are." Most of us like to feel that we are in control of our own lives, that we can escape from our upbringings and find new ways to live, and that we can revise our ideas of what gives meaning and purpose to our lives as we move through them.

Finally, like other conceptions of the Self, the Divided Self carries along with it its own moral universe. Sandel, who is a critic of the Rawlsian version of this self, nonetheless provides a good description of the space this self-inhabits:

> Bound up with the notion of the independent self is a vision of the moral universe this self must inhabit. Unlike classical Greek and Medieval Christian conceptions, the universe is a place devoid of inherent meaning, a world "disenchanted" . . . a world without an objective moral order. Only in a world empty of *telos* . . . is it possible to conceive of a subject apart from and prior to its purposes and ends. Only a world ungoverned by a purposive order leaves principles of justice open to human construction and conceptions of the good open to individual choice. [33]

He goes on to argue that "where neither nature nor cosmos supplies a meaningful order to be grasped or comprehended, it falls to human subjects to constitute meaning on their own. . . . What can no longer be found remains somehow to be created." [34]

Whether we see this shift as a tragic loss, or as an empowering and inspiring discovery, shapes how we view the Divided Self and the role played by the just state and its institutions, democratic choice, and the workings of the market, in facilitating individual conceptions of the good. Given the important role played by this self in bioethics, the way in which bioethicists address particular ethical issues will often be shaped by whether they endorse (some version of) this conception of the self and everything that accompanies it, or whether they find both it and the things it carries problematic.

THE DIVIDED SELF OF BIOETHICS: LOCATING MORAL ISSUES IN A POLITICAL CONTEXT

I now want to describe the Divided Self more completely, in light of the discussion above, and then say more about the role played by this self in bioethics. The Divided Self that emerges from Rawls's thought experiment, and whose characteristics are accepted in other liberal accounts is ghostly, existing somehow behind and apart from its particular characteristics, its conception of the good, and the commitments it makes. All of these things are either contingent or revisable, so who this self most fundamentally *is* exists apart from them. It is, therefore, separate from its commitments, personal connections, and conceptions of the good.

This self is individualistic; it is as an individual that it reaches agreements with others, and as an individual that it identifies life plans and acts upon them. Even if those plans encompass close connections to other people, it remains an individual, since these connections, too, are revisable. In keeping with its ghostliness, it is transparent to itself: it is not a self which is often torn between competing conceptions of the good, or unclear about what it wants; if it is uncertain, it can treat the choices it makes as experiments which are subject to revision if they don't work out. It is free to choose, and committed to the two principles of justice primarily out of self-interest: it does not want to be deeply disadvantaged if it turns out, once it emerges from behind the veil, that it is the worst-off person in the society. (But we can note that it may be a very different thing to be committed to the principles of justice *for their own sake*, and being committed to them for contingent and hypothetical reasons of self-interest.) Finally, this self is split into sharply contrasting private and public parts: when private commitments and values come into conflict with public obligations, the private self must defer to the public one.

It is striking to note the way that the characteristics of the Divided Self are mirrored in the requirements of the just liberal state. For example, the transparency of the self the way in which it is assumed that we can identify our desires and articulate our goals, relatively unencumbered by confusion, angst, or profound indecision, is reflected in the idea that the institutions of the just state should be equally transparent: citizens should be able to see what decisions were made, for what reasons, how they were reached, and by whom. Moreover, the lack of personal knowledge possessed by the individuals meeting behind the veil is mirrored in the neutrality of the state apparatus, and the value pluralism such neutrality supports. Finally, the public/private split required of liberal selves—the requirement that, in public, their actions must meet the demands of liberal justice—is mirrored in the claim that the just state must be neutral between (acceptable) competing conceptions of the good precisely *because* it recognizes the importance of individual and incompatible ideas about what gives meaning and value to life. Paradoxically, then, it is because private conceptions of the good are so important that they must give way to shared public values when the two conflict, and this importance also places an obligation on the just state to be neutral.

These features of the Divided Self, and their close connection to the framework of the liberal state, have profound implications for the way in which bioethical issues are discussed when this political-moral account is utilized. I want to consider two significant dimensions of this account that are particularly influential in bioethics. The first dimension is the central place held by autonomy; I will argue that positions that simply apply the Divided Self to bioethical problems often fit awkwardly with the issues they are meant to illuminate and resolve, and shrink the space in which moral questions can be asked and considered so profoundly that very little can be said about them. The second dimension is concerned with questions about the distribution of health care goods and services within a just society, and with procedural justice within health care institutions. The liberal framework (unsurprisingly, since Rawls and other liberals take questions of distributive justice very seriously) is helpful for considering these kinds of questions.

The Divided Self and its choices are placed in either an explicitly or implicitly political context, and, just as the private must give way to the public when the two conflict, so must the moral give way to the political when the two conflict. In fact, the moral is often subsumed into the political: what morality is taken to mean is that we respect one another's choices, and meet our obligations as liberal democratic citizens. This position is nicely demonstrated by Dworkin's sustained argument about abortion and euthanasia, as well as by other autonomy-based bioethical discussions that draw on the liberal approach.

In a book entitled *Law's Dominion*, Dworkin's argument demonstrates the importance of the political context within which the Divided Self moves, and against which its moral views must be balanced. Dworkin makes a claim about the nature of significant bioethical decisions that implicitly reflects Rawls's position, and which has been picked up, and echoed by, other bioethicists. His argument, simply put, goes like this: "beliefs about the inherent value of human life . . . [are] *essentially* religious beliefs."[35] As such, they fall into the category of private beliefs about which the state should remain neutral.

Dworkin uses this claim to defend procreative autonomy, and to assert that a respect for "procreative autonomy, in a broad sense, is embedded in any genuine democratic culture."[36] His argument then draws on the liberal conception of the self and the nature of its choices, and Dworkin places these things firmly within a political context: "The most important feature of . . . [Western political culture] is a belief in human dignity: that people have the moral right and the moral responsibility to confront the most fundamental questions about the meaning and value of their own lives for themselves, answering to their own consciences and convictions."[37]

The next step in Dworkin's argument draws on the public/private split that characterizes the Divided Self, and the obligations of citizenship that this split represents. While we should not be indifferent to the procreative choices other people make in our family, community, or society, we should be tolerant towards the religious beliefs of others (and we should note that the logic of the argument suggests that the same response would be made towards any private comprehensive beliefs which spill over into the public sphere), even when we profoundly disagree with them: "Tolerance is a cost we must pay for our adventure in liberty. . . . If we have genuine concern for the lives that others lead, we will also accept that no life is a good one lived against the grain of conviction, that it does not help someone else's life but spoils it to force values upon him he cannot accept but can only bow before out of fear or prudence."[38]

The implications of this position for bioethics are profound because both the range of ethical questions that can legitimately be asked, as well as the form that acceptable answers to them must take, are significantly reduced. Suppose, for example (to stick with the issue of procreative liberty), that someone who is opposed to abortion on moral grounds believes that these reasons are compelling, not just for him personally, but that they ought to be compelling for others as well, and that what follows from them are some restrictions of the conditions under which abortion is permitted. From the perspective of the liberal self-moral-political account, unless we can agree that abortion clearly violates the Harm Principle (with "clearly" meaning in a way that the majority can agree on without much thought or will come to realize after some discussion), anyone who makes this claim reveals himself to be either ignorant of, or insufficiently committed to, the requirements that liberal democracies place on their citizens because he is failing to recognize that his personal beliefs (in this case, about abortion) are private beliefs that have no implications for anyone else. In private, he can believe what he wants and conduct his own life accordingly; in public, however, he must allow others to make their own choices, in accordance with their own private beliefs. And the same is true for other controversial bioethical issues (such as euthanasia or the sale of organs): the fact that they are controversial demonstrates, in and of itself, that there is no widespread agreement about whether or not they violate the Harm Principle, and so objections to them must be considered to fall into the category of private beliefs as well. Just as we can be Nietzsche in private but must be J.S. Mill in public, so we can be opposed to abortion in private, but must not only, in public, allow others to think differently than we do, but also, as good citizens, be committed to the public provision of abortion services so that they can act on the basis of those beliefs as well. In short, if we don't approve of abortion ourselves, we shouldn't have one; but we also have no right to restrict the options that are available to others who don't share our beliefs.

Following this line of thinking, bioethicists who emphasize the importance of autonomy and understand this concept as it is articulated in the liberal self-moral-political framework tend to spend more effort on defending the freedom of individuals to choose than they do on a moral examination of those choices. It is, then, largely because the liberal self-moral-political framework has become so central to mainstream bioethics that bioethics has become so focused on procedural issues and so reluctant to make moral judgments about the choices people make, except about the value of free choice itself, and the necessity of respecting the Harm Principle. As we shall see in the next chapter, however, this perspective also contributes to a model of bioethics which, paradoxically, has very little to say about substantive moral issues, including issues connected to questions of distributive justice.

"THE AMBULANCE AT THE BOTTOM OF THE CLIFF": THE SOCIAL DETERMINANTS OF HEALTH AND EQUALITY OF OPPORTUNITY

Liberalism can be understood as, among other things, a theory of distributive justice that centers on questions of equality and what it means to treat citizens with equal concern and respect. Indeed, for many liberal theorists, a concern with equality and justice are prior to a concern with individualism and freedom: the reason why governments ought to leave citizens free to pursue their own conceptions of the good is that it is only by doing so that persons are treated as equals, and many of the arrangements of the liberal state are required in order to ensure that goods and services are distributed fairly. That is to say, it is only when equality is respected, and the requirements of fair distribution met, that individuals are even able to become autonomous and to pursue their own conceptions of the good. This is an aspect of liberalism that can be clearly seen in Daniels' discussion of the connection between health care and equality of opportunity.

Daniels places health care firmly within the context of social justice. When we understand the way in which social conditions affect population health we can, he believes, extend Rawlsian arguments so that health care, broadly speaking, is encompassed within the distributive framework that emerges out of the original position and the veil of ignorance: if we want to ensure that our society follows the two principles of justice, really does allow genuine fair equality of opportunity, and is, indeed, a society in which inequalities benefit the worst off, then we will pay attention to controllable social factors that affect people's health. As Daniels puts it, while he is not claiming that Rawls's theory is convincing in every way, it is the "most fully developed general theory of justice" that sets out arguments in support of fair equality of opportunity.[39] As such, Daniels argues, the fact that there is a "close fit between my account of health and health needs and Rawls's account of the needs of free and equal citizens enables me to borrow support from his view and simultaneously to extend its scope and power."[40]

Medical care, Daniels colorfully asserts, "is, figuratively speaking, 'the ambulance waiting at the bottom of the cliff.'"[41] By this phrase, he means to draw our attention to the fact (evident in every society) that health status is correlated with social conditions and income level, and the effects these factors have on individuals over the course of their lifetimes. In other words, by the time most people present themselves to medical professionals for treatment of particular conditions, preventable damage to their health has already been done.

Daniels observes that the fact that social factors (which he terms "the social determinants of health") that exist outside of what are normally understood to be the sphere of medicine have a profound impact on health is something which bioethics has largely ignored. The reasons for this lack of attention, Daniels believes, are complex, encompassing sociological factors, political arrangements, and ideological commitments. The media, abetted by scientists, encourage us to see improvements in health as resulting primarily from biomedical science, and this perspective is supported by economic interests (which affect bioethicists among others) which benefit from a widespread public understanding that this is, indeed, how medical progress is achieved. Moreover, I believe, this lack of attention results from the fact that many bioethicists now work with a conception of autonomy that largely detaches it from its political origins: as we shall see in the next chapter, the Divided Self is rapidly being replaced by its close relative, the Choosing Self.

To the extent that bioethics considers issues of justice, it focuses on questions of how to ensure equitable access to treatments, and what constitutes a fair distribution of goods and services within medical institutions. Larger questions of social justice, however, which have a profound impact on the actual health of individuals, tend to be ignored. As Daniels notes, "Challenging deeper inequalities in society . . . is divisive, not unifying, and it threatens those with the greatest power and the most to lose."[42] In order to address the issues raised by these deeper inequalities, Daniels asks one Fundamental Question: "As a matter of justice, what do we owe each other to promote and protect health in a population and to assist people when they are ill or disabled?"[43] He also asks three more specific Focal Questions, which are designed to help answer the Fundamental Question. The first Focal Question asks, "Is health and therefore health care and other factors that affect health, of special moral importance?"[44] The second asks, "When are health inequalities unjust?"[45] Finally, the third asks: "How can we meet health needs fairly, under resource constraints?"[46]

Daniels gives answers to these questions which either explicitly draw on Rawls's argument, or which are Rawlsian in spirit: health care, he argues, is of special moral importance because the "loss of function associated with disease and disability reduces the range of opportunities open to us compared to what it would be were we healthy or fully functional."[47] Ill health, in other words, adversely affects the ability of individuals to pursue particular conceptions of the good by restricting the range of possibilities open to them.

In response to the second question, Daniels argues that, while Rawls himself simplified his theory by assuming that the contractors in the original position would assume that they will have a normal lifespan free of disability and disease, other aspects of his theory—in particular the claim that social conditions which unfairly affect people's opportunities, should be addressed in a just society—suggests that the social determinants of health should be included. As Daniels puts it, the "general principles of justice as fairness that Rawls argues for in his theory of justice as fairness captures the key social determinants of health, especially if one includes . . . health care in the institutions that protect opportunity."[48] Consequently, "what justice requires in policy that affects health and the acceptability of health inequalities must be comparable with what justice requires in the distribution of a broad range of social goods."[49]

Finally, the third Focal Question asks us to consider what procedures are necessary to ensure that limited health care resources are distributed fairly. Since these goods are limited, any distributive choices we make will inevitably create winners and losers. What we need to do to achieve fairness, Daniels believes, is ensure that our distributive choices are made in accordance with the demands of procedural justice. They must be transparent: their rationales must be publicly available, and they must be reasonable. Furthermore, they must be open to appeals and revisions, and mechanisms must be in place to ensure that these conditions are met. While Daniels does not put it in precisely these terms, these procedures serve the same function that the veil of ignorance does in Rawls's thought experiment: they help ensure that, whatever decisions are ultimately made, they will be fair, and even those who end up being "losers" will (like the worst-off member of society) have no substantive grounds for complaint.

Daniels, I believe, makes a good case for the extension of Rawls's theory in such a way that the social determinants of health are included as items that a just society should concern itself with. Indeed, while Daniels does not make this particular argument in support of his extension of Rawls's theory, the *logic* of the thought experiment suggests that a knowledge of health and disability status would be one of the things that would be hidden behind the veil. Arguably, the set-up of the original position and the veil of ignorance could easily lead to more radical and far-reaching conclusions than Rawls himself allows.

CONCLUSION

"LIKE WEARING A TUXEDO TO A BEACH PARTY": THE AWKWARD FIT BETWEEN THE DIVIDED SELF AND THE ISSUES EXPLORED IN BIOETHICS

Liberal thinking generally, and Rawlsian-type thinking in particular, has been used in two very significant ways in bioethics, and both of these ways are predicated on the conception of the Divided Self. First, autonomy has become *the* dominant principle in bioethics: it trumps all the other principles, at least when we are dealing with competent persons, and is only constrained, on occasion, when resources are too limited to allow its exercise, or when harms resulting from its exercise can be clearly and controversially identified. Moreover, it is difficult to find any attribution of harm that is *not* controversial: *my* claim that human cloning would be harmful is seen by *you* to be nothing more than an expression of prejudice. We can call this the *moral* dimension of the self-moral-political liberal account, and I shall say more about the implications of the dominance of this form of autonomy in bioethics in a moment.

Second, as we can see in Daniels's proposals, Rawls's theory has played an influential role in addressing questions of distributive justice within health care systems, and in answering the question of what role health care provisions should play in a just society. Consequently, there is currently something of a consensus in bioethics that distributive decisions should follow liberal standards of procedural fairness, and that health care (including its social determinants) should be part of the package of goods available to citizens, because they protect equality of opportunity. As Daniels notes, even theorists who reject some of Rawls's claims agree "that we have an obligation to protect the range of opportunities open to us,"[50] and, as we saw in our earlier discussion of Beauchamp and Childress's principled approach, they develop the principle of justice in fundamentally liberal terms. This consensus on method and the widespread agreement that the social determinants of health are important, makes the failure of mainstream bioethics to robustly address issues of race, gender, and social justice in a sustained and challenging way both puzzling and noticeable. Far from critiquing present social arrangements, bioethicists working in the mainstream often provide arguments that justify the current status quo, and which, indeed, support the intrusion of the market into health care and the domain of personal life.

These views are predicated on the idea that there are diverse, competing, and incompatible conceptions of the good, and that the role of the just state is essentially twofold. First, to preserve as large a space as possible for citizens to pursue their own particular life plans, according to their own beliefs about what gives meaning and value to life, and, where possible, to ensure that social arrangements facilitate genuine choice. Second, to ensure that, when goods are limited, social institutions (including health care institutions) that are responsible for making distributive choices that create winners and losers will do so using procedures that are transparent. These two elements constitute the political side of the moral-political conjunction, as it is applied to bioethics.

However, the application of liberal thinking to bioethics fits better when applied to political questions (such as the place of health care in just societies) than to moral ones (such as questions about abortion, surrogacy, and the nature of the doctor-patient relationship). Why? Because liberalism is primarily a political philosophy, and the conception of the self that lies at its heart (as Rawls's own account makes clear) is designed to allow us to live together in democratic societies; but this conception leaves it up to each of us to determine for ourselves the nature of the good, which means that it simultaneously assumes that we have certain capacities. We must be reasonable, capable of conversing and reaching agreements with others; we must be tolerant of the choices made by other people, even when we disagree with them; and, most importantly for bioethics, it assumes that we have both the capacity to be autonomous, and that we have genuine choices open to us.

However, the most difficult cases in bioethics—the ones that generate dilemmas that are difficult and perhaps even impossible to resolve entirely satisfactorily—occur when someone's competency is questionable, or when competent individuals are seriously ill, and the only options open to them may be a choice between painful and possibly futile treatment, or no treatment at all. In short, the conditions which bring people into contact with medical professionals and health care institutions—which, that is to say, cause them to need the ambulance at the bottom of the cliff—have often already limited their options in such a way that it seems incongruous and even cruel to speak of the importance of respecting autonomy in order to allow these people to pursue their own conceptions of the good. If they are competent, of course their choices should usually be respected; but to say that the very ill are autonomous, as we normally understand the concept, arguably fundamentally misrepresents their situation. Moreover, the dominance of autonomy in bioethics does not help us determine what choices should be made for those who are incompetent or whose autonomy is questionable, even if we have no difficulty identifying an appropriate substitute decision maker. Finally, and also importantly, emphasizing autonomy in the way and to the extent that is required by the Divided Self does not help us determine, even for ourselves, what choices we ought to make in a medical or bioethical context.

We have already seen that the Troubled Self is in a state of confusion, and why this is the case. However, its confusions are not personally disturbing for most people using the ideas of Kant or the utilitarians in bioethics or elsewhere because very few people (outside of philosophy departments, anyway) describe themselves as "Kantians" or "utilitarians" and try to live their lives in accordance with these theories (although they may hold utilitarian or Kantian philosophical views). The presence of the Troubled Self, then, may create problems in our ethical thinking generally, and in bioethics particularly; but it seldom causes problems, it seems fair to say, for "real" people living their lives in the "real" world.

The Divided Self is different: it is, indeed, a dominant model of the self, not only in bioethics, but in North American political and social culture as well. As I noted above, it is arguably the case that most North Americans have been touched by it in their view of democratic politics, the place of freedom and the limits of legitimate government interference, in their ideas about their right to free speech, freedom of religion, and freedom of the press. Consequently, then, liberal claims about the importance of autonomy have become a part of many people's *self-conceptions*, even if they don't recognize the source of this concept, and even if they don't describe themselves as liberals.[51]

The very familiarity of the elements that compose the Divided Self make it difficult to see clearly, and, consequently, difficult to evaluate, which may explain why there are few, if any, competing contemporary accounts which are as comprehensive, as compelling, and as persuasively worked out as the liberal one is. Even critics of this account (or, at least, critics working within frameworks that are recognizable to most of us as modern, and democratic) have arguably been shaped by it.[52]

Despite the appeal of the Divided Self, with its emphasis on making choices and a life within the space provided by the just state, and despite the important role this self has played not only in our political and moral understandings, but also in our self-understandings, I want to argue that, at least within the context of bioethics and within the practice of medicine, a number of ethical problems are raised, not resolved, by this self. (These problems may extend beyond bioethics and medicine, but an exploration of this possibility would be well beyond the scope of this enquiry.) My contention is that the conjunction of self-moral-political in the liberal model sacrifices moral considerations to political commitments, and understands the self, its freedoms, and its choices, in primarily political terms.

First, the Divided Self doesn't fit well with how we actually understand our relationships with other people. This has implications for bioethics, which is concerned, often, with relationships (whether between health care professionals and patients, or patients and their families, or with taking care of people in a medical setting). Murray, for instance, argues that liberal defenses of (almost unlimited) procreative freedom, while not exactly wrong, seem tone-deaf; to describe familial relationships, and the reasons for which people create and value families, in terms of rights, freedom of choice, and political justice, is a "kind of mistake: it is slightly off-center; it misses something important. It is like wearing a tuxedo to a beach party. You might at first think the person in the tuxedo has a wry sense of humor; but when you realize that he is completely serious, that he honestly thinks this is what one wears to the beach, you might feel a little sorry for him. Obviously, he does not understand what beach parties are all about."[53]

Moreover, as Murray point out, this approach misrepresents the nature of many of our most important choices, including the choice to have a child. This choice, once made and acted upon, is not revisable (at least, not revisable without doing a great deal of moral damage: one shouldn't simply abandon a baby because being a parent turns out, in practice, not to be compatible with what gives meaning and value to one's life). It is a choice, moreover, which, if taken seriously and performed responsibly, will limit one's freedom in innumerable ways: the "responsibility of caring for an infant, then a child, then an adolescent, may be the most constraining thing a person can experience. Unless they have arranged for someone else to do it, the parents of an infant are not free to sleep late on weekends (or sleep through the night for that matter). They are not free to leave their young child home alone while they go out for a movies or a meal."[54] Viewing moral questions in the context of familial relationships through the lens of autonomy, freedom of choice, and the continual possibility of revising our decisions and remaking ourselves seems, in many ways, to miss the point. Familial relationships can, indeed, be a source of profound personal satisfactions and moral challenges, but these satisfactions and challenges occupy a moral space that is not easily encompassed by these concepts or well understood through an application of them.

Second, to describe the choices facing very sick people, who are often frightened, usually in pain, and possibly very heavily medicated, in terms of respecting their autonomy, seems to misdescribe their situation: of course, their autonomy should be respected, but we owe them much more than this—at the very least, compassion and kindness are also required. Indeed, as O'Neill notes, "because of the vulnerability and weakness of patients, even informed consent procedures, (let alone robust conceptions of individual autonomy) may be less apposite and less realistic in medical practice than in almost any other area of life."[55] In short, the Divided Self, in accordance with its divided nature, appears essentially disembodied, at a remove from the frailties and weaknesses that beset us as embodied beings, with which medicine is most concerned, and which make us fundamentally dependent both on other people and on physical characteristics and disease processes over which we have very little control. As we shall see when we explore illness narratives, an emphasis on autonomy in bioethics has not translated into a reduction in the suffering reported by patients—suffering, moreover, primarily generated not by their disease, but by a failure to be treated as persons within the medical context.

To put this point another way, we might say that this self is emotionally appealing and its mirroring of features of the just state as described by liberal theorists is intellectually elegant, but it appears unsatisfactory when it is applied to many of the issues with which bioethics concerns itself. In the bioethical context, the Divided Self is often unable to do what it purports to be able to do, which is provide us with the resources necessary to ensure as much as possible that each of us lives a meaningful and worthwhile (at least to us) life. What it does is defend the importance of choosing freely, but it fails to provide us with—as a moral theory arguably should—the resources to figure out what choices we *ought* to make, even given *our own* values, at least when we must make deeply difficult decisions.

Consider, for example, a woman who unexpectedly finds herself pregnant, just as she is about to begin a new dream job which involves advocating for the rights of her vulnerable ethnic community, a role which is important to her: her membership in this ethnic community constitutes an important part of her self-understanding, and gives her life meaning and value. She cannot possibly take the job and have the baby (it involves significant amounts of travel, and she lacks family supports and financial resources which would allow her to leave the baby when she goes out of town). However, she always saw herself as someday becoming a mother, and she sees reproduction as something that is also connected to her communal commitments (her ethnic minority needs new members if it is to survive). If she does not take up the job, someone else will, and her once-in-a-lifetime chance will be lost; but if she has an abortion, she will regret it as well. She is in her late thirties, and might not get pregnant again when her circumstances are more conducive to having a child.

What the conception of the Divided Self tells her is that the choice facing her is *hers*, and rightfully so (it is not one that anyone else should make for her) but it gives her no guidance in terms of what choice she should make or even in what terms she should think about it, and demonstrates very little understanding of the fact that some choices change our lives forever in irrevocable ways. Our most significant choices are not things we can stand apart from, and revise if they don't turn out the way we hope; they are, rather, things that can both shape who we are and send our lives off in new, and irrevocable, directions.[56]

Proponents of the liberal perspective in bioethics, of course, would respond to this objection by saying that this is why the democratic freedoms of thought, speech, religion, and the press are so important. They provide us with the resources to think about, and make, precisely these sorts of difficult choices. But the point here is that the choice is a lonely one; it is entirely up to each of us to determine not only what choices to make, but also which moral parameters to draw from, or to impose, on ourselves. This conception of the self, then, doesn't help individuals determine what to do with their freedoms, and it makes them absolutely responsible for the consequences of their choices without providing guidelines for how they ought to be made.

Third, and following from this, the liberal model shrinks the zone of what constitutes morality almost to a vanishing point in bioethics: as long as no one's rights are violated, consent is obtained, autonomy respected, and the requirements of the Harm Principle met, there is not much else to say. Consider, again, May's claims about the role of ethics committees within medical institutions in liberal societies. They ought to function, in his view, in much the same way that the liberal state does: as providing a framework through which the values and choices of individuals are respected and facilitated. "The clinical setting calls for a mechanism to protect patient autonomy in framing the evaluation of treatment according to the patient's own judgment. Health care ethics committees serve the role of providing this mechanism" by "refraining from imposing their own values" so "that the patient's own values can frame treatment decisions."[57] On this view (which is, arguably, if understood as a descriptive account, rather than the normative prescription which May intends, a pretty fair statement of the way in which ethics committees work, and bioethicists understand their role) "doing ethics" means little more than establishing what patient values are, and what treatment decisions follow from them. As May argues, within this framework, *nothing* can be understood as "medically necessary," recommended, or even straightforwardly reasonable treatment. The only standard that is acceptable in a liberal context is the subjective patient standard because it is only this standard that recognizes "at a fundamental level, the liberal idea of protecting an individual's right to author his or her own life."[58]

If ensuring that proper procedures are followed, and that the subjective patient standard for disclosure and treatment is met, it's not clear why ethics committees (or bioethicists) are needed at all: clear policies, procedural guidelines, and a hospital ombudsman to ensure that they are followed could do the job just as well. In short, a moral theory that simply tells us that we must be free to make our own choices, for our own reasons, constrained only by the Harm Principle and our democratic obligations, isn't really functioning as a moral theory at all.

However, if we go in the other direction (as an increasing number of bioethicists are doing), and detach the moral dimensions of liberal selfhood from its political and democratic commitments (the principles of justice that Rawls proposes, we should remember, place constraints on acceptable conceptions of the good, and the requirement that we must be reasonable in our encounters with other people so that together we can construct and maintain shared political space are meant to ensure not only that we seek what is good for us, but also what is good for the larger community), the result is even more unsatisfactory: what is generated is a conception of autonomy which revolves around the Choosing Self. This self takes for granted the liberal framework that the Divided Self articulates, defends against competitors, and works to maintain. The Divided Self has to respond to democratic requirements of good citizenship, needs to respect the Harm Principle in its choices, must allow its private conceptions of the good to give way to shared public conceptions when this is necessary to maintain political peace and social order, and ought to be concerned with issues of social justice, equality, and fairness. The Choosing Self, which is what remains when the Divided Self is detached from the liberal political framework, is not constrained in these ways, and its increasingly dominant presence in bioethics generates what I shall call the paradox of expertise.

NOTES

1. Thomas May, *Bioethics In A Liberal Society: The Political Framework Of Bioethics Decision Making* (Baltimore: Johns Hopkins University Press, 2002), 116.

2. Paul Root Wolpe, quoted in Onora O'Neill, *Autonomy and Trust In Bioethics* (Cambridge: Cambridge University Press, 2002), 36.

3. As Callahan observes, there has been the "almost complete triumph of liberal individualism in bioethics. I call this an ideology rather than a moral theory because it is a set of essentially political and social values brought into bioethics, not as a formal theory but as a vital background constellation of values. If it does not function as a moral theory, as philosophers have understood that concept, it is clearly present and pervasive as a litmus test of the acceptability of certain ideas and ways of framing issues. As a familiar constellation it encompasses a high place for autonomy, for biomedical progress with few constraints, for procedural rather than substantive solutions to controverted ethical problems, and for a strong antipathy to comprehensive notion of the human good." Daniel Callahan, "Individual Good and Common Good: A Communitarian Approach," *Perspectives In Biology and Medicine* 46, no. 4 (Autumn 2003): 496–507.

4. While "virtue" is a term that is not often used by liberal thinkers, Stephen Macedo persuasively argues that, when liberals make the case for pluralism, tolerance, and a respect for human rights, they are asking us to display a set of what can be called "liberal virtues." We must weigh liberal values against those values that are in competition with them, and make a self-conscious choice about which ones to support. "Is the freedom to debate, choose, and live one's life one's own way really more important than struggling to establish a common culture that supports piety and otherworldliness and punishes blasphemers? Is peaceful pluralism really more important than Christian unity?" Stephen Macedo, *Liberal Virtues* (Oxford: Clarendon Press, 1990), 60. If we believe that they are, we must acknowledge that "Liberal political values occupy the same space as personal comprehensive ideals, religious or otherwise." (Stephen Macedo, *Liberal Virtues* (Oxford: Clarendon Press, 1990), 60. Liberalism, then, not only makes a case for political freedom as something that ought to be protected by governments and state institutions, it also places obligations on individuals to act and think in ways which support those freedoms as well.

5. As Mill puts it, "the sole end for which mankind are warranted, individually or collectively, in interfering with the liberty of action of any of their number is self-protection. That is the only purpose for which power can be exercised over any member of a civilized community, against his will, is to prevent harm to others. His own good, either physical or moral, is not a sufficient warrant." J. S. Mill, *On Liberty* (London: Dent, 1984), 78.

6. Atul Gawande, *Complications: A Surgeon's Notes On An Imperfect Science* (New York: Metropolitan Books, 2002), 223.

7. As O'Neill observes, "Contemporary admiration for individual or personal autonomy still owes... far more to Mill than to Kant: although many of its admirers crave and claim Kantian credentials, they mostly seek an account of individual autonomy that fits within a naturalistic account of human action [such as the account provided by Mill]. Onora O'Neill, *Autonomy and Trust*, 29—30.

8. Macedo, *Liberal Virtues*, 204.

9. Macedo, *Liberal Virtues*, 204.

10. Ronald Dworkin, "Liberalism", in *Public and Private Morality*, ed. Stuart Hampshire (Cambridge: Cambridge University Press, 1978), 129.

11. May, *Bioethics In A Liberal Society*, 5.

12. Allen Buchanan, Dan W. Brock, Norman Daniels, and Daniel Wikler, *From Chance To Choice* (New York: Cambridge University Press, 2000), 382.

13. Allen Buchanan, Dan. W. Brock, Norman Daniels, and Daniel Wikler, *From Chance*, 382.

14. May, *Bioethics In A Liberal Society*, 121.

15. May, *Bioethics In A Liberal Society*, 122.

16. May, *Bioethics In A Liberal Society*, 125.

17. Robert B. Talisse, *On Rawls: A Liberal Theory of Justice and Justification* (Belmont, CA: Wadsworth, 2001), 4.

18. John Rawls, *A Theory of Justice* (Cambridge, Massachusetts: The Belknap Press of Harvard University Press, 1971), 96.

19. Rawls, *Theory*, 19.

20. Rawls, *Theory*, 18.

21. Rawls, *Theory*, 12.

22. Rawls, *Theory*, 302.

23. Rawls, *Theory*, 302.

24. Rawls, *Theory*, 44.

25. Rawls, *Theory*, 152.

26. Rawls, *Theory*, 432.

27. Rawls, *Theory*, 433.

28. This is ironic, because one of Rawls's most famous criticisms of utilitarianism is that it "fails to take seriously the distinction between persons. The principle of rational choice for one man is taken as the principle of social choice as well." (Rawls, *Theory*, 187).

29. John Rawls, *Political Liberalism* (New York: Columbia University Press, 1993), 32.

30. Richard Rorty, *Contingency, irony, and solidarity* (Cambridge: Cambridge University Press, 1989), 85.

31. Michael J. Sandel, *Liberalism and the Limits of Justice* (Cambridge: Cambridge University Press, 1982), 105.

32. Sandel, *Limits*, 105.

33. Sandel, *Limits*, 175.

34. Sandel, *Limits*, 176.

35. Ronald Dworkin, *Life's Dominion: An Argument About Abortion, Euthanasia, and Individual Freedom* (New York: Vintage Books, 1994), 155.

36. Dworkin, *Life's Dominion*, 167.

37. Dworkin, *Life's Dominion*, 166.

38. Dworkin, *Life's Dominion*, 167—168.

39. Norman Daniels, *Just Health: Meeting Health Needs Fairly* (New York: Cambridge University Press, 2008), 63.

40. Daniels, *Just Health*, 64.

41. Daniels, *Just Health*, 79.

42. Daniels, *Just Health*, 102.

43. Daniels, *Just Health*, 11.

44. Daniels, *Just Health*, 11.

45. Daniels, *Just Health*, 11.

46. Daniels, *Just Health*, 11.

47. Daniels, *Just Health*, 21.

48. Daniels, *Just Health*, 23.

49. Daniels, *Just Health*, 22.

50. Daniels, *Just Health*, 64.

51. For example, even religious conservatives who emphasize the importance of having a personal relationship with God can be said to be drawing on elements of this individualistic conception of the self.

52. For example, while Sandel makes a thorough and careful case against the Rawlsian project in *Liberalism and the Limits of Justice*, it's not clear what he would replace it with, apart from his assertion that a better account would be one which allows for a richer and more communal conception of the self, and a politics which is open to the possibility that "when politics goes well, we can know a good in common that we cannot know alone." (p. 183). This is arguably a claim that many liberals could make, although they might be pessimistic about the likelihood of achieving that good. Indeed, some liberals have argued that liberalism itself offers an account of the shared goods we need to acknowledge if we are to live peacefully together, such as a commitment to tolerance, liberal principles of justice, and the role played by democratic institutions in just societies. See, for example, Joseph Raz's *The Morality of Freedom*

(Oxford: Oxford University Press, 1986) and Stephen Macedo, *Liberal Virtues* (Oxford: Clarendon Press, 1990).

53. Thomas H. Murray, *The Worth of a Child* (Berkeley: University of California Press, 1996), 28.

54. Murray, *Worth*, 19.

55. Onora O'Neill, *Autonomy and Trust In Bioethics* (Cambridge: Cambridge University Press, 2002), 40.

56. I owe this example to one of my colleagues, Réal Fillion, and I thank him for letting me use it in a new setting, as well as for the stimulating discussions about the strengths and limitations of the liberal account.

57. May, *Bioethics In A Liberal Society*, 125—126.

58. May, *Bioethics In A Liberal Society*, 19.

Chapter Four

The Choosing Self

Bioethics and the Paradox of Autonomy

INTRODUCTION: THE PECULIAR NATURE OF BIOETHICAL EXPERTISE

The cultural role occupied by philosophy today is, in many respects, both minor and marginalized. Philosophers are often seen to occupy themselves with esoteric questions, and to offer little in the way of guidance for the practical resolution of social and political problems. Even within universities, administrators often have to be persuaded of the merits of a discipline that has limited potential to attract research funding or large numbers of students. There is, however, one general exception to this state of affairs, one area of philosophy that students, university administrators, the media, and the general public, all seem to believe that philosophers can offer something significant and important, and that is in bioethics. As we have seen, those who specialize in bioethics are widely considered to have (and often see themselves to possess) a particular kind of expertise not available to non-specialists. As a result, bioethicists are invited to serve on ethics committees in health care institutions, advise government policy makers on bioethical questions, and work as ethicists within hospitals. In short, it is primarily as "bioethicists" (not as metaphysicians, epistemologists, or even moral theorists) that philosophers are invited to make the move from the ivory tower to the bedside of the patient. In addition, bioethicists are often asked by the media to make public comments when stories of a bioethical nature generate headlines; philosophers, in contrast, are not often thought by journalists to have anything of interest to say. The disconnect between the low cultural value attributed to philosophy today, and the elevated place currently occupied by

109

bioethics is both odd and striking, and it at least partially explains the resentment some philosophers display towards bioethics, and the defensiveness with which many bioethicists justify and defend their own positions.

Bioethicists, then, are understood by others (and understand themselves) to be professionals who can provide objective, educated, and specialized expertise about ethical theory and practice, and who can give helpful guidance with respect to the particular problems that arise within healthcare institutions, are generated by medical and scientific research, or raised by legal and political developments. As Brannigan and Boss point out, "since 1970, healthcare ethics has become one of the most, if not the most, prestigious and lucrative fields in philosophy. Many colleges and universities have centers devoted to the study of healthcare ethics. Most large hospitals and medical schools have professional medical ethicists on their staff to act as professional advice givers when moral problems arise."[1] The elevated social role occupied by the bioethicist, that is to say, is entirely predicated on the possession of a unique, powerful, and useful kind of expertise.

A profound paradox, however, lies at the heart of these claims to bioethical expertise, a paradox generated by the nature of the self that increasingly animates contemporary bioethics, and which suggests that these claims to expertise are illusory. At the center of much contemporary bioethics stands the figure of the Choosing Self. Indeed, this self is becoming so dominant that it may eventually come to replace all the conceptions of the self that we have so far considered. Its presence can be discerned in every area of bioethics, from debates about the nature of the physician-patient relationship, the morality of euthanasia, or the requirements for ethical experimentation on human subjects, to questions about how the supply of organs for transplantation might be increased, how reproductive technologies should be regulated, and the appropriate use of genetic enhancements. Despite its ever-increasing ubiquity, however, what is most striking about the Choosing Self is its formlessness. It is defined as much by what it is not as by what it is, and its nature is seen more clearly by its critics than by those who simply assume its presence. It is characterized not by what it does, what it believes, or through its connections and interactions with others, but simply by its capacity to make autonomous choices. This self combines elements present in the philosophies of Kant and Mill, but its central characteristics are drawn from liberal conclusions about the nature of human flourishing which we explored in the last chapter. However, even though the Choosing Self has what might be termed a noble ethical and political lineage, it is set apart from its ancestors by its lack of ethical and political commitments. Moreover, the dominance of this conception of the self in much contemporary bioethical discussion undermines the public recognition enjoyed by bioethicists, as well as the social prestige conferred by the widespread public belief that bioethicists do, indeed, possess a variety of specialized ethical expertise that allows them to make educated judgments that go beyond those that could be made by non-experts examining the same questions and issues.

Consider, for example, the responses of professional bioethicists to headline-grabbing cases generated by the use of reproductive technologies. One was the birth of octuplets to an American woman (now dubbed 'octo-mom' in the popular press), who was reported to already have six children (all conceived through IVF), no job, and no partner, all elements of her story that received much media attention. The other case, which was widely discussed in Canada, concerned a sixty-year-old Indo-Canadian woman—at the time believed to be the oldest woman to have given birth in Canada—who had twins after undergoing IVF treatment in India using donor eggs. (The cutoff age for IVF treatments in Canada at the time was fifty.) She reportedly suffered from hypertension, placenta previa, and gestational diabetes, and was hospitalized for the last four weeks of her pregnancy. After their birth, her sons spent time in the neonatal intensive care unit.

Predictably, along with the publicity these stories received, bioethicists, as recognized experts in these sorts of ethical matters, were asked to comment on the concerns these cases raised. The tone and content of their responses, however, raises questions about the nature of expertise in bioethics, about what it is that the bioethicist is offering, and why bioethicists play such prominent institutional roles, and occupy such a visible place in the larger culture. In short, the responses made by bioethicists largely consisted in the assertion that it would be wrong to make judgments about the reproductive choices individuals make because no one other than the persons involved are well placed to understand the meaning and significance of their own reproductive choices. Moreover, the confidence with which bioethicists who spoke publicly asserted this position was interesting because they seemed oblivious to the fact that, in making these assertions, they were undermining their own claim to possess a specialized form of professional expertise.

This chapter will explore the possibility that a form of bioethics predicated on the Choosing Self becomes self-defeating, because it undermines the claim that bioethicists possess specialized expertise and can, therefore, offer unique ethical guidance, upon which the existence of bioethics (and bioethicists) is predicated. I will argue, further, that the problem is not so much that such specialized knowledge in ethics is unavailable or unobtainable (although it might look different from the form it takes in the approaches we have been considering), but, rather, results from the particular way in which the concept of autonomy that both provides the characteristics of the Choosing Self and justifies its actions has been applied in many bioethical discussions. As long as bioethicists cite this model of autonomy in their responses to ethical issues *as though it is essentially the whole story*, their claims to ethical expertise will be suspect, and their belief that they possess it will be self-deceptive.

This conclusion, however, raises important concerns that will be considered in the rest of the book. The issues considered under the rubric of bioethics are among the most important and serious that philosophers can consider, and bioethicists, who consider such fundamental issues as death, reproduction, and illness, have the potential to make a contribution not only to the general public as they grapple with ethical questions, but to the discipline of philosophy itself. As R. M. Hare puts it, "I should like to say at once that if the moral philosopher *cannot* help with the problems of medical ethics, he ought to shut up shop. The problems of medical ethics are so typical of the moral problems that moral philosophy is supposed to be able to help with, that a failure here really would be a sign either of the uselessness of the discipline or of the incompetence of the particular practitioner."[2] The increasing dominance of the Choosing Self in contemporary bioethical discussions demonstrates not that bioethicists are better equipped to deal with issues of bioethical concern, but that bioethics has endorsed a conception of the self that gives bioethicists nothing of real significance to say about them.

ETHICAL EXPERTISE AND SELF-DECEPTION

The paradox generated by a commitment on the part of bioethicists to the Choosing Self is that their defense and use of this conception of the self undermines their claim to possess specialized expertise because this self embodies the idea that each of us should be able to decide for ourselves what choices we want to make, and on what grounds. While the idea that no one should tell us how to live or what to do (at least in matters which primarily concern ourselves) is widely assumed in contemporary western society, it is odd that so many bioethicists promote it because it suggests that, in ethical matters, there can be no objective answers to questions of right and wrong, and that ethical expertise is unavailable. (This model of the autonomy is also in tension with the important place given to principles in mainstream bioethics, the role played by the concept of rights and cost-benefit analysis, to a commitment to liberal principles of justice, as well as, of course, the certainty with which bioethicists claim that this conception of autonomy is correct, objectively speaking.) A comparison of some representative statements on reproductive issues made by bioethicists as they were quoted in the media with those made by non-specialists on the same subject reveals the paradox generated by an acceptance of the Choosing Self. The challenge here is to identify which claims bioethicists made, and which were made by non-experts.

1. "Infertility is a medical problem, and all couples have the right to reproduce;"[3] consequently, whatever medical techniques make reproduction possible are morally acceptable.
2. "We need more than gut reaction when we're proposing to limit the reproductive liberty of . . . women or otherwise interfere with people's freedom to make decisions about what's best for them and their families."[4]
3. "Are we saying that doctors should decide which women are desirable for IVF treatment and which are not? That they should limit the choices of those women who are 'unmarried, unemployed' and who already have kids at home? Since when did it become acceptable again to imply that poor women should not procreate and that doctors should do everything in their power to stop them?"[5]
4. "If we say it is OK for an older person to adopt children, is it a double standard to say that an older person can't give birth to children, if the argument... is that the older person may not be around long enough to raise that child? . . . Then, we need to start looking at the age of anyone who is a parent and their behaviors. If the parent is a skydiver, for example, or engaged in high altitude mountaineering . . . should we preclude them from being patients for IVF, given the likelihood that they may not reach 60?"[6] (The answer to this rhetorical question, of course, is meant to be "No," because making such value judgments about other people's choices is inappropriate.)
5. "Far be it from me to argue in favor of denying a woman the joys of motherhood—even post-menopausal woman—if the technology exists to cheat nature. . . . The ethicality of their choices should be . . . [theirs] alone to judge."[7]
6. "Mr. Bowman [speaking about post-mortem sperm retrieval] said hospitals should refrain from imposing their value judgments. 'Where do we start and stop if we go down that road?' he asked. 'Do you really want a society where health care workers are weighing in very heavily on reproductive questions?'"[8]

Comments 2, 4, and 6 were ascribed to bioethicists; comments 1, 3, and 5 were made by non-specialists. When these perspectives are considered, however, it is difficult to see any significant difference between the two groups: far from adding a dimension of expertise to the discussion that would otherwise be lacking, the responses of the bioethical experts seem merely to reinforce the general public consensus that individuals should be left free to make their own choices, in the way that best fits their own beliefs about value—and what is significant about this is not only that bioethicists don't seem to have anything further to add to the conversation, it is *also* that they do not even need to make the case that this is the correct approach to take to difficult ethical issues. The acceptance of the Choosing Self is so complete that it has become, for many, invisible: for them, this conception of the self simply describes what humans being are.

The advantage of this approach, and the reason why so many bioethicists promote its widespread acceptance, is that it gets rid of many of the dangers inherent in paternalism, in the belief that doctors knew what was best for patients, and were not even ethically obliged to tell them the truth about their medical condition if this was deemed to be harmful to them. This is arguably a significant advance in our ethical thinking: none of us wants to be told how we should think, or what we should do. Moreover, as we saw in the last chapter, the move to autonomy as both a central moral value and an ideal of human flourishing provides one way of avoiding the difficulty generated by the fact that we have no good way to choose between utilitarian and Kantian commitments *and* are unable to fully reconcile them because it largely allows us to avoid these theories altogether. However, this position is a difficult one for a bioethicist to advocate: she seems to be claiming a kind of expertise in ethics that consists primarily in making the case for letting people make decisions for themselves because there is no possibility of reaching a consensus on ethical questions, and no objective answers to them that can be given. Contemporary bioethical expertise, in short, often appears to consist of telling non-experts that ethical expertise is impossible to obtain.

THE CHOOSING SELF AND REPRODUCTIVE TECHNOLOGIES

We have seen that bioethicists who work with a conception of autonomy drawn primarily from liberal political theory find themselves caught on the horns of a dilemma. If they work explicitly within the political framework provided by liberalism, they risk conflating ethical questions with political considerations, in a way that can make their discussions and conclusions odd and unconvincing: to use Murray's image, it is as though they are arguing that a tuxedo is an appropriate outfit to wear to a beach party. It was this side of the dilemma that was explored in the last chapter. However, if they assert the correctness of the liberal model of the autonomous self, but detach it from its home in liberal political theory, the result is even less satisfactory. What follows is that the value of individual choice must be endorsed, but the larger political context that provided a reason to accept this approach, and which required that acceptable individual conceptions of the good must accord with the requirements of liberal principles of justice, is lost. It is this side of the dilemma that will be explored in this chapter.

The Choosing Self of contemporary bioethics is very similar to the Divided Self envisaged by political liberals; it is, it might be said, the Divided Self taken out of a political context and placed in an ethical one. Because the

Divided Self is a conception that was intended to illuminate political questions about the nature of the just state, the transparency of its institutions, and the obligations of its citizens to one another, this self is required (even if only out of self-interest) to demonstrate respect for liberal principles of justice. Consequently, the Divided Self, whatever its weaknesses, is well designed to explore political questions, and can be appropriately used to answer at least some of them. However, political questions are distinct from ethical ones, and when the Divided Self is detached from a political framework and placed in an ethical context where it becomes the Choosing Self, it becomes logically problematic and practically unhelpful.

First, it encourages bioethicists to conflate political questions with ethical ones. Like liberal political theorists, bioethicists who assume the Choosing Self as their model of personhood are often concerned about the power of the state and the importance of limiting that power in order to ensure that individuals are largely left free to make their own choices. It is for this reason that bioethicists frequently concern themselves with questions of regulation (Should human cloning be banned? Should age restrictions be placed on women who want IVF treatment? Should governments regulate the fertility industry?) rather than on the logically prior questions that are relevant to an exploration of the ethical issues raised by at least some choices made by individuals: Is this (or that) a good thing? How should we think about the choices people make, and the desires that drive those choices? How should we think about *our own* choices and desires? How, in short, should we live, and what role might medical technology and practice have in our living well or living badly? It is only after asking and considering these kinds of questions that we can even begin to answer the question of whether or not particular activities should be encouraged, regulated, restricted, or forbidden.

What distinguishes the arguments of bioethicists who make reference to the liberal framework in their ethical arguments and rely on this framework to justify their conclusions from the arguments of liberal theorists (like Rawls and Dworkin) who articulate and promote this perspective, is that the former, unlike the latter, do not see the need to defend this approach against its rivals, or to make a case for it against competing conceptions. Instead, they simply assert its correctness, as though they are stating a clear and uncontroversial fact about the world that all democratically committed, fair-minded and rational individuals must recognize. (Those who fail to do so, therefore, are either not committed to democratic principles, not fair-minded, not sufficiently rational, or exhibit a combination of these moral failings.) Moreover, the Choosing Self that animates these arguments, unlike its progenitor, the Divided Self, is largely unconstrained in its choices by a commitment to liberal principles of justice. While the Divided Self can only legitimately pursue private conceptions of the good that are compatible with liberal justice, and must allow its private values to give way to shared public ones when the two come into conflict, the Choosing Self faces no such limitations. The influence of liberal political theory on contemporary bioethics and the way in which the Choosing Self emerges largely out of this political context but is ultimately detached from it can be seen in the following arguments.

In his famous defense of the importance of procreative liberty, John A. Robertson states that, even when our ambivalence about the uses to which reproductive technologies are put exists on both the personal and social level, reproductive decisions are so important and so personal, that those who make them should largely be left free to make them for themselves in accordance with their beliefs about value: "those who would limit procreative choice have the burden of showing that the reproductive actions at issue would create such substantial harm that they could justifiably be limited . . . A closely related reason for protecting reproductive choice is to avoid the highly intrusive measures that governmental control of reproduction usually entail."[9] Almost nothing, Robertson argues—not posthumous reproduction, not a market in reproductive materials, not reproductive methods that may cause children to be born with disabilities—meet the test of substantial harm, since no one can logically claim that he would have been better off had he not been born.

Likewise, Nicholas Agar extends the arguments around reproductive choice to include the freedom to choose genetic enhancements for one's offspring. In a recent book defending what he calls "liberal eugenics," Agar makes a case for leaving individuals free to make whatever choices they want, with respect to shaping the genetic makeup of their offspring. He makes his case by drawing a contrast between the morally unacceptable eugenics of the Nazis (which he calls *authoritarian eugenics* because it was imposed on individuals by the state) and a morally defensible eugenics which is predicated on personal choice: far from limiting reproductive choice in any way, the liberal state ideally would encourage the development of a wide range of enhancement techniques which prospective parents, drawing on their own personal conceptions of the good, could freely choose to employ. These eugenic freedoms should be, he argues, defended in just the same way that other liberal freedoms are: "Liberal societies are founded on the insight that there are many different, often incompatible ideas about the good life. Some seek huge wealth, others enlightenment; some devote themselves to their families, others to their careers; some commit to political causes, others to football teams; some worship God(s), others would rather go fishing. . . . Living well in a liberal society involves acknowledging the right of others to make choices that do not appeal to us."[10]

In this perspective, reproductive and genetic technologies are seen as simply part of the package of freedoms that liberal societies would make available to their citizens: they will allow people not only to reproduce, but also to reproduce offspring who reflect their particular beliefs about what is valuable in life: "Prospective parents may ask genetic engineers to introduce into their embryos combinations of genes that correspond to their particular conceptions of the good life. Yet they will acknowledge the right of their fellow citizens to make completely different eugenic choices."[11] There is scant recognition in Agar's account that there may be more options open to us than either the authoritarian imposition of particular choices upon individuals, or the almost unlimited acceptance of any choice made by parents, however controlling, ill advised, or idiosyncratic.

Finally, John Harris takes a similar approach in his defense of allowing individuals to choose for themselves whatever methods of reproduction they desire, including those that involve cloning and genetic enhancements. Harris makes it clear that, in his view, the most important task for the bioethicist is not to guide individuals through their reproductive deliberations, but, rather, to argue in support of their freedom to choose. As he puts it, "the burden of proof is not on those who would exercise this liberty or right to enhancement to show what good it does; rather, it is on those who would limit it to show how and to what extent its denial is necessary to protect either the exercise of a like liberty for all or is required to protect others or society from real or present harms and dangers."[12]

In Harris' view, none of the arguments made by those who are critical of developments in reproductive technology or genetics present a case that meets this burden of proof test adequately. For example, he responds to Leon Kass's argument against human cloning—an argument which depends, in part, on the belief that one of the features of human experience that contributes to our flourishing is our recognition of our own frailty and mortality—by stating, "When he seeks to defend limitations he trespasses on the freedom of others and seeks to shackle the human spirit within the confines of the limits of his own desires and imagination. This is something those who defend freedom will wish to oppose."[13] Likewise, in response to Sandel's concerns about genetic enhancement technologies on the ground that they represent "a Promethean aspiration to remake nature, including human nature, to serve our purposes and satisfy our desires,"[14] it is the protection of the freedom to choose that Harris believes is most morally fundamental: "I am happy for Sandel to welcome the unbidden and accept all the gifts that come his way, including the 'slings and arrows of outrageous fortune' which characteristically come out of the blue. But I wonder if he will let me and others choose the enhancements we prefer for ourselves, and those we judge best for our children. . . . Sandel can have the unbidden and welcome, but on condition that he will let me and others have access to the bidden."[15]

While the presence of the Choosing Self is visible in all of Harris' arguments, he does not appear to recognize that this conception of the self, far from being a straightforward and objectively true description of human beings, is actually a highly theoretical construct, as are the political and regulative arrangements that necessarily follow from its acceptance. He does not seem to understand that those whose arguments he so quickly dismisses on the ground that they do not adequately respect the right of individuals to make their own choices are not simply ethical elitists who wish to impose their views upon others and so restrict their freedom, but are, rather, employing different conceptions of the self, the ways in which selves are connected to others, and the role played by human limitations and frailties in our ethical sensibilities and judgments, than he is. Their concerns are easy to dismiss because they arise from features of the moral landscape that are either meaningless or invisible from the perspective of an advocate of the Choosing Self.

There are several striking features about the arguments presented by Robertson, Harris, and Agar. First, their arguments simply *assert* the legitimacy of the neutral liberal framework, and the conception of autonomy, value, and choice, that it articulates, rather than, as in the case of the arguments presented by liberal political theorists, making a case for its superiority over its competitors. Second, they assume that we will always, and must necessarily, disagree about the nature of "the good life," and that rational conversation about ethical issues *cannot* lead to agreement. Just as this provides the reason that the just state must be a neutral one, because any other model of the state will *necessarily* involve the imposition of value upon at least some citizens, so, too, it requires that the bioethicist be neutral between competing conceptions of the good, and refrain from making moral judgments about the choices that individuals make. We should note, however, that far from it being objectively and uncontroversially true that we cannot reach agreement on the nature of the good, while such agreement may be difficult to achieve, the claim that it is necessarily unobtainable is one that has a relatively recent philosophical history. This account of the nature of human good, for example, is very different from the one held by Aristotle, who believed that "whereas each of us by nature seeks to be happy and live well, one may be mistaken about what happiness consists in and hence pursue the wrong things in life."[16] (Aristotle's claims will be considered in more detail in chapter 6.)

Third, their approach detaches the Choosing Self from moral obligations: what is most important is that each individual be left free to make her own reproductive choices, not that these choices fit with prior ethical commitments. While a Kantian would argue that the choices we make must fit with what duty requires of us, and a utilitarian would require individuals not to do what will benefit only themselves, but, rather, what will produce the greatest amount of happiness for the greatest number of people, the Choosing Self is under no such obligation. Even the requirement that the choices individuals make must not violate the Harm Principle provides almost unlimited scope for action because any attribution of harm is itself likely to be controversial and contentious, not straightforward and clear cut. While one person might think that being brought into existence in a disabled state has harmed a child, or, conversely, that a child would be harmed if it were designed by its parents to possess certain features that those parents think desirable, another might see life itself as a blessing, and the designer features as things that confer wonderful advantages on the child.

Fourth, despite the contribution of liberal political theory to the construction of the Choosing Self, the Choosing Self is abstracted from political and social commitments, apart from a commitment to a particular conception of freedom. While the Divided Self discussed in the last chapter is committed to social and procedural justice, the Choosing Self is detached from such obligations. What is most important to the Choosing Self is that it be left free to choose, not that it contribute to the creation and sustenance of a just state. For example, the Divided Self would have to take seriously the possibility that genetic enhancement technologies, which are likely to be available only to the rich, will further entrench inequalities between rich and poor, and would have to ask hard questions about whether providing expensive reproductive and genetic enhancement services in a society in which the social determinants of health remain inadequately addressed can be morally (or politically) justified. Could a just liberal state, for example, really support expensive and elective medical treatments for the few, while the basic health care needs of the many go unmet? (Indeed, one reason, arguably, for the failure of mainstream bioethicists to address issues of social justice in the distribution of health care resources is that, while they refer to the framework of liberal justice in defense of their claims, they don't take the moral and political requirements it imposes on citizens seriously enough.) The Choosing Self that is revealed in these arguments faces no such concerns. For her, the hallmark of good citizenship consists *simply* in a willingness to respect the rights of others to make whatever choices fit best with their conceptions of the good, of what gives meaning and value to their lives, which has the effect of making questions about the moral legitimacy or acceptability or advisability of particular choices *politically* suspect and *personally* offensive: good citizens shouldn't make these kinds of judgments about other people and their choices. Moreover, since we have no shared, rational way of reaching agreement on questions of meaning, value, and the nature of the good, *any* such judgments must be nothing more than expressions of personal preference, for there is nothing else that they could be.

Fifth, while this perspective powerfully articulates the moral obligation to respect the choices that people make, even choices we deeply disagree with, it offers little guidance for helping any of us discern what choices we ought to make, what conceptions of the good we ought to endorse, or what values should be important to us. The widespread acceptance of the Choosing Self makes many bioethical discussions confused and confusing, as the arguments presented with respect to reproductive technologies and genetic enhancement

demonstrate: are bioethicists primarily concerned with arguing against
governmental restrictions on the freedom of people to make their own reproductive and genetic choices? Or, more fundamentally, with the inadvisability
of *making ethical judgments* at all about the reasons, and the means, for and
by which people reproduce because such judgments depend on particular
conceptions of "the good life" which not everyone shares, and that, therefore,
they can be nothing more than an attempt to impose one person's preferences
upon others? While we should notice that the second claim—that conceptions of the good life differ from person to person—can be used to support
the first—that governments should be neutral among conceptions of the
good, and should not regulate procreative choice in any but the most limited
circumstances—these two claims are logically distinct. We can believe that
something is ethically unclear, ethically questionable, or even immoral, without demanding that governments regulate or restrict it (for example, some
sexual practices that many consider immoral are not regulated, as long as
they occur between consenting adults); likewise, governments do regulate
many things, from the side of the road we drive on to whether or not we are
permitted to keep chickens in cities, which have no moral content.

Finally, perhaps the most striking feature of the Choosing Self that is
revealed in these arguments is its complete detachment from natural norms.
The Choosing Self, as envisaged by bioethicists like Robertson, Agar, and
Harris, is a figure that can transcend human physical limitations, triumph
over frailty and death, and even step outside evolution in order to control it.
Most conceptions of the self connect ideas about who we are as human
beings to at least some inescapable features of our embodied status. Feminists, for example, emphasize the role that gender plays in how our lives go,
while those who have written about the experience of serious illness observe
that physical weakness, pain, and death are an inescapable part of our existence as embodied creatures. The disembodied nature of the Choosing Self,
and the claim on the part of those who use it in their bioethical arguments
that it can overcome almost all limitations imposed by nature, arguably make
this particular conception of the self the most artificial and theoretical of any
of the conceptions considered in this book. Consequently, it is a conception
of the self that offers little help to real, embodied people as they live their
lives and grapple with their physical limitations.

HOW DOES THE CHOOSING SELF MAKE ITS CHOICES?

None of the arguments in support of reproductive autonomy that have been
considered give individuals a morally sound basis on which to make reproductive decisions. While it might be argued (as liberal theorists persuasively
do) that a just state will leave as much room as possible for individuals to

make their own decisions, ethicists should to be able to help them determine what decisions they ought to make, not simply echo political philosophers in a robust assertion of their right to make them. Bioethicists have frequently endorsed, and now often assume, a model of autonomy embodied in the figure of the Choosing Self which largely *gives them nothing to say* about the ethical merits of particular reproductive choices. Instead, they have treated ethical questions as though they were political and social ones, and have said that what matters *most* is that personal choice be respected. There are two reasons for thinking that this approach is problematic. First, it substantially undermines any claims bioethicists might make to possess a special expertise (namely, the sort of expertise which allows them to be respected as media commentators and ethics committee members, and to be people who have a legitimate place at the bedside of the patient). Second, and as a consequence, they have little to offer to those who are in the process of making difficult ethical choices. While bioethicists are very good at explaining why the choices that people make should be respected, they offer little guidance and few tools to people as they try to determine what values they should endorse and how they might live.

In an engaging account of her experiences trying to have a baby, Peggy Orenstein demonstrates how few resources there are for those who look for such guidance. Orenstein appears to meet all the requirements for moral agency and autonomy that form the basis of the Choosing Self. She is thoughtful, well educated, and appears to have made the decision to repro-duce freely: not as a result of societal expectations or pressure from her husband, but because she has reached a point in her life at which she is ready to become a mother. What is striking about her story, however, is how few resources she had as she struggled, first, with the decision of whether or not to become a mother, and then as she moved through an increasingly complex technologically and physically demanding set of steps in her attempt to have a child. She is able, that is to say, to clearly articulate a plan for herself, to think about what her values are, and to engage in the actions necessary to achieve her goals; what she is lacking, however, are any guidelines for decid-ing what she *should* want, and whether the choices she makes should be *different* ones. She is simultaneously fully autonomous, and at a loss to know what to do with her autonomy.

Orenstein details her difficulty in deciding whether or not she wanted to become a mother. There are so many possibilities open to her, so many things that she wants to do, and she is ambivalent about the sacrifices that motherhood will impose: "Maybe I wanted children, maybe I didn't. My own mother was no help. . . . 'Your life is so unlike mine,' she'd say. 'I can't even imagine it.' I longed for a mother who could be a mentor, someone I could turn to for wisdom and guidance. Her limits made me short-tempered."[17] Later, when she finally makes her decision to pursue parenthood and encounters difficulties, her anguish is exacerbated by the thought that, if she had made up her mind earlier, she might have conceived more easily.

Her desire becomes so acute that she risks her health to achieve her goal. Despite having had breast cancer, Orenstein decides to go on Clomid, a drug that might increase her chance of getting ovarian cancer: "Swallowing that little white pill was the first time I did something I swore I wouldn't in order to get pregnant: I willingly put my health on the line. It was at that moment that desire and denial merged to become obsession; it was then, right then, that doing anything to get pregnant, regardless of the consequences, became possible."[18] "Anything" included using donor eggs, which were presented to her as a logical next step when IVF failed. Orenstein comments on the contradictory messages she was sent by her doctors "after implying that a genetic link to our baby was so important that it was worth going to physical and financial extremes to attain, they whipped around and implied that the link, at least my link, was no big deal: the key to motherhood was carrying the child, not conceiving it,"[19] and she eventually realizes that her fertility doctors are essentially salesmen. Where she originally saw compassion and concern in their caring brochures and friendly smiles, she now observes that she is more consumer than patient: "I was undergoing a procedure, but I was also making a deal and they were making a buck."[20] She also notes that there is something insidious and deceptive about infertility treatments and the options they seem to provide: "the very fact of their existence, the potential, however slim, that the next round might get you pregnant creates an imperative that may not otherwise have existed. If you didn't try it, you'd always have to wonder whether it would've worked. That's how you lose sight of your real choices, because the ones you're offered make you feel like you have none."[21]

Bioethicists have done a very good job and, many would argue, a very necessary job of defending the rights of individuals to make their own choices, in accordance with their own values, goals, and conceptions of the good. Where they need to do more work, however, is in providing people with at least some of the tools to determine what choices they should make, and why; to help them, to use Orenstein's phrase, discover what their "real choices" are. By this, I don't mean that bioethicists should *tell* people what to do, impose particular ways of life upon them, or prevent them from making choices particular bioethicists may personally disapprove of. I mean, instead, that we should try to find a space for ethical discussion that falls somewhere between the fear that asking hard ethical questions will lead to unjustifiable regulation by governmental or medical bodies *and* the normal response to this fear which consists in the assertion that, as long as the Harm Principle is not violated in some clear, uncontroversial, and serious way, that whatever choice someone makes is simply up to them, and that nothing more should, or needs, to be said. I want to argue, further, that in this space bioethicists should use all the resources provided by moral philosophy in their deliberations. If bioethicists cannot help people decide which of the possible choices open to them might be better and which might be worse, then their claims to bioethical expertise are both suspect and delusional: they might as well, as Hare asserts, shut up shop!

Bioethics, as currently structured, can go in two directions: it can become ever more procedural in orientation, and see the appropriate role played by the bioethicist in much the way Thomas May does, as a kind of ombudsman whose role is to ensure that autonomous choices is respected and that procedures designed to ensure this are followed; or it can embrace a rich moral language, one that both considers what resources are available to us to help us make substantive moral judgments, and endorses the view that such judgments can be responsibly made. Each path has dangers. While the first approach fits well with larger cultural beliefs about the importance of freedom and free choice, adopting it makes it difficult for the bioethicist to justify his claims to expertise, and, ultimately, his professional existence: any appropriately trained administrator can ensure that procedures are followed and choices respected, and doing so does not require a particular kind of ethical professionalism. The second approach carries with it very different dangers; if we are required, on occasion, to make moral judgments, it's quite clear that we might sometimes get them wrong; moreover, this approach will suggest, to some people, a return to paternalism, to one person (the bioethicist) imposing his views upon others. In short, the risk of making moral judgments is that one will be perceived as both paternalistic and judgmental.

I don't believe, however, that bioethicists can avoid taking the second approach, despite these dangers—not if they want to be able to justify the claim that they possess the kind of ethical expertise upon which their professional credibility and respected public position are predicated. The key to embracing a richer moral language than the one currently employed in mainstream bioethics, and minimizing the dangers of a paternalistic or idiosyncratic imposition of values by bioethicists upon those who don't share them, is twofold. First, we need to conceive of the moral framework we are using to address moral issues differently, moving from a model in which bioethicists understand their role to involve constructing abstract moral frameworks that are then applied impersonally to specific issues, to one in which bioethicists recognize that they are themselves participants in moral life, and that the moral life involves much more than simply the application of rules, procedures, or principles when ethical dilemmas appear and must be dealt with.

Second, we need to maintain an important place for respect for autonomy, but conceive of autonomy differently than the models presented by the Divided Self and the Choosing Self: like justice, autonomy is a concept that can generate multiple and distinct conceptions. In what follows, I will consider one way in which moral space might be opened up, and propose a model of autonomy that differs in a fundamental way from those we have been considering, because it connects the value of autonomy itself to the value of the things chosen, and which places the autonomous individual within a particular social, political, and ethical context. Both this conception of autonomy, and the context within which it is placed, assert that the development of the capacity for autonomy requires others, and that the contexts within which autonomous choices are made and evaluated are social rather than individual. The various facets of this conception of autonomy will be put in place over the course of the rest of this book.

TWO MODELS OF MORAL THEORY

Given the framework that currently composes mainstream bioethics, it is difficult to see where it might go next, how it might find a space for the sorts of substantive ethical explorations and judgments it has so strikingly excluded from its purview. Moreover, bioethics arguably possesses fewer theoretical resources than it did thirty or forty years ago when it was a new field, and the form it might take was wide-open. In addition, the increasing dominance of the Choosing Self not only contributes to a form of bioethics which is primarily procedural, it also marks the point at which the market becomes a largely unquestioned mechanism for determining which choices are actually available to individuals: if few substantive moral judgments can legitimately be made, and if, consequently, government regulation that restricts choice on the basis of such judgments becomes problematic, then the only thing left is the market. A Kantian argument against allowing commercial surrogacy would now be difficult to take seriously, as would a utilitarian argument that proposed limiting the financial compensation paid to fertility doctors so that nurses working in chronic care could be paid more. Even questions about distributive justice which have traditionally preoccupied liberal theorists have largely given way, in mainstream bioethics, to a concern that the exercise of free choice should not be limited for goods which have both willing buyers and willing sellers: if that means buying reproductive materials and services from individuals in third-world countries, then this should be seen as an exchange that benefits both parties, not as something which might raise questions about those who have the power to buy and those who feel that they have no choice but to sell. Once the Choosing Self and the market, that is to say, begin to set the terms of the debate in bioethics, it becomes difficult to make a case for any other perspectives, if those perspectives suggest that individual choices should be judged or restricted, or markets, which provide a mechanism for facilitating such choices, should be regulated for moral reasons.

How, then, might a space be opened up which would allow us to ask ethical questions without falling into the terms set by the Choosing Self and the market-based moral universe that it brings with it? We need to find a model of moral reasoning that falls outside of those that we have so far been considering because, in mainstream bioethics, they have led to a place in which substantive moral discussion becomes largely impossible, and the making of moral judgments largely unacceptable. Margaret Urban Walker's distinction between two templates for moral theory can, I believe, help us find this philosophical space; her approach asks us to consider basic questions about what it is that moral philosophers are trying to do when they engage in their characteristic activities, and why they are trying to do it.

"Morality," Walker argues, "is woven through the way people live; it both shapes and is shaped by the rules, roles, and assumptions that constitute a social world."[22] Moral philosophers are engaged in trying to answer the question posed by Socrates, namely, "how should we live?" Walker suggests that there are two distinct pictures of morality into which our explorations of this question might fall. The first envisages morality (and moral theory) as falling into what Walker terms a theoretical-juridical model. This approach "is not itself a moral theory; [rather], it is a kind of template for organizing moral inquiry into the pursuit of a certain kind of moral theory."[23] According to this template, morality can be represented in the form of a "compact, propositionally codifiable, impersonally action-guiding code within an agent, or as a compact set of law-like propositions that 'explain' the moral behavior of a well-formed moral agent."[24]

It is this model of morality that has been seen as the form that "serious" moral theorizing should take, especially in the twentieth century in North American philosophy. Since this is a *template*, rather than a *theory*, many approaches to moral questions that are incompatible with one another—such as Kantian, utilitarian, contract, and rights-based theories—"can be seen to realize or approximate the theoretical-juridical model."[25] All the approaches that we have so far considered fall within the domain marked out by this template, and, arguably, all the central features of mainstream bioethics are modeled upon its requirements. This model, Walker argues, is implausible because it asserts that moral philosophers can stand apart from their own moral assumptions and commitments when they set out moral theories and make moral claims, as though they are outside or above the ideas they are considering. However, she argues, moral philosophers are always *part of* (and, consequently, cannot stand *apart from*) the moral world they are exploring: "Moral philosophers reflect on morality, moral judgment, and moral responsibility as they are familiar with it from their own moral training, formed characters, and social experience."[26]

Moreover, since moral philosophers are perceived by themselves and by others to be experts in morality (understood as consisting in a particular kind of abstract knowledge) what they say carries substantial weight: "When they say certain features of morality are true ones or certain interpretations of moral life important, or when they mention them at all, they give these features or interpretations visibility and legitimacy."[27] We can note that there is a clear similarity between the kind of expertise claimed by moral philosophers working within this theoretical-juridical framework, and the kind of expertise claimed by mainstream bioethicists: since both see themselves as standing apart from the claims that they make, as objective observers rather than as protagonists, they consequently believe that when they exclude competing theoretical perspectives that emphasize different features of the moral life than they would choose to draw attention to, they are doing so on purely rational grounds.

Walker contrasts the theoretical-juridical picture of morality with a model she terms expressive-collaborative. Like the theoretical-juridical model, it is not itself a moral theory; rather, it is a template for moral inquiry. This picture of morality is very different than that set out in the theoretical-juridical framework: it sees morality as arising from, and reflected in, particular roles, identities, and relationships, and understands the moral theorist to be part of the moral world she thinks about and tries to represent in her theorizing. We learn what is expected of us (and what we can expect of others) through what Walker calls "practices of responsibility": "morality consists in a family of practices that show what is valued by making people accountable to each other for it."[28] Moral accounts that fall within this expressive-collaborative template view morality in a messier and less clear but potentially richer and more creative way than views that fall into the competing paradigm. As Walker puts it, "Practices of making morally evaluative judgments are prominent among moral practices, but they do not exhaust them."[29] In addition, there are "habits and practices of paying attention, imputing states of affairs to people's agency, interpreting and re-describing human actions, visiting blame, offering excuses, inflicting punishment, making amends, refining and inhibiting the experience or expression of feelings, and responding in thought, act, and feeling to any of the foregoing."[30]

What is crucially important about expressive-collaborative approaches, which are expressed, demonstrated, and reinforced through practices of responsibility, is that morality is *not* understood as resulting from one individual's exercise of reason, from some place above the moral fray and apart from other persons (as it is with approaches that fall within the theoretical-juridical template) but is, rather, fundamentally collaborative and interpersonal: "we construct and sustain it together. . . . What goes on morally between people is constrained and made intelligible by a background of understandings about what people are supposed to do, expect, and understand."[31] While all human societies demand participation in the practices that constitute social life, particular societies will shape these practices in different ways, and the forms of moral life, therefore, will differ at different times and in different places.

But this does not mean, Walker argues, that we are only able to make empirical reports about the forms these practices take; ethical reflection is required as much by philosophers working within the expressive-collaborative framework as it is by those working with theoretical-juridical perspectives. However, instead of comparing existing moral conceptions to some ideal correct account that exists beyond and apart from the things that human beings actually do, advocates of expressive-collaborative perspectives see moral reasoning and judgments as "intrinsically comparative; in other words, when we ask ourselves what can be said for some way of life, we are asking whether it is better or worse than some other way we can know or imagine."[32] This intrinsic comparative aspect makes expressive-collaborative approaches necessarily more open to diverse viewpoints than their theoretical-juridical competitors: "moral philosophy should not arbitrarily select or presumptively disqualify some moral experiences; for those neglected are experiences of human beings who are fully parties to the moral understandings that furnish their ways of life."[33]

In short, Walker argues, morality consists in practices of responsibility, not in theories, and moral philosophers who believe that they can find some place outside of, or apart from, these practices are deceiving themselves; the theories they present, and the reasons they provide in their support, reflect not simply the exercise of abstract reason but are, rather, themselves responsive to the life experiences, commitments, and practices engaged in by those moral philosophers. If we cannot find a place (or a space) apart from particular moral commitments and practices, as they are expressed in particular times and places, we can, however, play accounts off against one another, make judgments about particular moral expressions and commitments and the actions that flow from them, and consider a wide range of human experiences, ways of interacting, and imaginative descriptions of what we are and what we might become as sources of moral knowledge. And we can, moreover, (as I shall do for the remainder of this book), self-consciously situate ourselves outside the expectations imposed by the theoretical-juridical template, in order to find an external standpoint from which its assumptions, methods of reasoning, and conclusions can be seen more clearly than they would be seen from the inside, begin to explore a moral terrain that is less "certain," but potentially more satisfying, richer, simultaneously more realistic and more imaginative, more open to a greater range of perspectives and a wider variety of evidence about ways in which human beings experience the moral dimensions of life.

My argument, so far, asserts that the rise of the Choosing Self in contemporary bioethics, and the paradox of expertise the dominance of this self within bioethics generates, demonstrate that bioethics, as currently framed, has largely exhausted the moral resources available to it and become primarily a procedural activity directed in large part to ensuring the protection of a certain conception of autonomy that detaches the value of autonomy from substantive considerations of the value of the things chosen. Moreover, this emphasis has contributed to giving the market a large place in bioethics, since it is the market—not the policies of the state, or other social institutions—which is seen to provide the main source of the options from which people can choose. The exercise of freedom, then, becomes largely the freedom to buy and sell—whether what is being bought or sold is medical services, reproductive materials, drugs, or organs. This is a lonely and thin conception of what autonomy might come to, and it does not explain why autonomy understood in this way is important, either as a model of human flourishing, or as a conception of a self whose choices are worthy of protection. The resources I will draw on are already available to bioethics; they just have not been fully incorporated into the mainstream, and, indeed, the likelihood of their being so incorporated decreases as bioethics becomes ever more procedural in orientation, and increasingly willing to let the workings of the market determine the nature of the choices that are available to individuals. In what follows, I will introduce some additional ethical approaches which already have a small role to play in bioethics; they are approaches that fall clearly within the expressive-collaborative template of morality, and I shall argue that they should play a much larger role than they currently do in bioethical deliberations; that they should not be understood as competitors with one another, but as different facets or components of what I shall call the Situated Self; and that from them, we can generate a conception of autonomy that is more satisfactory than the conception embodied in the Choosing Self.

CONCLUSION: FINAL THOUGHTS AND FINAL JUSTIFICATIONS

I have argued that the dominance of a conception of autonomy drawn primarily from the liberal self-moral-political framework, and then detached from its political context, is ultimately unsatisfactory. This model draws many of its features from political philosophy, and, far from being a simple factual description of what human beings actually are and how bioethicists ought to respond as a result, is actually a largely vacuous construct, as is the figure of the Choosing Self that underpins it. While the idea that the political structures of a society must allow for the free choice of individuals and must allow for diverse plans of life to be explored and lived is an appealing one, the Choosing Self needs more than this freedom if it is to determine for itself what good choices consist in. What bioethicists need to consider is what more and what else might be said about our choices and how to make judgments about them. We need to consider the Socratic question of how we should live, particularly given the frailty of our bodies, the inescapable fact of our own mortality, and the need to make good choices in a medical context in which technology plays an increasingly important role. Bioethicists need to employ a conception of what autonomy comes to that allows them to ask and consider this question, not one which renders it either invisible or morally suspect.

Carl Elliot suggests that all answers to the question of how we should live are played out against a particular historical and cultural background, and this, in turn, generates a subset of related questions, such as "What gives my life meaning?" "What is the purpose of it all?" and "How does it all fit together?" Elliot calls these kinds of questions "final justifications," and believes that questions of this sort require us to think not simply about the particular choices we might make but, rather, about "the shape and sense of . . . life as a whole."[34] Seeing a life as a whole allows us to "articulate a kind of moral description that lies somewhere between the domains of moral philosophy and psychology"[35] which is not composed of moral criticism, but which does allow us to consider different ways of life and make judgments about which might be better and which worse: "some of us might criticize or look approvingly at a person who devotes his life to the accumulation of material things, or who is single-mindedly focused on advancement in the company at the expense of family. Others might look with sadness or even pity at someone immersed in a life of quiet suburban desperation, a soul-deadening sequence of watching television, shopping at the mall and obsessively tending the lawn."[36]

The concept of final justifications suggests that, when we think about autonomy, we need to think not only about which choices available to us are genuinely valuable, but, also, how choosing *this* thing rather than *that* will contribute to, or detract from, the overall shape of our lives. Connecting autonomous choice to final justifications, that is to say, gives our thinking about the value of particular choices a context within which we can ask significant philosophical questions in the context of bioethics *without* (a) imposing ways of life on people that they do not endorse (there is no expectation that everyone will answer these questions in the same way); or, (b) supporting governmental or institutional regulations that restrict autonomy (questions about legitimate and illegitimate forms of regulation occupy a different social and political domain); or (c) saying (as we seem inclined to do now) that almost any way of life is as good as any other as long as it is harmless and freely chosen, a response which raises questions about the nature of bioethical expertise and whether bioethicists have anything significant to add to public or private discussions of ethical issues.

NOTES

1. Michael C. Brannigan and Judith A. Boss, *Healthcare Ethics in a Diverse Society* (Mountain View, CA: Mayfield Publishing Company, 2001), 5.

2. R.M Hare, "Medical Ethics: Can The Moral Philosopher Help?" in S. F. Spicker and H.T. Englehardt, Jr., eds., *Philosophical Medical Ethics: Its Nature and Significance* (Dordrecht: Kluwer, 1977), 49.

3. Lindy Forte, quoted in "Fund IVF, Experts Urge Governments," by Stuart Laidlaw, *Toronto Star*, Feb. 11, 2009.

4. Arthur Schafer, "The Case For Postmenopausal Mothers," *Globe & Mail*, Feb. 9, 2009.

5. Brendan O'Neil, *Spiked* online, athttp://www.spiked-onlinecom/index phn?/site/printable/6172/. (Accessed Feb. 12, 2009).

6. Shaun Winsor, quoted in "Mother's Age Raises Ethical Concerns," by Matthew Coutts, *National Post*, Feb. 6, 2009.

7. Lorne Gunter, "Cheat Nature, But On Your Own Dime," *National Post*, Feb. 11, 2009.

8. Kerry Boman, quoted in "Squalling Life After Death," by Tom Blackwell, *National Post*, March 9, 2009.

9. John A. Robertson, *Children of Choice: Freedom and The New Reproductive Technologies* (Princeton: Princeton University Press, 1994), 24–25.

10. Nicholas Agar, *Liberal Eugenics: In Defense of Human Enhancement* (Oxford: Blackwell Publishing, 2004), 5.

11. Agar, *Liberal Eugenics,* 6.

12. John Harris, *Enhancing Evolution: The Case For Making Better People* (Princeton: Princeton University Press, 2007), 79.

13. Harris, *Enhancing Evolution,* 137.

14. Michael Sandel, quoted in Harris, *Enhancing Evolution,* 112.

15. Harris, *Enhancing Evolution,* 122.

16. Robert B. Talisse, *On Rawls: A Liberal Theory of Justice and Justification,* (Belmont, CA: Wadsworth, 2001), 8.

17. Peggy Orenstein, *Waiting For Daisy: A Tale of Two Continents, Three Religions, Five Infertility Doctors, An OscarM, an Atomic Bomb, a Romantic Night, and One Woman's Quest To Become A Mother* (New York: Bloomsbury, 2007), 10.

18. Orenstein, *Waiting For Daisy,* 60.

19. Orenstein, *Waiting For Daisy,* 85.

20. Orenstein, *Waiting For Daisy,* 193.

21. Orenstein, *Waiting For Daisy,* 224.

22. Margaret Urban Walker, *Moral Understandings: A Feminist Study In Ethics* 2nd Ed. (Oxford: Oxford University Press, 2007), ix.

23. Walker, *Moral Understandings,* 7-8.

24. Walker, *Moral Understandings,* 8.

25. Walker, *Moral Understandings,* 8.

26. Walker, *Moral Understandings,* 4.

27. Walker, *Moral Understandings,* 4.

28. Walker, *Moral Understandings,* 10.

29. Walker, *Moral Understandings,* 10.

30. Walker, *Moral Understandings,* 10.

31. Walker, *Moral Understandings,* 10.

32. Walker, *Moral Understandings,* 13.

33. Walker, *Moral Understandings,* 14.

34. Carl Elliot, *A Philosophical Disease* (New York: Routledge, 1999), 137.

35. Elliot, *A Philosophical Disease,* 138.

36. Elliot, *A Philosophical Disease,* 138.

2

Introducing the Situated Self

Chapter Five

The First Component of the Situated Self

Gender

INTRODUCTION: MAKING GENDER VISIBLE

When I was in my final year of undergraduate studies in the late 1980s, I encountered philosophical feminism and feminist philosophers for the first time. The experience was stimulating, heady, and confusing. Stimulating, because it forced me to examine new ideas which were previously unimaginable, such as the possibility that gender expectations were nothing more than social constructions, that biological sex and gender identity were distinct, and that ordinary people could experiment with the tropes of androgyny (something previously understood to be limited to exotic British rock stars). It was heady as well: if gender was something mutable, what other parts of my identity (or anyone else's) might be up for grabs? And, finally, the experience was confusing: what was being challenged in these encounters was not only social expectations about how women ought to behave, or religious norms as I had experienced them (I went to a college at which people had serious debates about whether men and women had souls that were qualitatively different, with advocates of this position making the case that *this* was the reason why the concept of female priests was an oxymoron, like military intelligence or jumbo shrimp, and why women who desired to take on such roles were sad creatures, more to be pitied than condemned, because what they desired was contrary to built-in natural laws), but, even more fundamentally for me, all the philosophical training I had had up to that point, with its emphasis on objectivity, detachment, and clear-headed reason, undistracted

133

by the demands and weaknesses of the body, uncontaminated by questions of sex and gender, and unsullied by personal reflections or observations, was up for grabs. Autobiographical narratives of the sort I am writing now suddenly had a legitimate, even honored place in philosophical explorations and discussions (indeed, I sometimes felt in my feminist philosophy course that discussions revolved entirely around personal narratives), and emotions occupied the respected epistemological role of providing insights that would otherwise go ignored and unseen. (This was the only philosophy class I had been in where students actually cried, and were seemingly not embarrassed by this breakdown of classroom etiquette.) Instead of Descartes's mechanistic body-machine, Plato's astoundingly abstract forms, or Rawls's divided and genderless selves meeting behind the veil of ignorance which had previously populated my philosophical mental landscape, I was thinking instead about Gilligan's abortion studies and what they revealed about the presence of a distinctive female "voice," Noddings's feelings as she looked at her sleeping child and responded as one-caring to her students, and Firestone's contention that female liberation was unattainable until women were freed from the tyranny of reproductive biology.

This feminist world was simultaneously a world much more like the world I actually lived in and experienced than a Platonic or Cartesian one, and a world made strange, in which familiar things were turned on their head, social expectations revealed themselves to contain insidious and pernicious gender expectations, and previously invisible lines of power began to reveal themselves. In graduate school, the feminist voice grew louder, and feminist philosophy played an ever-increasing role in the philosophy departments in which I studied, and in the workings of the university itself. It was only a matter of time, it seemed, until society as a whole was transformed by feminist thought in the way in which departments of philosophy and the institutions of the university had been transformed.

Let me flash-forward twenty-plus years, and consider the state of bioethics as I practice it and observe it. Several decades of feminist thought have, of course, had an impact on bioethics. But what sort of impact has feminism had?

Sidney Callahan recounts, "Twenty-five years ago I co-led bioethical workshops with a philosopher colleague who would hold up two flow charts displaying formulas for making ethical decisions. One chart laid out the steps in a decision tree to reach a deontological solution and the other demonstrated how to reach a utilitarian answer."[1] Callahan notes that she had her doubts about this approach: "'Can it really be so simple?' I would protest."[2] Today, she argues, the theory and practice of ethics (including bioethics) has been transformed by new approaches, including feminist and care ethics.

I'm not so sure that such a transformation has taken place. I have observed presentations of the sort Callahan describes; indeed, I have been asked to give them. The health care institutions on whose ethics committees I have been a member are all led by men and staffed largely by women. In the local hospital, professional roles tend to fall along traditional gender lines, with physicians usually being male, and nurses, personal support workers, and administrative assistants female. Likewise, in the other organizations; while I meet the occasional male nurse or female program director, most roles, similarly, line up in traditional gender categories, with men occupying the higher levels of the organizational hierarchy and women the lower, with the latter clustered in "caring" positions, and the former in "curing" and administrative ones.

What is both remarkable and philosophically interesting about this state of affairs is that it is taken for granted: it is never commented upon or, seemingly, even noticed. It is as though those stimulating, heady, and confusing feminist challenges never took place, or, at least, never hit their target in a lasting and damaging way. Even in theoretical bioethics, in which feminists have launched blistering attacks on standard assumptions (including assumptions about the individualistic nature of autonomy, the hierarchical power structures in medical institutions, and the inappropriately detached relationship between health care provider and patient that is fostered by an application of the principled approach, and the important place occupied by emotion within such relationships) standard or mainstream bioethics seems largely untouched by feminist critiques.[3] Abortion, for example, is still often discussed in terms of the moral status of the fetus rather than focusing on the feminist observation that it is only women who can get pregnant and their insistence that this fact is of fundamental moral importance; informed consent is built on liberal individualism rather than relational autonomy; hierarchical power structures within health care organizations remain largely untouched; and issues of social justice which affect the delivery of health care, and their overlap with gender issues, are largely ignored. (This is often the case, even in the liberal moral-political account that explicitly addresses some of these social questions. This approach often occupies itself more with issues of procedural transparency and ways to ensure that autonomy is respected, rather than with the transformation of health care institutions to ensure that they meet the needs of Rawls's worst-off member of society, and what it might mean that that person is probably female.)

The promise that feminist approaches to ethics seemed to offer, then, appear largely to have bypassed bioethics, to have come and gone, or not yet to have been fulfilled. The one place where feminist considerations have had the greatest impact in bioethics is clearly nursing ethics. Nursing ethics, Oberle and Bouchal argue, places feminist thought and an ethics of care "at the center,"[4] and is shaped along all its dimensions by the relational commitments identified in this ethical approach. However, they note, many nurses experience moral distress, an uncomfortable feeling that arises when one knows what one ought to do but is prevented from acting on that knowledge by institutional constraints: "a nurse being asked to continue treatment on a patient whom the nurse believes would prefer to die with dignity suffers moral distress."[5] It is likely that moral distress will be exacerbated if nurses, who occupy a lower position in the power hierarchy in medical institutions, rely on an approach to ethics that is largely ignored by their superiors.

I will argue in this chapter that feminist approaches have important contributions to make to bioethics, both practically and theoretically: they draw our attention to features of health care that other approaches ignore and which might otherwise remain invisible; they remind us that medicine is concerned, at its heart, with caring for the sick and vulnerable and trying to address their suffering, rather than with the exercise of autonomy, the accumulation of wealth, or advancing knowledge through medical experimentation; and they properly remind us that the medical universe is permeated by emotion. As Vacek puts it, "The world of medicine is charged with grandeur and gore, with relief and regret, with triumph and tragedy. The world of medicine is propelled by noble aspirations and narcissistic ambitions and power-seeking preoccupations, by bored salary-seekers and compassionate do-gooders."[6] This is not a world in which rational ethical calculations predominate, or a world in which the procedural policies, even if rigorously followed, will prevent the emergence of moral dilemmas. Further, feminist approaches offer a relatively well-worked-out example of what an expressive-collaborative ethical approach might look like when applied to bioethics.

In bioethics, then, the challenge feminist approaches offer to standard or mainstream accounts remains acute and potentially transformative. I will endorse the position advanced by many that these feminist approaches, while ultimately not entirely capable of replacing principlism, Kantian, utilitarian, or liberal-based theories, stand as a corrective to them, and, moreover, that feminist approaches can help us identify features that a more adequate account of the self (and of bioethics) should contain. I will argue that this more adequate account is one rooted in virtue ethics, but a virtue ethics updated and transformed by contemporary commitments to social justice, a recognition of the role that gender plays in our conceptions of who we are (even if gender roles and expectations can be challenged and gender lines blurred); that our personal conceptions of the self are ultimately at least partially social creations, not entirely individualistic ones, and that emotions have an important role to play in shaping and maintaining the relationships that make social connections (and our lives) not only meaningful to us, but possible at all; and that it is the stories we tell, the narratives within which we place ourselves and through which we make sense of our lives, that allow us to hold all these elements together.

GENDERED BIOETHICS: FEMININE AND FEMINIST CRITIQUES

Criticisms of bioethics written from a perspective informed by feminist philosophy fall (roughly) into two groupings: what I will call *feminist* ethics and what I will call *feminine* ethics. Both feminist and feminine ethicists offer a critique of standard bioethics, with its utilitarian and Kantian roots, its current domination by the autonomous liberal self striding unencumbered across the moral landscape, and its employment of ethical principles that require of us primarily a rational analysis of moral problems, rather than one that both reflects and makes central to our ethical evaluation the role that relationships play within health care. The difference between what I am calling *feminist* and *feminine* approaches to bioethics, despite these similarities, is quite profound. Roughly speaking, feminine bioethicists tend to take these features of selves (embodiment, gender, relational identities) as givens, and then work to explore what they mean, and how they might be applied in the medical context. Feminist bioethicists, in contrast, tend to view these features critically: gender expectations, for example, arguably rely to a large extent on social constructions, and these can be pernicious; likewise, even if it is the case that women (still) end up doing much of the work of nurturing others (particularly children), and even if there may be some biological basis for this, (perhaps) it doesn't follow that the social and personal expectations that arise from this are necessarily to be applauded or treated as inevitable. Rather, they are aspects of our world that need to be critically examined and then altered, if the critical examination reveals them to be problematic.

While feminist and feminine ethics differ in important respects (which I will consider in more detail below) they share some central features when it comes to the conception of the self they assume and work with. These features are lacking or truncated in the competing conceptions explored in the first four chapters of this book. Most importantly, these approaches and, therefore, mainstream bioethics itself fall into Walker's theoretical-juridical template of morality. What this model of morality ignores is the fact that ethics comes from somewhere and that particular ideas about ethics can benefit some people at the expense of others; consequently, approaches that fall within this framework tend to pay inadequate attention to the role played by power structures in human experiences, relationships, and institutions. What feminist approaches to ethics share, despite their differences, is a willingness to put "the *authority* and *credibility* of representative claims about moral life under harsh light and challenge epistemic and moral authority that is politically engineered and self-reinforcing."[7] Rather than being an approach which can be "added on," one which provides insights that can be incorporated within utilitarian, Kantian, principled, or liberal moral-political approaches (all of which share features of the theoretical-juridical model), feminist ethics, Walker and other feminist ethicists argue, offers a strikingly different take on ethical thinking that stands in fundamental opposition to these other approaches: to think that feminist ethics can be somehow subsumed within these theories, then, is to fundamentally misunderstand the nature of feminist critiques of these approaches. Of particular relevance to bioethics are the following features.

First, these approaches share a recognition of the importance of embodiment, the role that this plays in our self-conceptions, and in the way in which we are perceived by others: in part, the question of who we are can be answered by the response that I am the person who inhabits this particular body, and that the events which take place upon and within it profoundly affect how my life goes. (And even to phrase the matter in this way to suggest that we *inhabit* our bodies may be to concede too much to the Cartesian model; it is, rather, that whatever we are, we are fundamentally and inescapably embodied.) This recognition of the moral significance of embodiment emerges most clearly with respect to issues that arise around reproduction, including issues of contraception, fertility concerns, pregnancy, and childbirth, all of which make the reality of embodiment inescapable for women. Consequently, for example, while a robot or highly advanced computer might be able to meet the requirements of Kantian personhood, this is nothing more than an absurd male fantasy from the perspective of feminine and feminist critics. The denial of the reality, indeed, the necessity, that embodiment and moral personhood are closely connected, moreover, is not merely absurd, but revealingly so: it demonstrates that the conceptions of the self employed in much of bioethics are essentially *male*, not *genderless,* but this maleness is hidden behind the assumptions that structure these theories.

And this leads directly to the second point: to be *embodied* is to be *gendered* (even if gender itself contains elements that are socially constructed, and even if the lines between genders may sometimes be blurry and porous, and even though gender identity and the physical traits of particular bodies may not always coincide). Moreover, gender has a profound effect on almost everything that occurs in a medical context: from how people are treated and viewed, what events they can expect to have occur in and with their bodies over a lifetime, to how long that lifetime is likely to be. Gender, however, is seldom noticed or remarked upon by non-feminist or non-feminine bioethicists: indeed, a case can be made that the significance of gender is largely ignored in all of the competing mainstream accounts, whether Kantian, utilitarian, principled, or liberal. For example, the model of autonomy that dominates bioethics today is essentially disembodied and genderless.

Feminist and feminine bioethicists, then, must both make what is invisible (embodiment and gender) visible, and must, as Lindemann puts it, "reunite what non-feminists have put asunder,"[8] namely, embodiment, gender, and what this means, in particular, for human reproduction. As she puts it, "If you were a Martian unfamiliar with human life forms and you happened to be reading a typical nonfeminist bioethicist's assessments regarding abortion, you would have no idea that fetuses grow inside women's bodies."[9] But they do; and this is not a minor fact, but one with profound emotional, social, political, and ethical implications.

Third, and consequently, bioethicists who consider issues from a feminine and feminist perspective employ a conception of the self that is constituted through, and exists in, relationships with others. This conception of the self (however it is further filled out), by definition, cannot be individualistic in the way envisaged in the liberal account; nor can it be the benevolent, disinterested rational spectator described by Mill, or the emotionally disengaged Kantian self, who is appropriately moved to act, not by affection, sympathy, or love, but, rather, by a recognition of duty.

Finally, and in a point that is connected to the relational conception of the self, both feminine and feminist approaches encourage us to think about narratives: while not all narrative ethics frameworks encompass feminist and feminine concerns, because these approaches root the self in relationships with other selves, they encompass narrative conceptions of the self. The stories we tell about ourselves (and about our selves) to ourselves and to others, and the stories they tell about themselves to us, and about us, have a role to play in the construction of the self and the maintenance of self-identity, according to these approaches. For feminine bioethicists, who advocate what is often called an ethics of care, we can only be in caring relationships when we listen to the voices of others, and the stories they tell us about who they are. For feminists, Lindemann suggests, the picture is similar, though with an important difference. While first-person narratives about who we are—who each of us is—are central to personal identity, the stories that other people tell about who we are are equally important, and can be analyzed critically: "Identity-constituting stories aren't just *depictive* they're *selective*. Rather than representing every moment of your life, they cluster around the things about you that matter the most to you, as well as around the things about you that matter the most to other people."[10] And, she notes, "These aren't necessarily the same. . . . Because identities are often unchosen, the things about you that other people choose to emphasize might have a far greater impact on your life than your own, first person stories do."[11] The stories told by other people about us, that is to say, may distort our identities, diminish the things that are important to us, or emphasize accidental features that we believe are unimportant.

Walker suggests that feminists must take the narrative components of moral identity seriously because narratives are connected to our ability to make our selves and our actions intelligible to others, and to their ability to make themselves and their actions intelligible to us. In her view, we make sense of, work through, and perhaps even resolve, moral problems, by seeing that they have a narrative form. As she puts it, "a *story* is the basic form of representation for moral problems,"[12] because such problems have histories that led to them, and sequels which follow from them, and this history is "constituted by patterns of action and response over significant periods of time, and actions themselves . . . [are] conceived and reconceived in terms of their relations to what precedes and what follows them."[13] Our narrative identity conveys "intelligibility over time" and helps make our lives meaningful because it allows us to "read and reread actions and other events backward and forward, weaving them into lives that are more than one damned thing after another."[14] It is only when we have a narrative identity of this sort that we can be held responsible for our moral attitudes, actions, and choices, and we need a mutually shared language of value itself embedded in moral narratives if we are to make sense both of who we are and of what a commitment to the moral life requires of us: "So the narrative of 'Who I am' (or 'Who we are') and the narrative of 'how we have gotten here together' is threaded through by another story, one about 'what this means.' The last involves a history of moral concepts acquired, revised, displaced, and replaced, both by individuals and within some communities of shared moral understanding."[15] The three roles played by narratives identified in these feminist approaches—that of creating identity and holding us together as one person over time, that of making our actions and choices intelligible to others and theirs to us, and that of helping to articulate what moral responsibility might look like in particular situations and how we might understand what it is to live a moral life—will be important for a reconfigured bioethics of the sort I am proposing.

CONCENTRIC CIRCLES OF CARE, LINKED CHAINS OF ATTACHMENT, LINEAR HIERARCHIES, AND RELATIONAL WEBS: THE GEOMETRY OF CARE

Proponents of what is often called an ethics of care sometimes claim to offer a *feminine* analysis. The critique of bioethics offered by ethics of care theorists is what I shall call "soft," not in the sense of being "weak," but, rather, in the sense that they primarily focus on the nature of human relationships, particularly as they exist between those being cared for, and those doing the caring. Noddings, for instance, even uses hyphenated terminology—the one-caring and the cared-for—to illustrate the centrality of caring relationships to our ethical life. These relationships and the emotions that they generate are not *manifestations* of our morality, she argues; they are, rather, its very *foundation.*[16]

Proponents of the ethics of care take the nurturing capacities that they often correlate with the female gender as lying at the heart of an adequate moral account. Consequently, their conception of the moral space through which their selves move, is full of people, and the air is thick with emotion; multiple connections exist between us, and we are both enclosed within concentric circles of care, and tied to one another through what Noddings calls "chains of caring." As she puts it, in "the inner intimate circles, we care because we love . . . as we move outward . . . we are guided by at least three considerations: how we feel, what the other expects of us, and what the situational relationship requires of us."[17] In these relationships, we must try to apprehend the other's concrete reality, to take him on his own terms, and to enter into the world as he perceives it.

But we are also linked through chains of caring to those who are currently strangers, but people with whom we have the potential to live with in relationship: "Beyond the circle of proximate others are those I have not yet encountered. Some of these are linked to the inner circle by personal or formal relations . . . chains of caring are established, some linking unknown individuals to those already anchored in the inner circle and some forming whole new circles of potential caring."[18]

This sense of being connected to others through concentric circles and linked chains of caring is echoed in first-person accounts of illness written from within the perspective of care. For example, in his narrative about preparing for, and recovering from, heart surgery, Paul F. Camenisch identifies (to use Nodding's terms) concentric circles of care in the communities of which he was a part (work, church, and family) and linked chains of attachment (particularly as he developed relationships with those in the health care system who were responsible for his medical care). He observes that facing a serious illness challenged his conception of who he was, and put his sense of self in jeopardy. These people, he claims, quite literally helped him to heal by re-membering and re-constructing him, so that his sense of self ultimately remained intact.

They did this by emphasizing not his individuality, but, rather, his connections to others: "They did not . . . come to comfort the individual, Paul, floating in regal and devastating isolation in some otherwise uninhabited universe of his own."[19] Rather, they "came as persons, to me as a person, one to whom they were already connected, with the message that we were still connected to each other and simultaneously to numerous others, and that the life we all enjoyed was not a fragmented life parceled out separately to each incidentally connected but ultimately individual entity, but a life that flowed between, among, and around us, so that the loss of any one of us was a loss for all."[20] The people who cared for him, he concludes, were "living lifelines"[21] of reciprocal connection, and the severing of any of these lifelines would diminish everyone who was attached through them.

Camenisch's account demonstrates another feature of the ethics of care, namely, that while care may be built on natural instincts, those instincts can be developed and enhanced through attentive practice. This is particularly

important within a health care setting because it means that health care workers can be taught to care for patients in a way that reduces the toll that illness
takes on them. Moreover, even if medical treatment is not always successful
in restoring physical health, this kind of care can nonetheless keep the patient
whole and recognizable to himself: it can, in short, preserve him as a self.

The origins of the ethics of care are usually traced to investigations undertaken by Carol Gilligan, who observed that psychological studies of moral
development were typically done by male researchers, used males as research subjects, took them to provide the normal standard of personhood, and
then defined females as "deficient" because they did not reach the highest
levels of moral development as described by their theoretical models. Gilligan decided to focus on girls and women instead, and famously observed that
males and females seem to use different "voices" when they describe themselves as moral agents, and appear to view moral problems and their possible
solutions very differently. As Gilligan puts it, "When one begins with the
study of women and derives developmental constructs from their lives, the
outline of a moral conception different from that described by Freud, Piaget,
or Kohlberg begins to emerge and informs a different description of development."[22]

The models based on males saw moral development as hierarchical, as
consisting in moving up a ladder of moral competency in which subjectivity
is exchanged for objectivity; emotion for reason; relationships for individualism; attachment for separateness; concreteness and specificity for abstraction; and which culminate in the discovery of universally applicable general
rules. In this model, moral dilemmas arise when competing rights come into
conflict. This approach has been called an ethics of justice, or an ethics of
rights and justice (and we should notice that many of its features are incorporated into mainstream bioethics).

When Gilligan interviewed girls and women, however, she discovered
that females speak in the language of responsibility, which "provides a web
like imagery or relationships to replace . . . [the] hierarchical ordering"[23]
which characterizes male moral development. Not only is this web like image not hierarchical, but within the web, many of the orderings that charac-
terize the male view are reconstructed or reversed: emotions, for example,
become fundamentally important to descriptions of the moral life, and individualistic conceptions of the self that suggest that each of us is independent
of other selves become untenable.

In this web, moral problems arise not from competing rights but from
conflicting responsibilities, and can only be resolved by "a mode of thinking
that is contextual and narrative, rather than formal and abstract."[24] In this
process, we must listen attentively to one another; as Gilligan puts it, she is
interested in (and, one assumes, those in favor of an ethics of care should be
interested in) "the interaction of experience and thought, in different voices

and the dialogues to which they give rise, in the way we listen to ourselves and others, in the stories we tell about our lives."[25]

Interestingly, even though Gilligan "aimed for findings that would be empirical and descriptive of the psychological outlooks of girls as they became more mature in their thinking about morality,"[26] the ethics of care quickly took on normative dimensions. For many theorists, it became not merely a descriptive account of the different voices of males and females as they spoke about morality, it provided an alternative model—and in many respects a superior model—to already existing ethical theories.

For many of those working within health care professions, particularly nurses, the ethics of care seemed both to capture something of the nature of their own experience, and to offer a more satisfactory account of the ethical dimensions of their work than that offered by mainstream bioethics based primarily on the principled approach. Nurses are often women (still) and physicians are (still) often men; nurses are lower in the organizational hierarchy than physicians; and nurses are more likely than physicians to see their relationship with their patients as one centered on care, in all its dimensions, and not just on medical treatment. As a result of the work of Gilligan and Noddings, in particular, nursing scholars began to ask whether their analysis and proposals were more applicable to the experiences of nurses than other ethical models. These scholars "began to question . . . whether bioethics, which in many ways reflects a male or androcentric point of view, was the most appropriate theory for nursing ethics."[27]

Bioethics, many concluded, reflects a male perspective and ignores the voices of women, in much the same way that Kohlberg's studies did. Indeed, from the perspective of an ethics of care, Kantian, utilitarian, liberal, and principled contributions to bioethics are more similar than their apparent differences might initially lead us to believe: all reflect a male perspective, all assume an individualized self, all give reason a much more important place than emotion, and all treat moral dilemmas as things which can be resolved through the application of abstract moral theories, principles, and rules. Given that the relationship between nurses and patients is central to nursing practice, many of those now working in nursing ethics believe that some form of relational ethics is required in any adequate moral approach applicable to nurses: "nursing ethics as such must be relational. In other words . . . the basis of nursing ethics is relationship with others: patient, family, community, colleague, or environment."[28] As Andolsen notes, the ethics of care has been "eagerly embraced" by nurses because it "seems to describe accurately the fundamental dynamic of their professional lives. . . . The feminine ethics of care coheres nicely with nursing as a quintessentially feminine profession."[29]

While some form of the ethics of care has found a home in nursing ethics, and from that perspective it offers a challenge to mainstream bioethics, we should note, however, that the model of care proposed by an ethic of care must encompass more than this if it is to offer a robust challenge to mainstream bioethics. Which is to say: if an ethics of care poses a real challenge to bioethics, that challenge cannot be restricted to the relationship between patient and nurse, or nurse, patient, and family; rather, it must extend to hierarchical organizations (such as hospitals and long-term care homes) in their entirety, and to ethical approaches that emphasize the role of reason over the expression of emotion, abstraction over concreteness, and individualistic conceptions of autonomy over considerations of the dynamics of particular caring relationships.

An ethics of care arguably contains important elements necessary for a critique of mainstream bioethics, including an emphasis on listening to the "voices' of people as they tell their stories in a way that goes beyond merely respecting their autonomy; it makes a place for the emotions within descriptions of the ethical life, and suggests (rightly, I believe) that only descriptions of that life which make a place for the emotions are adequate; and it recognizes the reality that human lives are lived out within the context of relationships with other people. However, I shall argue that an ethics of care is ultimately unsatisfactory in important ways, and that its strengths can be captured without the weaknesses by a version of virtue ethics that is expressed through practices and centered upon a conception of autonomy that relates the value of choice to the value of the things chosen, and connects both to the ongoing development of moral character.

THE NEED FOR JUSTICE AND DERIVING AN 'OUGHT' FROM AN 'IS': WEAKNESSES OF THE ETHICS OF CARE

It is something of a banal truism in modern moral philosophy to proclaim that "You can't derive an 'ought' from an 'is'": which is to say, a description of how things *actually* are or a description of how people *actually* think tells us little or nothing about how things *ought* to be, or what *ought* to go on in people's heads. While Gilligan is clear that she is engaged in a psychological study that contrasts the way in which girls and women tend to think about morality with the ways in which boys and men tend to think about morality, the reliance on Gilligan's study as an important source of our thinking about an ethics of care sometimes appears to blur the line between an "is" and an "ought." Some advocates of the ethics of care, that is to say, seem to draw too many *normative* conclusions about her psychological discoveries, and seem to assume, for example, that care is necessarily morally good, and that caring relationships provide a sound ethical model for how we ought to treat one another. Noddings, for instance, is clear that she believes that "natural caring" is more fundamental than "ethical caring": "Our priority . . . is on natural caring, and our efforts at ethical caring are meant to establish or reestablish the more dependable conditions under which caring relations thrive."[30] She goes on to claim, in defense of her position, that "it is important . . . to recognize that there is empirical evidence for much of what has been claimed."[31]

Some advocates of the ethics of care, then, seem to mistake empirical evidence for philosophical justification, and they (arguably) miss asking some important ethical questions as a result. Even if it were empirically the case, for example, that males and females tend to approach ethical dilemmas differently, this does not tell us how such dilemmas ought to be approached; and by locating an ethics of care in empirical evidence about how women view themselves (and their selves), there is little space or impetus to ask questions about whether these differential approaches might not be at least partially socially constructed, and whether the expectations of nurturing and care placed on women might not be, in fact, pernicious and limiting. That is to say, even if it is the case that a contrast can legitimately be drawn between an ethics of rights and justice and an ethics of care and responsibility, and even if it can be empirically demonstrated that men tend to endorse the former and women the latter, this does not show that women (or anyone) should embrace an ethics of care: perhaps we would all be better off with an ethics of justice; or perhaps both approaches have merit and need to be balanced with one another. While "caring" does have an *aspirational* element—the "ethical self," as Noddings puts it, "is an active relation between my actual self and my vision of my ideal self as one-caring"—the care approach doesn't leave much space for asking whether we ought to understand the "ethical self" as being constituted solely or primarily by a commitment to care for others.[32]

Second, and following from the contrast between an ethics of rights and justice and an ethics of care, by locating the ethics of care in "caring relationships" modeled on the ideal nurturing relationship between mother and child that lies at the very center of the concentric circles of care, it is difficult for proponents of such an ethic to clearly identify ways in which relationships can be stifling and constraining as much as they can be rewarding and empowering (for both the one-caring and the cared-for). In short, the theory itself doesn't seem to contain elements, apart from our emotional responses, which might be used to judge the *quality* of the relationship. At the very least, this suggests that even if an ethics of care captures something important about the nature of the moral life, it needs to be supplemented by elements drawn from other ethical approaches.

Third, and consequently, there are good reasons to think that an ethics of care needs to be supplemented by, or work in conjunction with, some version of an ethics of justice. Interestingly enough, this is something that Gilligan herself recognizes: the ethics of care and the ethics of justice, she says, engage in a dynamic dialectic with one another, in which "the tension between responsibilities and rights sustains . . . human development. . . . This dialogue between fairness and care not only provides a better understanding of relations between the sexes but also gives rise to a more comprehensive portrayal of adult work and family relationships.[33]

Without supplementation by an ethics of justice, an ethics of care provides few resources to identify, let alone deal with, larger questions of sexism or racism within society, issues of social justice, or power differentials within relationships, organizations, and political arrangements. This is particularly important in bioethics: just as parents have more power than children, so physicians have more power than nurses, nurses have more power than unlicensed assistive personnel, and all health care workers, at least on occasion, have more power than patients. Andolsen, for example, argues that an ethics of care is unrealistic in an era of managed care unless it is "supplemented by attention to the value of justice in order to address all the questions arising from the reorganization of nursing labor as the health care system is restructured,"[34] because only an ethics of justice allows questions about the ethical implications of power differentials within health care organizations to be addressed. Gudorf argues, moreover, that even in cases in which nurses "care" for patients as they should according to an ethics of care, they need to remain cognizant of the principles that animate an ethics of justice. In an extensive case study exploring the treatment her son Victor received during a five-month hospital stay after he contracted Guillian-Barre Syndrome, Gudorf recounts an incident in which the line to Victor's catheter was clamped for a test and then forgotten. This led to urine reflux, which caused intense pain, and the eventual destruction of Victor's kidney. Because the nurses were distracted by Victor's pain, they put off doing an assessment of the lines attached to the patient. Gudorf believes that "One of the best indications that an ethic of care needs to be coordinated by a more systematic, principle-based model of treatment is the catheter incident. Had the lead nurse and incoming nurse of the afternoon shift followed normal procedures, instead of being absorbed in sympathy for Victor's pain, the clamp would have been discovered much earlier, and the kidney possibly saved."[35] She concludes that the "ethic of care is not an alternative to a system that implements a theory of justice,"[36] and argues that the two approaches must work together.

Finally, there is another way in which the ethics of care is "soft": it is ambiguous, its boundaries undefined and amorphous. It is not always clear, for example, what care is: is it an attitude? A feeling? An orientation? A series of actions? A virtue?[37] Is it primarily a relational ethic (because it focuses on relationships and suggests that selfhood can only be understood in relational terms), or is it a kind of narrative one (because it asks us to listen to the voices of those we care for as they tell their own stories), or does it simply encompass both approaches?[38] As Held observes, "There is not yet anything close to agreement among those writing on care on what exactly we should take the meaning of . . . [care] to be, but there have been many suggestions, tacit and occasionally explicit."[39] This lack of consensus on something as basic as the meaning of the term "care" makes it difficult for an ethics of care, however described, to stand alone; any description will be incomplete, have serious rivals, and be subject to ambiguity and challenge, to an even greater extent than is usually the case with competing moral conceptions.

FEMINIST ETHICS: FROM THE MARGINS TO THE CENTER AND BACK AGAIN

There are many different feminisms, and, consequently, many different feminist approaches to bioethics. However, they are tied together by a shared overarching emphasis on the role played by (often invisible) strands, networks, and forces of power and oppression which are embedded in societal and class structures, in the practice of medicine and in health care institutions, and within the discipline of bioethics itself. One of the most important contributions made by feminist bioethicists to bioethics is that even as they actively engage in bioethical discussions and address central bioethical questions, they simultaneously challenge bioethicists who take the assumptions of mainstream bioethics as givens to justify their moral commitments, and ask themselves whether they are able to persuasively do so. Because (to use Walker's helpful analysis) feminist bioethicists offer a critique that stands outside the theoretical-juridical framework that encompasses all the mainstream approaches to bioethics, they remain outsiders who can see more clearly than insiders what is *really* going on, and they can ask questions about the exercise of power, who possesses it, and what role it plays in maintaining the dominance of particular positions within the discipline of bioethics.

We saw in chapter 1 that bioethics has a center (which is occupied by particular people and shaped by their ideas), which means that it also has margins (and, consequently, persons who are considered marginal and whose views are marginalized). We also saw that an important theme of many philosophers' accounts of how they came to be bioethicists—to be recognized as persons who have a legitimate place at the bedside of patients, to have a voice that is listened to in a medical setting, to be taken seriously by health care professionals—was that they were offered an invitation to come down from the ivory tower located on the periphery and to enter into the "real world" of practical bioethics which lies at the center.

Many feminist bioethical accounts, as the title of this section suggests, also play with the idea that there is a bioethical center (occupied by certain people, and shaped by particular ideas), and that there are other people (and their ideas) who are on the margins.[40] However, unlike the triumphant tales of the movement to the center that we explored earlier, feminist bioethicists tend to see this journey as generating a profound professional and personal conundrum. In order to be heard and taken seriously by those at the center, feminist bioethicists, too, must be invited in; however, once they are there, they are very conscious that they must not challenge the medical and the bioethical status quo too intensely or provocatively or their invitation will be rescinded, and they will be pushed out to the margins again. However, at the same time, in order to do their jobs as feminist bioethicists, both standard medical practices and dominant bioethical paradigms must be forcefully challenged and vigorously critiqued. Mainstream bioethics, moreover, has been successful in resisting the feminist critique precisely because it uses the strategy of marginalizing it and the feminist bioethicists who make it whenever it threatens to actually change the way in which things are done. As Wolf puts it, in bioethics, there "are satellite ethics discussed for various ethnic groups and women, but at the center, mainstream bioethics remains undisturbed."[41]

This conundrum has political, professional, and personal implications for feminist bioethicists. On one hand, it is only when they remain on the margins that they can clearly see what goes on at the center, as one can see a city more clearly when one views it from a distance than when one sits down in a central square; moreover, it is only when one is on the margins that one is fully aware of others who are also marginalized and can have some insight into their perspectives, and so it is only from this marginal position that one can claim to legitimately speak (carefully and respectfully) for others who are keeping one company at the edge. In addition, considering those on the margins, and the moral significance of their experiences within the medical system, some feminist bioethicists argue, is something that mainstream bioethics has been woefully negligent in addressing.

Holmes, for instance, argues that the rise of bioethics as a recognized discipline, and of the bioethicist as a respected and often well-paid professional, coincides with a period in which lower level health care workers have seen their salaries drop, and the poorest and most vulnerable members of society have had an increasingly difficult time accessing medical care, and she asks why bioethicists at the center have paid so little attention to issues of social justice and their connection to health care. (Even if bioethicists working within the liberal framework, for example, have paid attention to the social determinants of health, their approach has focused less on challenging existing power structures than on developing procedural methods that can easily be incorporated into standard medical and bioethical practices.)

Holmes wonders, "What can feminist bioethicists do to close the gap?"[42] In answer to this question, she concludes, "Unfortunately, we can do very little. Those who wish to get tenure, and to have papers published—that is, to get paid for 'doing' ethics—can write and speak only within accepted paradigms. We can't rock boats. The deep structure of bioethics needs to be changed. . . . And this is unlikely to occur, because so many people *enjoy* the status quo,"[43] and benefit from the professional and financial privileges it affords them.

This tension between having important ethical insights that come from one's presence on the margins that need to be heard and taken seriously by those with power, and the fact that one is only invited into the center and encouraged to speak there when one does not use this as an opportunity to challenge the status quo, is identified by Barbara Nicholas as one of the most important dilemmas facing feminist bioethicists. As she puts it, "I believe that one of the challenges for a feminist bioethicist concerns how to move from the margins to the 'center,' to lose one's marginal status, to claim the power that it gives without selling out, losing one's critical edge, becoming absorbed, assimilated, or domesticated."[44]

The movement from the margins to the center, then, allows feminist bioethicists to gain power—the power which benefits those at the center, and which is reflected in their professional prestige and demonstrated by the fact that they, as Holmes puts it, get paid to do ethics—but only if they temper their feminist views, make them less radical, less threatening, and more congenial to the medical and bioethical status quo. However, of course, to make these views less radical and threatening, and more congenial, is precisely to make them less feminist and to silence the distinctive voice offered by feminist bioethicists, and to sustain the marginalization of the particular (and particularist) concerns that feminist thought considers important and makes visible. As Nicholas observes, "Not only are we [feminist bioethicists] negotiating the place of bioethics within medicine, we are also negotiating the place of feminism within bioethics."[45]

It is this constant negotiation and re-negotiation between the center and the margins of bioethics, I believe, that shapes feminist responses to, and critiques of, the dominant ethical approaches in bioethics. To put this point slightly differently, the space occupied by feminist bioethicists within the discipline of bioethics is neither at the center nor at the margins, but within the shifting and constantly re-negotiated border zones between them, and the feminist self of bioethics that lies beneath these negotiations and re-negotiations is a self that is similarly negotiated and re-negotiated: sometimes an insider, sometimes an outsider, sometimes weak and sometimes powerful, sometimes able to speak for those whom existing power structures render voiceless, sometimes aware of the arrogance and condescension implicit in the claim that any of us can speak for anyone other than ourselves. (Given my claim that this conception of the self is a negotiated and renegotiated one, of course, any claims I make about it are themselves open to challenge and renegotiation.)

The specific features of the feminist self that I wish to draw attention to include the following: First, it often makes explicitly political claims, not merely analytic, procedural, or theoretical ones. Second, because feminist bioethicists are aware that bioethicists speak, write, and think from somewhere (which is to say, they have particular experiences, beliefs, and moral commitments), there is a merging of the self of the feminist bioethicist and the feminist self of bioethics. While a bioethicist working within the mainstream approaches can use utilitarian or Kantian reasoning (for example), without ever becoming a Kantian or a utilitarian, feminist bioethicists must incorporate their personal feminist commitments into their bioethical reasoning if they are to remain feminists. And, finally, the feminist self of bioethics conceives itself to be autonomous or sets the achievement of autonomy as a goal, but understands this concept in a way that is very different than the independent, self-reliant, and self-directed conception characteristic of principled, liberal, and bioethical accounts.

First, feminist bioethics is *political*, in a way that standard approaches (even approaches built on the liberal model) are not. Consequently, the feminist self of bioethics is located in political as well as moral space. A central point of ethical theorizing and analysis for feminist bioethicists (to paraphrase Marx) is not merely to create theories and analyze existing situations that have generated moral dilemmas, but to argue for change when such explorations reveal that the status quo is unjust. Purdy, for instance, argues that at the heart of what she calls "core feminism"—a set of beliefs shared by all those who call themselves feminists—lie two simple judgments: "First, women are, as a group, worse off than men, because their interests routinely fail to be given equal consideration. Second, that state of affairs is unjust and should be remedied."[46]

Purdy notes that to say that feminist bioethics is "political" is often to invite the response from bioethicists working in the mainstream that feminist bioethics is not *real* ethics, that ethical thinking requires a neutral and detached theoretical analysis. Purdy argues that the categories of "political" and "ethical" overlap with one another, and a bioethics that ignores political questions is limiting itself in a significant way: "ethics that turns a blind eye to particular forms of unfairness is broken and in need of repair."[47] Feminist bioethicists often extend their political analysis to encompass other categories of vulnerable persons (most of which also overlap with categories of gender), such as race, ethnicity, class, and disability.

Feminist inquiry in bioethics is political in another way as well: feminist bioethicists challenge mainstream bioethicists not only to enlarge the scope of their inquiry from a relatively narrow perspective which focuses on things like the health care professional-patient relationship, informed consent, research, and the distribution of scarce medical goods within a health care system, to the larger political questions of who is oppressed and by whom, but also to examine the ways in which the discipline of bioethics itself may reinforce and maintain oppressive ways of thinking and acting. As Fitzpatrick and Scully note, feminist inquiry in bioethics "makes explicit, and critiques, oppressive and exclusionary practices in mainstream bioethics and seeks to provide non-oppressive non-exclusionary alternatives."[48]

In her consideration of the issues facing lesbian couples who wish to have children, Murphy forthrightly locates her philosophical analysis in her own experiences and those of her partner: "A few years ago, my partner and I began using assisted reproduction to conceive our first child, and it occurred to me as I wondered about lesbians' access to reproductive services, insurance coverage, and parenting rights for non-birthing partners that there was little difference between us and the many infertile couples for whom reproductive services were designed."[49] This openness about the way in which the life experiences of the feminist bioethicist not only shapes her responses to ethical questions, but even prompts the questions themselves, is a second important feature of feminist bioethics that is largely absent in mainstream approaches. It is, of course, a feature which is shared with proponents of the ethics of care; what distinguishes the way in which those I have designated care ethicists from those I am calling feminist ethicists is that the latter connect it to the explicitly political agenda discussed above. The personal experiences reported by feminist bioethicists not only illuminate ethical questions in a new way (which, arguably, care ethics does as well), but their analysis is often tied to transforming the structures that make those experiences worthy of analysis in the first place: for example, the situation facing lesbian couples seeking assisted reproductive services is only a subject for ethical analysis when lesbian couples are treated differently than heterosexual couples. Because feminist bioethicists not only place the ethical concerns raised by medicine within a larger political framework, but also focus on identifying the ways in which bioethicists may be complicit (although not always consciously) in maintaining oppressive practices in medicine, feminist bioethicists tend to be more self-aware of their own moral assumptions and commitments than most bioethicists, and self-conscious and self-reflective about the way in which they analyze bioethical issues.

As Rehmann-Sutter points out, feminist bioethicists have made some key contributions to bioethics, including this self-conscious awareness of their own perspectives: "Moral philosophy does not happen in a pure, rational superworld. 'Good practice' in moral philosophy and bioethics means first of all being prepared to reflect and try to free oneself from prejudice and partiality."[50] And, he notes, it is not only the fact that all philosophers begin their reasoning from somewhere rather than nowhere, in the "real" world rather than in the "superworld" that is important, it makes a difference whether they are self-consciously aware of their own assumptions and commitments and how they may affect ethical analysis: "Even after recognizing the unavoidable perspective of ethics itself, it makes a difference whether somebody is seeing/thinking/speaking from a standpoint with or without being aware of this fact, and with or without including this fact in his or her reflections."[51]

This self-conscious awareness of their own context and how it may affect their philosophical judgments on the part of feminist bioethicists means that the feminist conception of the self that operates in bioethics is significantly different than its rivals. The feminist self of bioethics and the self of the feminist bioethicist simultaneously merge with one another (when feminist bioethicists write about bioethical issues, they not only employ a conception of the self that is gendered, relational, and embodied, but reflect on their own particular context, and on how this might shape their analysis) and somewhat paradoxically because this merging is made explicit, both selves are made visible.

Feminist bioethicists, that is to say, make visible aspects of their own lives because they understand that even the questions that interest them result from their own particular life experiences, and that their own perspectives shape the answers they give. Far from pretending that the conception of the self employed in their bioethical explorations was drawn from a neutral model that can fairly represent all adequate moral agents, feminist bioethicists acknowledge that their conceptions are shaped by their own experiences, and may not even be true of all women, let alone of human beings more generally. In this perspective, then, reference's to one's own life, and considerations of the way in which one's experiences might be implicated in one's bioethical judgments are not only permitted, they are also understood to be morally important and philosophically significant.

Finally, like other bioethicists, feminist bioethicists emphasize the importance of autonomy, the importance of people being able to live lives of their own choosing, and to have their choices respected in a medical context. However, given their political and epistemic commitments, feminist conceptions of autonomy are fundamentally different than the individualistic, self-directed, and unsituated model envisaged in principled, liberal, and mainstream bioethical approaches that are dominated either by the Divided Self or the Choosing Self. I want to draw attention to three features of most feminist conceptions of autonomy that are distinctive. These feminist claims about autonomy provide an important contribution to the expressive-collaborative model of autonomy I am proposing, and out of which the figure of the Situated Self is built.

First, feminist bioethicists emphasize connections between persons, and note that autonomous persons come into being in particular families; are raised in particular cultural, racial, and social contexts; and their self-conceptions are shaped by their experiences as gendered and embodied creatures. Feminist bioethicists often call their conceptions of autonomy "relational" (to highlight the contrast with standard individualistic conceptions), a name that Mackenzie and Stoljar identify as an "umbrella" term: "These perspectives are premised on a shared conviction, the conviction that persons are socially embedded and that agents' identities are formed within the context of social relationships and shaped by a complex of intersecting social determinants such as race, class, gender, and ethnicity."[52] Relational autonomy, then, however it is further articulated or developed, will be intersubjective and social, often elaborated in terms of narrative, and part of the intellectual task facing the feminist bioethicist is to analyze the ways in which these social determinants affect the ability of particular individuals to shape their own lives and make choices which are genuinely their own. Feminist bioethicists will also, of course, consider the ways in which these elements—race, class, gender, disability—affect the treatment of women and other vulnerable people in a medical context.

Second, and following from this, feminists who advocate a relational autonomy perspective argue that individuals are situated in particular contexts—familial, cultural, economic—and that any adequate discussion of what it means to see oneself as autonomous, and to exercise autonomous choices, must take these contextual features into account. Even if autonomy is an ideal, that is to say, it is not one that is equally open to everyone, in terms of their self-understandings (which are distinct from their intellectual capacities), their ability to exercise their choices, or even whether they have genuine options open to them at all. Which is to say: given that power structures are most beneficial to those who already possess power, any conception of autonomy that takes their privileged experience of having genuine choices open to them as its model (as standard bioethical accounts of autonomy tend to do) ignores the way in which persons who are disadvantaged because of gender, race, poverty, or disability, among other possibilities, is hardly an account of autonomy at all. Rather, such conceptions simply disguise unjust social and political arrangements by, as Wolf puts it, straining "for universals, ignoring the significance of groups and the importance of context."[53] And, she argues, a bioethics that tries to speak for everyone ends up speaking for no one (although it may privilege certain people over others): "There is no such thing as a patient without race, ethnicity, and gender,"[54] and a bioethics that ignores these differences misses much that is important in real cases.

A third important feature of accounts of autonomy that are relational, situated, and contextual, is recognition of the fact that selves develop in time as well as space. Selves, that is to say, have pasts as well as futures, and develop through fluctuating and ongoing relationships with others, are held together by memories (their own, and others of them), and must be able to imagine different possible futures, different ways in which their lives might go. As Lloyd poetically puts it, "A self is born into a future in which it will make individual decisions, for which it will be held responsible, praised or blamed. But it has also been born into the past of its communal life a past that both precedes it and awaits it; a past of collective memory and imagination which must be reckoned with in the present."[55]

Since the relational self is situated not only in space but also in time, the role played by the imagination in envisaging possible futures (arguably, a necessary part of the capacity to exercise autonomy on any plausible account of what autonomy might look like) connects to feminist concerns about who has power and who doesn't—who, that is to say, is able to both envisage different possible futures and choose from among them, and who is deprived of such imaginative resources and denied real choice. As Mackenzie observes, "in self-reflection and deliberation, our own imaginative activities, our abilities to imagine ourselves otherwise, draw on a cultural repertoire of images and representations. When the cultural repertoire is predominantly phallocentric, the culturally available images on which women can draw seriously constrain their imaginative possibilities and their self-conceptions."[56]

Relational autonomy, and the corresponding contextualized and particularist conception of the self that accompanies it, arguably provides a richer theoretical model of autonomy than that commonly used in individualistic accounts, and reflected in the principle of respect for autonomy employed in bioethics that draw extensively on either the Divided Self or the Choosing Self. It locates persons in a web of relationships, and explores how those relationships can both help and hinder the exercise of choice; and, since this self is located in time as well as space, past events which generate present options need to be considered, as well as the imaginative resources available to envisage future possibilities; and, finally, because existing social arrangements affect the degree to which individuals can act on their choices, no plausible conceptions of autonomy can be detached from a consideration of issues of oppression and social justice.

CONCLUSION: FROM FEMINIST ETHICS TO VIRTUE ETHICS

Feminist bioethics offers an important corrective to the central assumptions of mainstream bioethics. Because it stands outside the theoretical-juridical framework into which mainstream bioethical approaches fall, it allows us to notice features of the moral landscape that are overlooked or insufficiently accounted for in standard bioethics. Of particular importance are two things: an understanding of autonomy that is relational rather than individual; and, second, a recognition of the role played by narratives in descriptions of the ethical life, the construction of the self, and as sources of moral knowledge and insight. We learn to become autonomous only through the assistance of others, and the autonomous choices of particular persons are helped, hindered, and played out in conjunction with the autonomous choices made by others. In addition, as in the liberal account, autonomy has an inescapably political dimension because the exercise of autonomous choice requires political and social conditions that allow individuals to have a sense of the possibilities open to them and provide them with the freedom to act upon particular choices.

As feminist accounts make clear, however, any form of bioethics that takes autonomy seriously must take issues of power, economic inequalities, and exploitation as central concerns because these things hinder, in profound but often nearly invisible ways, the ability of some individuals not only to act autonomously but even to conceive of themselves as persons who are, or could be, autonomous. It is not enough, that is to say, for bioethicists to insist that choices ought not to be interfered with, or even that positive freedoms are sometimes necessary for the exercise of autonomy. Rather, unless issues of inequality and power are addressed, some people will be able to live autonomous lives, and other people will not be able to do so. Any form of bioethics, then, which makes a central place for autonomy but which fails to take these things adequately into account, and to work hard to identify ways in which they can be addressed, will be deceptive: what it will support, as in the case of bioethical arguments that, for instance, take it for granted that the market is the appropriate mechanism for facilitating choice, is the exercise of autonomy on the part of some at the expense of the autonomy of others. Consequently, one of the great contributions of feminist thought to bioethics is the challenge offered to bioethicists themselves to be aware of their own place in the world, and to be self-reflective about the ways in which this may shape their own moral assumptions and theoretical commitments.

Second, the concept of autonomy and the concept of narrative are importantly connected to one another. One useful way of conceiving of autonomy is to see it as (metaphorically) meaning that we are the authors of our own lives (rather than bit players or minor characters in the stories of others), that we can tell our own stories on our own terms, and that we have some control over how these stories might develop in the future. When this conception is connected to the feminist assertion that selfhood is narratively constructed, we can identify four distinct dimensions that narratives play in constructing an autonomous self and in placing that self in a moral universe that closely connects autonomous choice to ethical choice. First, we can understand the internal stories we tell ourselves about who we are, what we are doing, what is important to us and why, as narratives that play an important role in the construction of the self. Second, the stories we tell about other people, and the stories they tell about us, link these internal stories to external and shared narratives. Selfhood, as we have already seen, has a reciprocal dimension: I am a self, in part, because I can recognize your selfhood, and you are a self, in part, because you can recognize mine. However, as feminist bioethicists remind us, not all forms of recognition are benign: some stories do damage, diminish, or marginalize others.

Third, ethical issues themselves are narratively constructed. No issue exists on its own, apart from a narrative context which helps explain how it appeared, why it is thought of as something that raises ethical concerns, and how it might be resolved. Following Walker's claim that we can identify better and worse ways of living and acting only by comparing various possibilities that we are aware of to one another, we identify moral problems, their implications, and their possible resolutions, by comparing and contrasting different narratives to one another. For example, whether we fall into the pro-choice or the pro-life camps in the abortion debate, and whether we believe that laws against euthanasia are necessary to protect the vulnerable or an unacceptable interference with autonomous choice and a denial of dignity at the end of life, often comes down, in the end, to the stories we have heard and which of those stories have moved (or failed to move) us. Finally, narratives themselves (whether fictional or factual) serve as important sources of moral information, insight, and knowledge; indeed, they sometimes reveal aspects of the moral life that are largely invisible or inaccessible through straightforward philosophical argumentation. These are all claims that will be more fully developed in subsequent chapters.

However, as Walker notes, feminist ethics is not the only well-developed ethical perspective that exists outside the theoretical-juridical framework: virtue ethics also occupies this position, "and contemporary authors find ways, including feminist insights, to refresh the ancient view."[57] As is the case with feminist ethics, virtue ethics has had surprisingly little impact on the dominant bioethical views which occupy the center; like feminist ethics, when it is paid attention to at all, it is usually treated as offering insights which can be added on to particular aspects of the dominant framework, rather than as a moral perspective that construes the moral life in a fundamentally different way than it is envisaged in mainstream accounts, and which revolves around a strikingly different conception of the self and the moral universe through which it moves than these accounts do.

I will argue that the strengths of feminist ethics can be captured within a contemporary version of virtue ethics, and that feminist insights attached to the ethical framework provided by a neo-Aristotelian version of virtue ethics can do a better job than feminist ethics considered alone can of helping individuals make sense of their own lives, particularly in the face of difficult life challenges, including illness. While feminist bioethics offers tools that are useful for the theoretical analysis of some bioethical issues, it is not so clear that it provides an ethical framework within which individuals can easily make sense of their own lives, particularly when confronted by illness and suffering, or what form of justice it should be supplemented with when a feminist analysis reaches the limits identified by Gilligan and experienced by Gudorf during the care of her son Victor.

As noted, while virtue ethics has played a surprisingly minor role in mainstream bioethics, I shall argue that it can provide a conception of the self and a description of the moral universe that is more satisfactory than its competitors, not only for the theoretical exploration of issues that are of concern to bioethicists, but in helping individuals cope with what Aristotle called the *peripeteia*, the unexpected event that turns someone's life upside down or sets it on a new course, and which is a fundamental part of the human condition. The issues of concern to bioethicists have the *peripeteia* at their heart, although this is a fact that is seldom apparent in the way in which these issues are discussed. As Bruner observes, in the context of medicine, the unexpected event can be the stark announcement of "'I've got news for you, you're on the brink of death.' The ordinary canonicity is that you'll go on living forever, and then someone tells you it's finite and you're going to be dead."[58] In terms of reproductive technologies, the unexpected event can be the discovery by someone who wants children that he is infertile; in the context of our discoveries in genetics, it can be the diagnosis of a fetus with a genetic disorder and the need to make a difficult decision; and in the case of organ transplantation, the need to decide what to do with the organs of a much-loved family member immediately after being told that she has suffered an unexpected accident. Moreover, conceptions of autonomy that fail to consider the impact of the unexpected event on individual self-conceptions, perceptions of choice, and the limitations on the options available imposed by the reality of embodiment, illness, and mortality may preserve freedom but provide few resources for individuals when they must face the *peripeteia*. These are all events that mainstream bioethical approaches have a difficult time making sense of, and which are not reducible to issues of choice, gender, power, and oppression (although the pain they cause can, of course, be exacerbated by these things.) Virtue ethics, moreover, underpins a new approach to ethics called revolutionary Aristotelianism, which pays attention to issues of power, manipulation, and exploitation, which feminists correctly identify as important matters of ethical concern, as well as providing a coherent moral approach that can provide an alternative to mainstream bioethics, and a perspective from which to evaluate bioethics itself.

NOTES

1. Sidney Callahan, "The Psychology of Emotion and the Ethics of Care," in *Medicine and the Ethics of Care*, ed. Diana Fritz Cates and Paul Lauritzen (Washington, DC: Georgetown University Press, 2001), 141.

2. Callahan, "The Psychology of Emotion," 141.

3. In this regard, it is instructive to note that the 7th Edition of Beauchamp and Childress's *Principles of Biomedical Ethics* which came out in 2013, makes only a few, short references to feminist ethics, and feminist insights are largely subsumed into the framework provided by their principled approach. Feminist ethics are not considered at all in the chapter on moral theories.

4. Kathleen Oberle and Shelley Raffin Bouchal, *Ethics In Canadian Nursing Practice* (Toronto: Pearson-Prentice Hall, 2009), 18.

5. Oberle and Bouchal, *Nursing Practice*, 21.

6. Edward Collins Vacek, S.J., "The Emotions of Care in Health Care," in *Medicine and the Ethics of Care*, ed. Diana Fitz Cates and Paul Lauritzen (Washington, DC: Georgetown University Press, 2001), 105.

7. Margaret Urban Walker, *Moral Understandings: A Feminist Study In Ethics*, 2nd ed. (New York: Oxford University Press, 2007), 23.

8. Hilde Lindemann, *An Invitation To Feminist Ethics* (Boston: McGraw-Hill, 2006), 121.

9. Lindemann, *An Invitation*, 121.

10. Lindemann, *An Invitation*, 47.

11. Lindemann, *An Invitation*, 47–48.

12. Walker, *Moral Understandings*, 116.

13. Walker, *Moral Understandings*, 116.

14. Walker, *Moral Understandings*, 116.

15. Walker, *Moral Understandings*, 119–120.

16. Nel Noddings, *Caring: A Feminine Approach To Ethics and Moral Education* 2nd ed. (Berkeley: University of California Press, 2003), 42.

17. Noddings, *Caring*, 46.

18. Noddings, *Caring*, 47.

19. Paul F. Camenisch, "Communities of Care, of Trust, and of Healing," in *Medicine and the Ethics of Care*, ed. Diana Fritz Cates and Paul Lauritzen (Washington, DC: Georgetown University Press, 2001), 256.

20. Camenisch, "Communities of Care," 256.

21. Camenisch, "Communities of Care," 256.

22. Carol Gilligan, *in A Different Voice* (Cambridge, Massachusetts: Harvard University Press, 1982), 19.

23. Gilligan, *Different Voice*, 173.

24. Gilligan, *Different Voice*, 19.

25. Gilligan, *Different Voice*, 2.

26. Virginia Held, *The Ethics Of Care* (Oxford: Oxford University Press, 2006), 27.

27. Oberle and Bouchal, *Nursing Practice*, 39.

28. Oberle and Bouchal, *Nursing Practice*, 41.

29. Barbara Hilkert Andolsen, "Care and Justice as Moral Values For Nurses In An Era Of Managed Care," in *Medicine and the Ethics of Care*, ed. Diana Fritz Cates and Paul Lauritzen (Washington, DC: Georgetown University Press, 2001), 41.

30. Noddings, *Caring*, xv.

31. Noddings, *Caring*, 67.

32. Noddings, *Caring*, 49.

33. Gilligan, *Different Voice*, 174.

34. Andolsen, "Care and Justice," 41.

35. Christine E. Gudorf, "The Need For Integrating Care Ethics Into Hospital Care: A Case Study," in *Medicine and the Ethics of Care*, ed. Diana Fritz Cates and Paul Lauritzen (Washington, DC: Georgetown University Press, 2001), 96.

36. Gudorf, "Integrating Care Ethics," 97.

37. Oberle and Bouchal, for example, describe an ethics of care as a "type of virtue ethics" (17); Noddings, however, states that "caring is not itself a virtue" (96), and warns that "we must not reify virtues and turn our caring toward them" (97).

38. Bouchal and Oberle, for example, distinguish the ethics of care from both relational and narrative ethics, and make the case that each has features that make it distinctive. Bouchal and Oberle, *Nursing Ethics*, 43.

39. Held, *Ethics of Care*, 29.

40. This idea that there is a contrast between the center and the margins is so strong that it forms the title of a recent book: *Feminist Bioethics: At The Center, On The Margins*, edited by Jackie Leach Scully, Laurel E. Baldwin-Ragaven, and Petya Fitzpatrick (Baltimore: The Johns Hopkins University Press, 2010).

41. Susan M. Wolf, "Erasing Difference: Race, Ethnicity, and Gender in Bioethics," in *Embodying Bioethics: Recent Feminist Advances*, ed. Anne Donchin and Laura M. Purdy (Lanham: Rowman & Littlefield Publishers, Inc, 1999), 73.

42. Helen Bequaert Holmes, "Closing The Gap: An Imperative For Feminist Bioethicists," in *Embodying Bioethics: Recent Feminist Advances*, ed. Anne Donchin and Laura M. Purdy (Lanham: Rowman & Littlefield Publishers, Inc, 1999), 57.

43. Holmes, "Closing The Gap," 57.

44. Barbara Nicholas, "Strategies For Effective Transformation," in *Embodying Bioethics: Recent Feminist Advances*, ed. Anne Donchin and Laura M. Purdy (Lanham: Rowman & Littlefield Publishers, Inc., 1999), 239–240.

45. Nicholas, "Strategies," 242.

46. Laura M. Purdy, *Reproducing Persons: Issues In Feminist Bioethics* (Ithaca: Cornell University Press, 1996), 5.

47. Purdy, *Reproducing Persons*, 18.

48. Petya Fitzpatrick and Jackie Leach Scully, "Introduction To Feminist Bioethics," in *Feminist Bioethics: At The Center, On The Margins*, edited by Jackie Leach Scully, Laurel E. Baldwin-Ragaven, and Petya Fitzpatrick (Baltimore: The Johns Hopkins University Press, 2010), 3.

49. Julien S. Murphy, "Should Lesbian Couples Count As Infertile Couples? Anti-lesbian Discrimination in Assisted Reproduction," in *Embodying Bioethics: Recent Feminist Advances*, ed. Anne Donchin and Laura M. Purdy (Lanham: Rowman & Littlefield Publishers, Inc., 1999), 103.

50. Christoph Rehmann-Sutter, "'It Is Her Problem, Not Ours': Contributions of Feminist Ethics To The Mainstream," in *Feminist Bioethics: At The Center, On The Margins*, ed. Jackie Leach Scully, Laurel E. Baldwin-Ragaven, and Petya Fitzpatrick (Baltimore: The Johns Hopkins University Press, 2010), 39.

51. Rehmann-Sutter, "'It is Her Problem, Not Ours,'" 39.

52. Catriona Mackenzie and Natalie Stoljar, "Introduction: Autonomy Refigured," in *Relational Autonomy: Feminist Perspectives On Autonomy, Agency, and the Social Self*, ed. Catriona Mackenzie and Natalie Stoljar (New York: Oxford University Press, 2000), 4.

53. Wolf, "Erasing Difference," 70.

54. Wolf, "Erasing Difference," 70.

55. Genevieve Lloyd, "Individuals, Responsibility, and the Philosophical Imagination," in *Relational Autonomy: Feminist Perspectives On Autonomy, Agency, and the Social Self*, ed. Catriona Mackenzie and Natalie Stoljar (New York: Oxford University Press, 2000), 122.

56. Catriona Mackenzie, "Imagining Oneself Otherwise," in *Relational Autonomy: Feminist Perspectives On Autonomy, Agency, and the Social Self*, ed. Catriona Mackenzie and Natalie Stoljar (New York: Oxford University Press, 2000), 126.

57. Walker, *Moral Understandings*, 30.

58. Jerome Bruner, "Narratives of Human Plight: A Conversation With Jerome Bruner," in *Stories Matter: The Role of Narrative in Medical Ethics,* ed. Rita Charon and Martha Montello (New York: Routledge, 2002), 4.

Chapter Six

The Second Component
of the Situated Self

Virtue

INTRODUCTION: WHAT'S THE REAL PROBLEM, ANYWAY?

The issues that draw the most attention to bioethics are exciting, intriguing, and thought provoking: will the genetic revolution change what it means to be human? Can frozen embryos inherit property? Should they be sold over the Internet? Is a woman in her sixties too old to give birth to a child? Should euthanasia be legalized? These issues garner headlines in newspapers, spark lively debates in bioethics classes, and generate numerous journal articles. However, most of the issues dealt with by ethicists and by ethics committees are far more mundane and far less provocative than this list might suggest. Indeed, often the topics of discussion and the issues of concern explored in the various ethics committees of which I have been a member are not actually ethical *dilemmas* at all, not situations in which we genuinely aren't sure what "the right thing to do" would be; rather, they are problems that appear because of the behavior of the persons involved and their failure to act virtuously.

These problems include: physicians sitting on research ethics committees that approve their own research projects; patients who get violent after waiting in the emergency room for twenty-six hours; personal support workers who don't speak to residents when they bathe them, or do speak to them, but in condescending or humiliating ways; physicians who read charts and talk to nurses (although they don't always listen to what they have to say) but never directly address the patients they are treating; families who insist that their

161

"loved ones' deserve to be moved to the top of the waiting list for the newest and most desirable long-term care homes, and threaten to call their important friends if this does not happen; administrators who are more concerned with good publicity than with ensuring that their institutions are run in a way that is focused on patient care; and friends of certain residents who bring alcohol and even illegal substances into long-term care homes.

These are not ethical dilemmas because it is clear what should (or should not) be done: of course, physicians should not approve their own research projects, and should speak to patients; of course, friends shouldn't smuggle marijuana or alcohol into long-term care homes; of course, personal support workers should treat residents with respect and dignity; and of course family members should recognize that their loved one is not the only person on the waiting list, and that they don't deserve special treatment simply because of who they know.

Despite the fact that these concerns are easy to resolve, ethically speaking, they remain intractable problems; it's very easy to say what people should do, or what they should have done, and very hard to get them to change. Furthermore, it is very difficult to know how one would even begin to address these issues, what one should say, or even whose responsibility it is to state the obvious: is the issue one of risk management, policy, or professional responsibility? Moreover, while these activities clearly raise ethical questions, they are not ones that a bioethicist working within the standard framework can easily address. Interestingly, then, what these discussions often reveal is that such occurrences are both recognized as moral failures *and* that we lack a moral language that allows us to describe them as such. They do not arise, that is to say, from a failure to respect autonomy, or from a clear-cut conflict between beneficence and justice; rather, they arise because someone was callous, insensitive, selfish, rude, domineering, impatient, or thoughtless—all things that we are not allowed to say because they imply, not that we are making justified moral judgments, but that we are being inappropriately judgmental.

The fact that we simultaneously recognize the source of the problem, but are unable (at least when working within the framework provided by mainstream bioethics) to accurately describe, it creates practical and conceptual problems. We want people working in health care to behave ethically, which is why ethics committees spend so much time discussing ethics education and creating ethical tools, but the standard ethical approaches and terminology present a conceptual scheme that may help the user address certain kinds of ethical questions (for instance, what an adequate consent form should look like, or who should decide whether life support can be removed from a particular dying patient), but which is largely unable to encourage people to internalize ethical values and act on them in their encounters with patients.

Moreover, as some of the examples just cited demonstrate, it is not only health care workers who need to behave ethically, it is patients and family members as well: beyond asserting that their autonomy should be respected, it is not clear what standard bioethics offers in terms of articulating which moral expectations of these persons are legitimate. So we are faced with some intractable questions: how can we encourage personal support workers to be kind as well as efficient when they bathe residents? How do we prevent staff from developing inappropriately intimate relationships with residents or patients, while encouraging them to get to know, and to care *about* the people they are caring *for*? Indeed, where (and how) do we draw the line between one kind of relationship and the other? What should we do about the technically proficient neurosurgeon who is so lacking in social skills and empathy that some of his patients call him "Dr. Asshole," and believe that he is responsible for exacerbating their fear and suffering?[1] And how ought patients to respond when they have been stuck in emergency for twenty-six hours?

In order to try to address these kinds of questions, ethics committees create values statements, patient bills of rights, codes of conduct, and mission statements, and what all of these things reveal, as the problems remain despite the existence of these documents, is that there is a persistent gap between the way we want our institutions to be, and the way people working within them and making use of their services actually behave, and this gap *never* seems to be narrowed or bridged, no matter how many ethics workshops we offer, how often we refine our ethics tools, or how frequently we rewrite our mission statements.

In short, the issues faced by ethics committees are almost never about genuine ethical dilemmas, in which we are at a loss to know what ought (morally speaking) to be done, or intellectual puzzles concerned with what principles ought to be applied in a particular case, or about what values the institution ought to uphold, but about something far more difficult and fundamental: how to get people to *behave* ethically, to *notice* when they are faced with a situation in which ethical judgment is called for, to *recognize* that all of their encounters with other human beings have an inescapably ethical dimension, and to *care* about how they respond. No matter how helpful these principles might be for addressing certain kinds of issues, or how carefully we identify values, these activities are useless if individuals lack an ethical sense (and sensibility): they must already want to behave ethically before they will turn to the principles, and they must recognize that they are in a situation in which their application is called for before they will think of using them.

Moreover, unless individuals are already ethically oriented, they will always have to be reminded to use the ethical tools, and are likely to see them as nothing more than a workplace requirement, like the obligation to respect a dress code or to follow health and safety measures; not, that is to say, as a set of values and commitments they internalize, but, rather, as an external expectation imposed on staff by their employer. Furthermore, if individuals lack an ethical sense and sensibility, even if their actions meet the obligations set out by the principles, something will still be lacking in their encounters with others, as illness narratives make clear. As Fitterer notes, "Argument alone will not make someone good."[2] Moreover, we are not good even if we respect autonomy, but fail to demonstrate compassion and kindness.

There is one approach to ethics that focuses extensively on the question of how to make people good, and that is virtue ethics. Virtue ethics is a strangely underused resource in mainstream bioethics; if it is mentioned at all, it is usually treated as an add-on or supplement to the principled approach, and as subordinate to the individualistic and liberal autonomy-based assumptions that underpin the standard framework.[3] However, Walker's useful identification of the theoretical-juridical template helps explain why virtue ethics should not be seen as something that can simply be added to, or incorporated within, theoretical-juridical ethical theories, but, rather, as something that (like feminist ethics) provides a genuine alternative, one which asks us to think very differently about ethics. From the perspective of virtue ethics, mainstream bioethics leaves out almost everything a virtue ethicist considers important, misconstrues the nature of the moral life, draws our attention to the wrong things, and forces us to work with an impoverished and unsatisfactory ethical language.

According to Aristotle, arguably the best-known proponent of this approach, living an ethical life requires us to develop virtuous habits and avoid vicious ones, to demonstrate ethical discernment that allows us to see clearly what is required of the virtuous person in this precise set of circumstances, to act on that recognition, and to feel the emotions that are the proper accompaniment to action. Both the emotions felt by a virtuous person and the actions she performs ought to aim to hit the mean, the middle point between excess and deficiency, and learning how to do this is more like learning how to swim, or read, than it is like a science: if we are to become virtuous, we must learn "to feel [emotions] when one ought and at the things one ought, in relation to those people whom one ought, for the sake of what and as one ought all of these things constitute the middle as well as what is best, which is in fact what belongs to virtue."[4] An education in ethics, then, ought to be concerned with three things: learning to feel what a virtuous person feels, so that one feels pleasure when behaving virtuously, and pain when behaving viciously; learning to act as a virtuous person would act; and developing the capacities required to exercise practical wisdom and moral discernment, so that one can recognize what is required in particular circumstances. Virtue ethics, then, is as flexible as utilitarianism, since it recognizes that each circumstance in which we find ourselves has elements which make it unique and to which we need to respond, but it is nonetheless predicated on a kind of objectivity: the mean is what it is, in any given context, and we can either hit it, or miss our mark.

From the perspective of a virtue ethicist, then, it is no surprise that bioethical education based on conveying the principles and demonstrating how they can be applied to cases is such a failure: it could hardly be otherwise, since it misconceives both the nature of an education in ethics, and the place of human beings within it: "Arguing ethical ends . . . does not mean simply hearing ethical facts and arguments. . . . Moral education is about instilling habits such that in their performance the student would come to know the intrinsic goodness and pleasantness of virtuous action. Argument and factual knowledge cannot impart or remove habits."[5] Further, because of the way in which autonomy is understood in standard bioethics, as well as the important role this conception plays, bioethics emphasizes our individuality and our freedom, rather than our social nature and our connections to others, and so it is ill-equipped to address substantive moral questions that focus not on freedom but on our interdependence: "Moral pedagogy is not . . . simply the imparting of a private intellectual skill at spotting right choices and objects. It is a social collaboration in which a taste for noble and virtuous actions is absorbed by the learner as one would acquire connoisseurship."[6]

In this chapter, I will explore some of the possibilities a neo-Aristotelian version of virtue ethics might offer to bioethics, and propose a conception of autonomy that fits within the framework provided by virtue ethics. Hursthouse describes neo-Aristotelianism as a term of art, one which indicates that the work of Aristotle is being drawn upon, but which does not compel the user to do this in any particular way, and I will adopt her usage: "The general kind is 'neo' [because] . . . its proponents allow themselves to regard Aristotle as just plain wrong on slaves and women, and also because we do not restrict ourselves to Aristotle's list of virtues. . . . It is 'Aristotelian' in so far as it aims to stick pretty close to his ethical writings wherever it can."[7]

THE VIRTUOUS SELF AND AUTONOMY: A NEO-ARISTOTELIAN APPROACH

I will argue that the language and moral framework provided by mainstream bioethics, if it is unable to do something as basic as bridge the gap between moral argument and moral character, is inadequate to deal with the issues that arise in the context of medical practice and within health care organizations, let alone address the larger questions raised by developments in biotechnology and the genetic revolution or their social implications. The most basic and fundamental task of any ethical perspective, arguably, is not to tell us what we should do, but to explain how people who desire to do the right thing are created in the first place. (That is to say, even if we accept for the sake of the argument that Beauchamp and Childress are right to assert that the principles they propose can all be located in what they term the "common morality," this does not explain where persons "committed to morality" come from, or why some people are not so committed. Are the latter evil, or improperly or insufficiently educated?)

Further, I will claim that mainstream bioethics has become part of the problem rather than part of the solution. The model of autonomy it employs, which asserts that the fact that something was freely chosen is of greater significance than what that thing is, not only fits poorly with the experience of illness and the suffering it engenders, but also flattens out our moral language to such an extent that we are no longer able to see ethical problems clearly, or discuss them productively, let alone resolve them. However, a conception of autonomy that connects the value of choice to the value of the things chosen, which allows us to conceive of the autonomous self as a virtuous self (and the virtuous self as an autonomous self), permits us to make the claim that there is no contradiction between choosing freely and choosing what is good. Once this conception is in place, a rich moral language, one that allows us to discuss virtues and vices, becomes available to us.

In this chapter, I want to draw on a version of neo-Aristotelian virtue ethics to lay the foundation for a model of autonomy that is oriented around virtues and teleologically aimed at the achievement of genuinely valuable goals. I shall argue that it is quite possible and even necessary to tie the value of autonomy to the achievement of genuinely valuable things *and* to the pluralistic requirement that we have multiple morally sound options open to us from which we can choose; and that, moreover, understanding autonomy in a way that is responsive to the requirements of virtue ethics better protects the interests of the weak and vulnerable than the value-free conception that currently prevails in bioethics.

A virtuous life can easily be—perhaps even must be—an autonomous one, as someone who still needs the moral guidance provided by others in order to know what to do is not yet fully virtuous nor fully autonomous, but still learning what both require. Moreover, there are many different ways in which a virtuous life can be lived, even though they all, as Aristotle argues, are ultimately directed towards the unitary goal of happiness or flourishing. Of course, since autonomy is a modern concept, the language of autonomy is not, itself, used by Aristotle (nor often, to my knowledge, by those who call themselves virtue ethicists). However, as Hursthouse notes, no neo-Aristotelian need consider herself committed to every detail of Aristotle's account, any more than deontologists inspired by Kant believe that they must accept his views on animals. (Indeed, some defenders of animal rights use versions of Kantian arguments to support their claims.) Instead, virtue ethicists believe that Aristotle's views "can fruitfully be adapted to yield what we now recognize as moral truth."[8]

We have been exploring the way in which different moral approaches revolve around distinct and incompatible conceptions of the self. It is these conceptions of the self, as we have seen, which are responsible for the identification of what the theory or approach takes to be morally significant and why; these selves, moreover, move through moral universes in which reality is described and mapped in distinctive ways. I want now to make explicit a claim which has been, up to now, largely implicit, namely, that our self-conceptions—mine and yours and everyone else's—are shaped by the ideas that surround us, including ideas about what human beings are and how we should live. If we inhabit a social and intellectual world that emphasizes individualism and choice, then we will come to understand ourselves as individuals whose flourishing consists in our freedom to choose.

In addition, the shared ideas that we internalize, that become part of our self-conceptions, will be reflected in the activities we engage in, and in the institutions we create. For example, if our culture emphasizes the importance of religion and of preparing for the afterlife, many of us will incorporate religious beliefs into our self-conceptions, will contribute to the building of pyramids and cathedrals, and will participate in the religious and social practices that result from this shared understanding. If our society places priority on the accumulation of wealth, and views those who are most successful in this enterprise with a mixture of envy and respect, then many of us, too, will come to believe that we would be happy if only we were as rich as they are. However, a virtue-based approach is predicated on the belief that some ways of living are genuinely better than others, and that most of us want to make choices that will actually help us live well. As we shall see, one of the strengths of virtue ethics is that it allows us both to recognize that we are shaped in this way without drawing the relativistic conclusion that there is nothing more to be said, no further judgments that can be made. In addition, such an approach provides us with a conceptual framework that helps us distinguish good ways of living from mediocre or bad ones.

Kleinman argues that we can understand the self as being like a rocky shoreline that seems, from one day to the next, largely unchanged, but which is in fact constantly battered by currents and storms so that, over time, channels move and markers shift. The limits of the self "are set by the principles and empirical reality of biology and psychology. The self is moored by the neurobiological hardwiring of rude sentiment and the rough genetic scaffolding of personality."[9] Like a physical shoreline, currents, sudden storms, and high tides batter the topography of the self.

We are, for instance, shaped by our encounters with other selves: "Remorse, regret, and other complexes of emotions and values are strongly influenced by interpersonal relations and meanings that contribute to the building of subtle and elaborated sensibilities that constitute who we are."[10] We are not only shaped by interactions with others, however, but also by the cultural landscape through which our lives move: "culture, politics, and economics transform each of us if not from day to day, then from year to year as jobs change, careers transmute, families undergo growth and collapse, marriages rise and fall, and the large historical forces that shape the destiny of nations and influence entire populations roll over our lives, grinding us, wearing away, shifting, making us let go and move on."[11] And, it is important to note, these changes are not morally neutral: some of them contribute to our flourishing and some inhibit it; some promote the development of an inner life which is rich and complex and support the creation of an outer world that is satisfying, just, and productive, others to inner lives that are flattened and impoverished, and a shared world that is exploitative, dangerous, and uncertain.

Kleinman worries that the world we live in now is not a world that contributes to our flourishing, but one which is increasingly superficial, materialistic, and devoid of public spaces within which moral values can be seriously discussed. In the process, we are becoming transformed as well, in danger of becoming something new and frightening, focused on consumption, choice, and pleasure, a world in which moral angst is transformed into psychological conditions that can be treated with pharmaceuticals, and one in which, moreover, we have an increasingly difficult time describing our own moral situation: "When this happens, the furnishings of our interior are no longer the same; we are not the same people our grandparents were, and our children will not be the same kind of people we are."[12]

The conception of autonomy employed by standard bioethics, as we have seen, is drawn primarily from the self-moral-political account, which directly generates the Divided Self and, increasingly in bioethics, indirectly spawns the Choosing Self. It is not a conception of autonomy that allows us to easily ask substantive moral questions in bioethics, because it is predicated on the claim that judgments of the worth of the things we choose are up to each of us to make for ourselves. As a result, not only is it difficult for bioethicists to discuss moral concerns in substantive rather than procedural ways, the kind of bioethics that results provides few resources for individuals facing difficult choices in their own lives, such as whether or not to have an abortion, or to be pre-symptomatically tested for Huntington's Disease. These choices are understood to be their own to make, but little guidance is provided for how they might be evaluated, or for considering what their long-term implications might be. Moreover, as long as persons make choices that do not violate the Harm Principle in some clear and uncontroversial way, no particular way of living can be judged better (or worse) than any other.

I have already argued that a bioethics predicated on this conception of autonomy, paradoxically, undermines the claim that bioethicists make that they possess a particular kind of professional expertise. I now want to argue, further, that this conception of autonomy is not one that contributes to our flourishing as individuals or as human beings; it does not, that is to say, help us experience rich and morally nuanced inner lives, provide resources that help us confront illness and suffering, or give us a reason to participate in the creation and maintenance of a just and satisfying outer world arranged in a way that contributes to human flourishing more generally. What it does, (contrary to the expectations of liberal theorists who have constructed and defended this conception of autonomy, and the self-image of bioethicists who employ it in their deliberations) is give us little reason to be confident that the choices we make are genuinely good ones, (good, that is to say, in two respects: good for us, and morally sound). Consequently, it leaves us vulnerable to manipulation and exploitation by others as a result because it does not provide any measure against which the options open to us might be examined, except our own desires and our internal reflections upon them. Consequently, if those desires are inculcated in us by (for example) advertisers or politicians, we will have few resources by which to evaluate either their source or their content. (This point will be discussed more fully below, and in chapter 9).

In addition, it provides very little in the way of a shared moral language that allows us to describe and explore features of the human condition that pull us beyond, or away from autonomy (such as the experience of illness, and the disintegration of the self that can sometimes result). In contrast, or so I hope to demonstrate, a conception of the autonomous self built on the moral framework provided by virtue ethics can contribute, in practical and straightforward ways, to our flourishing as individuals and as human beings because it provides us with a broader range of moral terms to employ, and draws attention not only to the characteristics that make each of us unique, but also to things that we share, simply in virtue of the fact that we are human beings. It is this conception of autonomy, or some version of it, that bioethicists should employ and defend.

Interestingly, the clearest way to see the difference between these two conceptions of autonomy is not to focus on examples of individuals whom virtue ethicists would consider to be vicious (the genocidal dictator, the serial killer, or the corrupt politician) because the behavior of such people can also be condemned on the liberal account: however autonomous their actions, their behavior clearly violates the Harm Principle. The more striking cases, then, are those that meet the requirements of liberal or bioethical autonomy (that is to say, could be endorsed by the Divided Self and the Choosing Self), but which would fail the virtue test because they are clearly not examples of flourishing lives lives which are teleologically aimed at the achievement of the good, filled with the things that human flourishing requires (friendships, accomplishments, families), and which demonstrate the exercise of the virtues as much as the avoidance of the vices.

One of the stranger characters we have encountered in our explorations is Rawls's example of the man who enjoys counting blades of grass. Recall that this individual enjoys spending his time engaged in only one activity, counting blades of grass in parks and in other places where grass is contained within geometrically shaped expanses—although he is of normal intelligence and psychology. Given that it is this activity that provides him with pleasure, the most rational long-term plan for him, Rawls says, is to shape his life around it because it constitutes his conception of the good. Since his activity harms no one, it meets the requirements of liberal justice, and since this man has freely chosen to engage in this activity after identifying that it gives him pleasure, there is little more that any of us could or should say about this choice. We might find it an odd way to live, perhaps, and even wonder why someone would enjoy counting blades of grass, let alone design his entire life around this activity since most of us would find it pointless and boring, but we would also have to acknowledge that other people might think the same thing about those activities that give *us* pleasure. *I* might enjoy reading philosophy texts, which *you* find almost as pointless and boring as counting blades of grass; *you* might enjoy selling mutual funds, something that would make my eyes glaze over and my brain freeze up. This man, then, should be left alone to count his blades of grass: we should recognize both his right to pursue the good as he sees fit, and our own epistemic inability to make objective and rationally grounded judgments about which ways of living are morally better and which are morally worse, as long as the lives we are considering don't involve clear and uncontroversial violations of the Harm Principle.

From the perspective of neo-Aristotelian virtue ethics, however, there is much more to say, both about the choice he is making, and about our capacity to distinguish good choices from bad ones. Aristotle argues that everything that exists has a goal or purpose, and that these goals or purposes are built in by nature. What is true of natural objects is true of human activities as well: "Every act and every enquiry, and similarly every action as well as choice is held to aim at some good. Hence people have nobly declared that the good is that at which all things aim."[13] Whatever we do, we have some end in mind, some goal that we want to achieve, even if we do not always explicitly articulate it to ourselves or to others. One way to identify this goal is to ask questions, such as: "Why are you reading this book?"; "Why are you sitting on this ethics committee?"; and "Why are you counting blades of grass?" and give answers such as "Because I am interested in the concept of the self"; "Because I want to contribute to making this hospital a more ethical place"; and "Counting blades of grass gives me pleasure."

We consider every end that we strive for, Aristotle believes, to be valuable, since no one strives for something that he considers to be bad. Further, he argues, there must be an ultimate or final goal, something which is valued for its own sake, not because it produces some particular good; he famously identifies this goal as *eudaimonia*, which is usually translated as "happiness" or "flourishing," and which means essentially living well or doing well. Happiness, as Aristotle understands it, is not a feeling, like pleasure or amusement; it is, rather, a way of living that requires us to live in accordance with what reason tells us is the proper purpose of human beings.

We can see, in this claim, that Aristotle's ethics is connected to his metaphysics, to his assertion that *everything* has a function or purpose, not only human activities or creations, but also natural things things like trees, dogs, and, of course, human beings. In fact, we do not really know what something is until we know what its function or purpose is. Acorns, for example, while they may resemble other seeds, have, as their built-in purpose, to become oak trees: "Thus, we may say that *what it is to be* an acorn is to be something that by nature strives to become an oak. In this way, the acorn is *defined* in terms of its purpose, its goal. Therefore, the oak is *prior* to the acorn in the order of explanation; that is, in order to understand what an acorn is, one must first understand what an oak tree is."[14] In short, we can distinguish some thing from other things, even other similar things, if we can find its essence, that feature which uniquely makes it what it is and which is not shared with anything else.

Moreover, something is a good example of what it is when it performs its function well. A doctor who keeps her patients healthy, who minimizes their suffering, who will put aside her own plans when this is necessary to help a patient, is a good doctor; a pen that writes well, which is well balanced and comfortable to hold, is a good pen; a heart which pumps blood well and keeps a regular rhythm is a good heart; and a human being who lives as a human being should, whose actions correspond to the requirements of the Mean and demonstrate the exercise of practical reason, is a good human being, both in the sense that he is doing what a person should *and* because, by performing in this way, he is behaving virtuously. Further, while the function of a doctor is to heal, a pen to write, a heart to circulate blood, and a human being to live in accordance with reason, the best examples of these things perform their functions not only adequately or well, but also with excellence. As Aristotle puts it, "So it must be stated that every virtue both brings that of which it is the virtue into a good condition and causes the work belonging to that thing to be done well. For example, the virtue of the eye both makes the eye and its work excellent, for by means of the virtue of the eye, we see well."[15] And what is true of organs like the eye is also true of living creatures: "Similarly, the virtue of a horse makes the horse both excellent and good when it comes to running and carrying a rider, and standing its ground before enemies. If indeed this is so in all cases, then the virtue of a human being would be that characteristic as a result of which a human being becomes good and as a result of which he causes his own work to be done well."[16]

In this picture, learning to become a virtuous person—fulfilling, we might say, our naturally built-in purpose, just as an acorn fulfills its built-in purpose if it falls on fertile ground and grows to become an oak tree—will make us happy. We should strive to become the best human beings we can be, which means, Aristotle believes, to become virtuous, because it is in this that our excellence consists: "the human good becomes an activity of the soul in accordance with virtue."[17] We learn to be virtuous in much the same way as Aristotle's horse learns to stand its ground in battle, and we learn to do other practical things, like read, ride a bike, use a computer, or drive a car: we initially need to have instruction from those who already understand what virtue consists in, and then we practice until we are able to do it ourselves, at first with difficulty and then with ease. Over time, we will no longer struggle to be courageous, generous, or honest, just as once we have learned to read, ride a bike, use a computer, or drive a car, we no longer find these things difficult. Indeed, as we become proficient and then excellent, it becomes hard to remember why we ever found these things hard to do.

As Lear observes, "For Aristotle, character is a developmental and psychological achievement. We are habituated into certain character formations by our parents, family, and teachers, who get us to act in certain ways repeatedly, before we can understand the reasons for doing so."[18] Over time, of course, "We thereby develop certain stable psychic dispositions to see and think about the social environment in certain ways and to act accordingly. This is our 'second nature.'"[19] Consequently, in this approach, there is an important connection between the roles we occupy and the virtues we need to be educated in so that they become, over time, our "second nature." As we perform the activities and engage in the practices that are characteristic of particular roles and do so in the proper way, we learn what it is that the role requires of us and are shaped accordingly. From this perspective, then, just as we can ask what features a good or excellent war horse must demonstrate, so we can ask about the virtues of a good or excellent teacher, politician, personal support worker, nurse, or physician ought to possess and demonstrate. An important part of learning what these roles require of us, then, goes far beyond learning a set of technical skills; rather, we need to learn how to think, feel, and act in the ways in which good or excellent exemplars of these roles think, feel, and act.

Importantly, what it means to be a good reader, an agile bike rider, a competent computer user, or a safe driver is determined by our ability to meet standards that are external to us, independent of our personal judgments, and widely recognized: an over-confident sixteen-year-old who just got his driver's license lacks the experience necessary not only to be an excellent driver, but also to correctly judge his own abilities. And so it is in the case of virtue: *my* believing that I am courageous, honest, and generous does not make me so, unless my actions, judgments, and emotional responses demonstrate that I am, according to criteria which are independent of my own evaluation, and do so consistently, over time. Likewise, what it means to be a good or excellent nurse, physician, and personal support worker are set out by standards that are external to the beliefs about their own capacities held by any particular inhabitant of those roles. Finally, the context in which virtue is learned, demonstrated, and perfected is, Aristotle makes clear, that of a whole life: "For one swallow does not make a spring, nor does one day. And in this way, one day or a short time does not make one blessed or happy either."[20] What this indicates is that, like autonomy, the capacity and achievement of virtue develop as we grow and learn more and more clearly what is required of us.

The flip side of this portrait of the virtuous person is, of course, the vicious one, and less starkly, the person whose character remains merely adequate, but who never becomes fully virtuous, never quite manages to act as virtue requires, or who often manages to act appropriately, but never does so with ease and pleasure. Such individuals are like the person who can read but only with great difficulty, or the driver who somehow manages to keep his license, but who gets into frequent fender-benders. People become vicious, or fail to develop fully virtuous characters, when their educations is inadequate, aimed at the wrong things, or they are not given sufficient opportunity to practice, so that acting virtuously never becomes their "second nature." Importantly, just as it is objectively the case that acorns need fertile soil, sunlight, and water to grow, and these things in the right amounts to flourish, so, too, human beings can become vicious or incompletely developed if the larger political and social contexts in which they are raised are wrong-headed, unjust, or distorted in some way, just as it is the case that social and political arrangements that are well structured can contribute to human flourishing.

The virtuous human being, then, is teleologically oriented: it is by determining what is the proper function of human beings that the good for human beings is identified, and the person who is educated properly will likewise make choices that are designed to bring her closer, as a particular individual, to achieving that good in her own life. This will not mean that her life will follow a preset pattern—she will live in a particular time and place, have particular strengths and weaknesses, and will pursue a particular career (or careers), will share her life with particular other people—but it does mean that she will ask herself not only the question "What do I want to do with my life?" but, also, "Which of the possibilities open to me will bring me closer to flourishing as an individual and as a human being?" Her autonomous choices will be informed as much by the latter question as by the former.

In addition, the virtuous person will not assume that living a virtuous life will necessarily mean living an easy life; rather, she will be aware that the lives of human beings always take place against a backdrop of things over which they have no control, and that, as embodied creatures, human beings are fragile and vulnerable. She will practice being virtuous, will recognize that it is primarily through interactions with other people that opportunities to be virtuous or vicious arise, and will look to those who provide good examples as a guide. She will recognize that what it means to display virtue or vice depends on criteria that are external to her, and against which her own actions, intellectual judgments, and emotional responses can be measured.

Finally, because the social, cultural, and political backdrop against which particular human lives play themselves out affects not only what possibilities are open to those persons, but also can be better or worse at promoting and permitting human flourishing, the Virtuous Self will take moral, social, and political questions seriously, and will seek to address political policies which are unjust and social arrangements which are manipulative, exploitative, or oppressive. The virtuous person can employ a rich moral language to describe her own choices and those made by others, and the social and political structures of her own society. Consequently, she will not only talk about what she wants, feels, or needs, but also about whether wanting, feeling, or needing those things is courageous or cowardly, selfish or generous, and whether they contribute to the living of a virtuous life and the creation of a better world, or whether they detract from these goals.

We are now in a position to identify more clearly what is wrong with the life of the man who enjoys counting blades of grass, and why a self-moral-political theory or bioethical framework which accepts his choice as a perfectly valid example of what it means to live an autonomous life embraces a peculiar model of what human flourishing comes to, and why a bioethics that understands autonomy in the same way is misguided. While this man is not vicious, he is clearly not fully developed, morally speaking. Perhaps his moral education was inadequate, in which case, the way he is living, far from demonstrating what it means to live an autonomous life, is a preventable tragedy. While his life is not harmful to others, it makes no contribution to them, either. If he really orients his entire life around this activity, then, when it is over, his life will have been wasted: he has accomplished nothing, added nothing to his community or the lives of those around him, and has not even fully developed his own capacities.

If this is not a life that one would want for oneself, one's friends, or one's child (and it would be hard to take someone seriously if he claimed that he would not be concerned if someone he cared about chose to live his life in this way), then it appears that we do have shared conceptions of what it means to live well (and of what a wasted life might look like), even if we cannot specify, in advance and completely comprehensively, all the details of those lives, and this minimal agreement can provide the basis for a further discussion about what it means to be virtuous, to be vicious, to flourish, and to fail to do so.

FIXING A BOAT WHILE AT SEA: VIRTUE ETHICS AND THE NEURATHIAN PROCEDURE

I have argued that there is no neutral, external perspective from which moral claims can be judged and moral issues evaluated. Rather, each contender for that external position, upon examination, actually reveals itself to be as much a highly structured work of the moral imagination as a product of the rational exercise of the intellect, as the identification of the various conceptions of the self which animate these theories reveals. However, the claim that such a neutral and external perspective can be found has an entrenched place in modern ethical thinking, and mainstream bioethics, which works primarily with approaches that fall within the theoretical-juridical model of moral theorizing, often asserts or implies that the principles it endorses and the conception of autonomy it employs, are ideas which are justified both *from* this neutral and external place, and *because* they can be found there. And these things are asserted or implied despite the inability of bioethicists to resolve long-standing moral issues such as abortion, or even to work through particular cases in the same way. The danger of this assumption is that it can encourage us to believe that we have already achieved this perspective, and that anyone who disagrees with us is wrong. In short, we can confuse our feeling of moral certainty with the attainment of moral truth. Moreover, it is ironic and even paradoxical that many of the ethicists who work within mainstream bioethics are so skeptical about the possibility of identifying the characteristics of good lives, when they are so certain about the principles they use, the importance of rights, the legitimate place of the market in facilitating choice, the correctness of the Harm Principle, and the nature of autonomy.

As Fitterer notes, modern Western culture including our thinking in ethics, "is beholden to a notion of objectivity ascribed to the empirical and theoretical sciences—bracketed emotions, identically trained colleagues, accurate and widely accepted standards of measurement, theoretical laws, absolute constraints, mathematical degrees of certainty, and so forth."[21] However, he argues, the attempt to apply the kind of certainty and objectivity proper to the hard sciences to our ethical reasoning has produced nothing but difficulty. "Ethically charged decisions such as which books I should permit my young children to read do not obviously call for such criteria as absolute precision, consensus among all parents, or inference from theoretical descriptions of the good or the right."[22] These things require judgment, and, as Aristotle reminds us, the degree of certainty and precision we can expect from our enquiries depends both on the subject in question and on what it is that we hope to discover about it: "one must not seek out precision in all matters alike but rather in each thing in turn as accords with the subject matter in question and insofar as is appropriate to the enquiry. For both carpenter and geometer seek out the right angle but in different ways: the former seeks it out insofar as it is useful to his work; the latter seeks out what it is or what sort of thing it is, for he is the one who contemplates the truth."[23] Consequently, what we need to make, Fitterer argues, "is a distinction between the kind of objectivity proper to the hard sciences and that proper to ethics."[24]

It is exactly this kind of distinction that the neo-Aristotelian virtue ethicist tries to make. The first thing we need to give up is the idea that the character of the moral agent is unimportant, and that it does not matter who is making the moral judgment. "There is no possibility of 'justifying morality from the outside' by appealing to anything non-moral or by finding a neutral point of view that the fairly virtuous and the wicked can share."[25] The virtue ethicist recognizes that there is nothing the virtuous can say to convince the moral skeptic, the morally indifferent, or the psychopath, since they do not even share the most basic assumptions on which such a conversation could be based.

Instead, we discover moral truth together, by engaging in conversations about the nature of morality with others who share our commitment to it. However, it is important to understand that it does not follow from this claim that we "make morality up," or that there are no objective criteria we can employ to guide our discussions: the virtue ethicist is not a relativist. Rather, we should keep in mind the Socratic point that it is through rational conversation of a particular sort, in which individuals are committed to examining, together, what morality comes to, that we are able to see more clearly what we ought to believe. The virtuous life is a shared life, and the pursuit of morally justified claims must be a shared pursuit (if the claims we make are, in the end, to have any authority over others). If we move away from the theoretical-juridical template of what ethical knowledge consists in (primarily, certain kinds of neutral propositions, which each of us could discover on our own and which both the virtuous and the non-virtuous can agree on in the same way that they can agree on scientific truths or mathematical calculations) and see them, instead, as existing externally to us but discovered together, and exhibited through shared forms of social life, we can recognize the social nature of ethics without succumbing to an "everything and anything goes" kind of relativism. We can, that is to say, find the kind of objectivity appropriate to ethics.

This kind of objectivity can be discovered, Hursthouse argues, through the application of what she calls, following Quine and McDowell, "a Neurathian procedure." The virtue ethicist assumes "that there is a space within which the rational validation of beliefs about which character traits are the virtues could proceed," in a way does not assume "either the excessive demands of ethical foundationalism" or that is reducible to "mere rationalizations of one's personal or culturally inculcated values."[26] The Neurathian procedure asks us to imagine a mariner who must fix and maintain, and over time, perhaps, even completely rebuild, his ship while at sea. He cannot, of course, do this all at once. Instead, he must replace a rotten plank here, a piece of wiring there. Our conceptual scheme is like this ship: we cannot replace it overnight or all at once. However, over time, we can replace the bits of it that don't work, improve the parts that could work better, and, ultimately, end up with something very different, something that reflects our better understanding and our improved judgment.

Neo-Aristotelianism, Hursthouse believes, allows us to think about ethics in radically new ways, through the application of this procedure, despite the fact that Aristotle's theory is one of the oldest in the Western ethical tradition. "Now once we have the Neurathian 'There's no basing knowledge on an *independent* foundation' image firmly in mind, we can see the possibility of *radical* ethical reflection, the critical scrutiny of one's ethical beliefs which could be genuinely revisionary and not merely a reiteration of an acquired ethical outlook, despite proceeding from within it."[27]

The Neurathian procedure helps us achieve the kind of objectivity appropriate to ethics because it allows us to distinguish between what we *currently* believe (which may well be mistaken) and what we *ought* to believe, without asserting that the latter can be discovered in some abstract place (whether we call that place "the common morality," "the original position," or the disinterested God's-eye view of the benevolent, rational utilitarian spectator) that exists apart from the particular experiences, beliefs, commitments, and deliberations of actually existing people.

TWO OBJECTIONS

There are two important objections to virtue ethics that need to be considered. The first is the conceptual claim that teleology is false—that there is no way that humans ought to live, no purposes built-in to anything by nature—and that, therefore, virtue ethics of any neo-Aristotelian form is a non-starter because it is built on an entirely untenable foundation. The second objection is a moral-political one, which holds that a belief in teleology is politically dangerous and morally problematic because it will permit some people to feel justified in imposing their moral beliefs on others who don't share them,

and will authorize politicians to construct the apparatus of the state on perfectionist lines. (The frequent concerns expressed by bioethicists about legislation and regulation itself, rather than about which of the options open to
individuals are morally sound, reflects this concern.)

While these two objections are logically distinct, they are often joined
together in a single claim which suggests that the belief in teleology is
politically and morally dangerous because teleology is false, which means
that an application of it within the spheres of politics and morality necessarily involves the imposition of particular views which are nothing more—
because they can be nothing more—than personal opinion. I will consider
each objection is turn, and then suggest ways in which a neo-Aristotelian
might respond.

The first objection holds that Aristotle was simply wrong to build a moral
scheme on a teleological foundation, and that any virtue ethicists who follow
in his footsteps are simply wrong as well. As Bartlett and Collins observe,
"In our time, a chorus of voices . . . protest, if not in unison then in perfect
harmony: there is no single greatest human good or best way of life! Everyone now knows that nobody knows what the good life is!"[28] Aristotle, in
short, was an idiot: "To undergraduate freshmen and sophisticated scholars
alike, this view of things is mother's milk, which means that the average
freshman is superior, in the most important respect and without lifting a
finger, to Aristotle himself."[29] However, they point out, Aristotle was well
aware that many people did not share his views; indeed, ancient Greece was
home to the Sophists, whose relativism was even "more radical and impres-
sive than our own."[30]

Why then, we should ask, are we so quick to assume that Aristotle was so
wrong that we do not even need to consider his approach seriously and work
to understand it, before we reject it? Individuals who have not conducted a
full enquiry into the question "must admit that they are guided less by knowledge than by sanctioned opinion, or by inherited prejudice, in a matter whose
importance goes well beyond the proper approach to an old book,"[31] because
the questions that Aristotle is considering—how we ought to live and what
human beings need to flourish—ought to be deeply significant for all of us.

If we put prejudice and received opinion aside, and remember that the
Nuerathian procedure does not require us to replace all of our conceptual
schemes at once, we can see multiple roles that a tentative acceptance of
teleology might play in helping us address ethical questions, including questions about the purpose of ethics. While the characteristics of human beings,
and therefore of the nature of human flourishing, may not be identifiable in
some hard, fast, and entirely uncontroversial way, as Kleinman's image of a
shore battered by winds and currents suggests, there are, nonetheless, consistent features which—like the rocks that make up the shoreline and the water
that shapes them—persist, but which we can only see once we accept the

possibility that they are there. There is a common scaffolding, built out of elements of physiology and psychology, DNA and physical embodiment, that all human beings share, and out of which shared conceptions of the human good can be articulated and explored.

Moreover, Hursthouse argues, we should notice that we evaluate other species all the time, and can identify, as we do this, instances of particular individuals that are flourishing, and others that are failing to do so. Gardeners do this, as they monitor the growth of their vegetables over the course of the summer (Are they getting enough water? Have they been attacked by aphids?); dog owners do this, when they buy a dog of a particular breed, and when they judge whether their animals are healthy or whether they need to see a vet; and ornithologists, who compile guidebooks for bird watchers to help them identify the kind of bird they are looking at, and where and when particular species might be found, have no difficulty distinguishing one species of bird from another, even though individual members of a species may differ in noticeable ways and be found far outside their expected habitat. "Looking at the evaluation of other living things, we should be struck by the extent to which they depend on our identifying what is *characteristic* of the species (and / or special members of it)."[32]

Moreover, she notes, "The other sophisticated social animals have a characteristic life expectancy, characteristic ways of continuing their species, characteristic pleasures, sufferings, and freedom from suffering, characteristic ways of going on in their social group, and it is in the light of what is characteristic of them that they are evaluated."[33] Again, while individual members of a species may differ in particular ways, our understanding of what, generally speaking, is characteristic of a thing of that sort, allows us to make an assessment of whether they are doing well or badly: "If they are good x's, they will, with a bit of luck, be thriving or flourishing in their characteristically x way, living well, as x's, unless something external to themselves is preventing it."[34]

And, Hursthouse asks, if we can do this with other species, why are we so reluctant to think that we can do it with human beings? If we are willing to try, what we might discover is that many people are *not* living well: "Does anyone think that, regarding ourselves as a collection of social groups or as a global one, we are flourishing, living well as human beings? Surely not."[35] Many people live in conditions that barely allow them to survive let alone to flourish, and many people, from greedy bankers, to genocidal tyrants and corrupt politicians behave viciously, worsening the lives of those around them. Virtue ethics, in Hursthouse's view, far from making us complacent about our current social and political situation and focusing only on our own moral development, has the potential to galvanize us to action.

There is a common misconception that endorsing virtue ethics requires the person making that endorsement to move in a conservative direction, to argue in support of old-fashioned and reactionary ways of thinking, and to justify current institutional arrangements rather than working to transform them. However, while some versions of virtue ethics may lead in conservative directions (just as some versions of liberalism end up providing support for existing institutions, political structures, and social arrangements) virtue ethics can be as revolutionary as Marxism and as transformative as feminism, since it requires that political, economic, and social arrangements be reconfigured if they do not, in fact, contribute to human flourishing. As Lisa Tessman argues, virtue ethics provides a very useful lens through which to think about "liberatory political struggles, for one might portray oppression as a set of barriers to flourishing and think about political resistance as a way of eradicating these barriers and enabling flourishing."[36] Indeed, she observes, "there is some notion of flourishing implicit in . . . [all] projects of political resistance for without some idea of what is a better and what is a worse life, there is no explanation of nor motivation for the commitment to change systems of oppression."[37] Virtue ethics, then, contains within it a measure against which existing social, political, and economic arrangements can be examined and critiqued, and articulates a goal—namely, creating the conditions that make human flourishing possible—that their activities should be working to achieve.

The virtuous self can only develop, act, and flourish when political, economic, and social circumstances are arranged so as to allow and encourage this flourishing, and, as a result, structures of oppression, domination, and exploitation can arguably be more clearly seen and easily evaluated when viewed through the lens provided by virtue ethics than through the lenses provided by most of its competitors. Moreover, vices, and the social, political, and economic arrangements that encourage their development and permit their exercise, can also be clearly seen and named, in ways that are impossible within most competing approaches. We can—and we must—not only consider (for ourselves and for others) whether choices are freely made in the sense that procedural requirements for non-interference are met, but also whether the context in which they were made actually allows individuals to make choices that are free and that genuinely contribute to their flourishing; moreover, we also need a moral language that allows us to describe some choices as greedy, callous, selfish, or cruel.

This claim is important, because the second objection—that accepting a teleological approach is politically and morally dangerous—is often connected to the first objection, that teleology is false, and that, therefore, the concept of human flourishing (understood in a teleological sense) when attached to the question of which political or social arrangements will promote or inhibit it necessarily requires the imposition of one person's (or group's) personal values on the larger citizenry. As Bartlett and Collins put it, "because we can know not the good but only the fact of its 'subjectivity' and 'relativity,' each of us really has no alternative but to pursue happiness according to whichever opinions of it propel us onward, while tolerating or celebrating as much as possible the differing opinions of others."[38] This belief, they add, "constitutes the orthodoxy of our time; it is for us the chief product of the modern revolt from ancient thought in general and from Aristotle in particular."[39]

Let us examine an articulate defense of this orthodox assumption, and then consider whether or not it is entirely convincing. In a spirited defense of liberal political morality that is built on this modern orthodoxy, Kymlicka defends the position that it is wrong to interfere with the judgments people make about their own choices and lives. His defense has moral implications as well, because, as we have seen, bioethicists who accept this orthodoxy are similarly disposed to defend the claim that it is impossible to make justified moral judgments about the choices that individuals make (even though they have no difficulty asserting, with a high degree of certainty, that the conception of autonomy that follows from this moral skepticism is itself correct).

The basic political morality espoused by liberals is, he argues, connected to claims about our essential interests: "Our essential interest is in having a good life, in having those things a good life contains."[40] This claim has certain consequences, one of the most important of which is that we may be mistaken about the value of the life we are presently leading: "leading a good life is different from leading the life we *currently believe* to be good."[41] We may discover, at certain points in our lives, that what we previously thought worthwhile, and the goods we were pursuing, are, in fact, valueless, or, at least, not as valuable as we thought them to be. We may, moreover, have deliberated long and hard about these goals, and even manage to achieve them, which means that "we may regret our decisions even when things have gone as planned."[42]

We deliberate, then, not only about how to achieve our goals, but also about whether those goals are really worth pursuing. However, Kymlicka argues that even if our belief in the value of what we are doing is *clearly* mistaken (we may have decided, for example, to spend our life counting blades of grass in public parks), it does not follow that others have the right to come along and alter our lives for us, in order to correct our mistakes: "On the contrary, no life goes better by being led from the outside, according to values the person doesn't endorse. My life only goes better if I'm leading it from the inside according to my beliefs about value."[43]

A life that is in fact good, then, Kymlicka argues, has two requirements: one is that we be allowed to revise our beliefs as we go along, in the light of experience and new information, and the other is that our life be led from the inside, "in accordance with our beliefs about what gives value to life."[44] These requirements provide an explanation for the traditional liberal concerns to protect certain civil and personal liberties, such as freedom of expression and freedom of the press because these liberties provide individuals with the tools necessary both to become aware of different conceptions of the good life, and to continually examine and revise (if necessary) their own views in the light of various sorts of information and new considerations. The basis of liberal self-moral-political theory, Kymlicka claims, is formed by this account of our essential interests. This means that, according to liberalism, "since our most essential interest is in getting these beliefs right, and acting on them, government treats people as equals, with equal concern and respect, by providing for each individual the liberties and resources needed to examine and act on these beliefs."[45] This, in a nutshell, "forms the basis of contemporary liberal theories of justice."[46]

Arguably, however, there are tensions within this "essential interests" account, tensions that reflect incoherencies within the larger liberal self-moral-political framework that Kymlicka is trying to defend (as well, of course, with the arguments that employ the Divided and Choosing Selves that emerge from it). The unproblematic claim (1) that a valuable way of life may *in fact* be quite different from the one we currently believe to be valuable and the (equally unproblematic) claim (2) that liberal freedoms are valuable because they enable us to come to reasoned conclusions about what *in fact* makes a life good, do not, even when combined, seem to support the claim that (3) what is crucially important is that our lives be led from the inside. What is more important: that our beliefs about value are (at least partially) valid, or that we endorse them, even if they are mistaken?

The first two claims suggest the former, while the last claim suggests the latter. But what arguments might be given in support of the claim that it is how we *feel* about our lives that is most important, even if our beliefs about the value of the pursuits we engage in is mistaken? It seems that one would have to give an argument that such a belief is valuable in itself. But why might this be the case? Might it not be argued that if this belief is mistaken (and we must keep in mind that it is a belief about a very important matter, namely, the value of what we are doing with our lives), then this is enough to render its value dubious? If it would be better for us to realize that we are mistaken as fast as possible (because we are *in fact* not making the most of our lives), why should it be thought impermissible for someone else to make us aware of our mistake?

If we follow the example set by Socrates, we do not treat persons with respect when we ignore the fact that we believe that their important choices are mistaken; rather, we treat them as fellow human beings who are capable of responding to rational arguments when we draw attention to why we believe these choices to be misguided. (And, of course, others should be expected to draw our mistakes to our attention when they observe them as well). What is important, arguably, when it comes to respecting other people is not that we endorse a principle of non-interference no matter what, but that we present sound reasons for the judgments that we make.

While this conclusion might make many of us uncomfortable, if we want to make a coherent defense of autonomy, it seems that there is no way of avoiding it. If we accept that the man who gets pleasure from counting blades of grass meets the requirements of liberal autonomy, as Rawls asserts, and that this choice should not be questioned by others, as Kymlicka's principle of non-interference holds, then it is arguably the case that the liberal self-moral-political framework not only does not provide sufficient resources to allow individuals to distinguish between choices that are *genuinely* good from those that are not, *and* becomes incoherent: as soon as we acknowledge (which the subject matter of ethics requires us to do, no matter what theoretical approach we are employing) that some choices we make are morally good and others morally bad, some are better at helping us live well, and others worse, and that reason can help us make these distinctions, then there is no justification for arguing that we cannot make similar judgments about the value of different ways of life when it comes to exploring questions about the nature and content of human flourishing.

We cannot, that is to say, defend autonomy itself without making the case that a life lived autonomously is better lived than a life that is not—and the same sort of arguments we give in support of this claim ought also to allow us to distinguish between better and worse conceptions of the good chosen by autonomous persons. Conversely, if we can't make justified evaluations of different conceptions of the good, then it's not clear how the superiority of a life lived autonomously over one that is non-autonomous can be demonstrated.

CONNECTING AUTONOMY TO VALUE

Given the sorry history of paternalism in medicine, bioethicists are understandably concerned with protecting the right of patients to make their own decisions. This concern has led to the central place now occupied by autonomy in contemporary bioethics. However, as I have been arguing here, the role currently played by autonomy in bioethics, coupled with the way in which the concept of autonomy is understood, undermines to a substantial degree the claim made by the bioethicist to possess a particular and specialized kind of expertise. Moreover, as we shall see when we consider illness narratives, an emphasis on autonomy has not translated into a reduction in the suffering experienced by patients. I want to argue that the issue here is not that the concept of autonomy itself is inherently misguided or problematic; it is, rather, that the particular conception of autonomy used in bioethics fits awkwardly with the questions and issues that bioethics examines. As we have seen, like the concept of justice, autonomy is a rich notion that can generate multiple and competing conceptions. The conception of autonomy used by bioethicists is drawn almost completely from the liberal self-moral-political framework and now increasingly detached from its political foundation, and it is one that is ill equipped to cope with either the realities of serious illness, or with the substantive moral judgments required by virtue ethics.

In the case of the former, it assumes capacities on the part of the person that simply may not apply to the seriously ill. In an examination of her own experiences as a critically ill patient who suffered ICU psychosis while being treated, philosopher Cheryl Misak observes that what she experienced was a kind of disintegration of the self. Since the concept of autonomy assumes a relatively stable self that persists over time, such disintegration poses a serious challenge: "As David Velleman put it, in truly extreme physical circumstances . . . a patient 'is already in the twilight of his autonomy, where self-determination is more of a shadowy presumption than a clear fact.' . . . The patient both is and is not a responsible agent in this twilight. For in such circumstances, one's self is quite literally falling apart, disintegrating, or coming undone."[47]

Arguably, then, bioethics needs to employ a richer and more complex conception of autonomy than the one it is currently using, if it is to be able to make sense of some of the most basic issues raised by illness and mortality. The situated model of autonomy that I am developing acknowledges that human beings are essentially social creatures, and that even our individual understanding of who we are is shaped by our social connections.

In this section, I want to begin the process of making a place within bioethics for this conception of autonomy by exploring the arguments Joseph Raz presents in support of an understanding of autonomy that is non-individualistic, connected to questions of well-being, and, nonetheless, pluralistic. His approach suggests that it is possible and, indeed, even necessary to connect the importance of autonomy as a model of selfhood to substantive moral questions about how we ought to live *without* thereby committing ourselves to answering those questions in a predetermined way, or imposing one person's or group's values on others who don't share them. I accept Raz's arguments, and will partially construct the figure of the Situated Self on the foundation his views provide.

There are four major components to Raz's view of autonomy. First, Raz argues that autonomy is only valuable if it is used to pursue *valuable* options. Second, he claims that autonomy can only be attained if a person has a *plurality* of valuable options to choose from. Third, the options chosen must be ones that the agent consciously endorses. The first and third claims can be understood as embodying the insight that, while conscious endorsement of one's choices is necessary if one's life is to have value, it does not follow that any life that is consistently endorsed is *therefore* valuable. Finally, Raz sometimes says that being autonomous means that we are the partial authors of our own lives.

Raz is a political philosopher, and his views demonstrate the important role played by the concept of autonomy in contemporary political philosophy. Since, as I have argued, mainstream bioethics imports a political conception of autonomy into its theoretical framework, and employs this conception extensively, Raz's views can be understood to provide a counterpart to those we have already seen, particularly the views expressed by Dworkin and Rawls. While Raz is a liberal, his account of autonomy and why we consider it valuable fits easily within the framework provided by a neo-Aristotelian account that considers both autonomy and virtue to be important components of human flourishing. Because his conception of autonomy allows us to hold both that autonomy is a central component of human flourishing and that its moral value is connected to the moral value of the choices it allows us to make, it fits better than the models that give rise to the figures of the Divided Self and the Choosing Self with the issues and questions explored by bioethics because it allows bioethicists to ask substantive moral questions about the choices people make rather than focus primarily on procedural issues, and allows them to make judgments about which choices are worth pursuing and which are not, while still recognizing that autonomous choice is important.

The first major component of Raz's view of autonomy is the claim that autonomy is only valuable if it is used in the pursuit of valuable options. While Raz affirms the value of freedom, he argues that its value does not lie in the fact that it is freedom as such, but because it allows us to do valuable things. In contrast to anti-perfectionist liberals like Rawls and Dworkin, who seem to rely on the intuition "that people's beliefs about how they should live their lives are worthy of respect purely in virtue of being their beliefs, and it is this respect for the moral opinions of her fellow citizens that leads this kind of liberal to exclude even valid ideals from politics,"[48] Raz believes that "[f]reedom to perform certain actions in certain circumstances is valuable only if it serves other values."[49]

In Raz's view, governments may be, under the right circumstances, a source of liberty because they "can create conditions which enable their subjects to enjoy greater liberty than they otherwise would."[50] Because liberals recognize that people have different conceptions of the good, most embrace anti-perfectionism because they believe that the state would be failing to treat its citizens with respect if it imposed perfectionist ideals upon them. Raz, in contrast, argues that one better treats another with respect when one "treats him in accordance with sound moral principles" than if one ignores morality in one's treatment of him, and governments (and, we might add, bioethicists) are no exception to this rule.[51]

This leads him to give three arguments against anti-perfectionism. First, while he acknowledges that much of the intuitive appeal of anti-perfectionism rests on the belief that anything else involves some individuals imposing their conceptions of the good upon others, he argues that this belief is mistaken. Practically speaking, perfectionism does not necessarily mean that the views of one group are imposed on the members of another: "Perfectionist political action may be taken in support of social institutions which enjoy unanimous support in the community, in order to bring them formal recognition, bring legal and administrative argument in line with them, facilitate their use by members of the community who wish to do so, and encourage the transmission of belief in their value to future generations."[52] Raz cites the role monogamous marriage plays in many societies as an example, and it is quite easy to think of many others, including the expectation that parents will take care of their children, the existence of hospitals that receive public money, and universally accessible educational systems. Second, as these examples show, not all perfectionist action involves the "coercive imposition of a way of life" by some groups on others.[53] Indeed, it may be primarily concerned with encouraging certain sorts of activities (by, for instance, conferring honors on those who engage in them) while discouraging others (through, for example, taxation). Third, Raz argues that "permitting governments to act on reasons that arise from ideals does not necessarily imply a rigoristic moral outlook, in that all but one morally approved form of life will be suppressed."[54]

Anyone who gives a central place in their moral scheme to the ideal of autonomy must recognize not only that we desire to be autonomous, but also that the choices we make must genuinely help us to become autonomous, and they cannot actually do this, Raz thinks, unless they are *actually* valuable, actually a means for bringing us to this goal. As Raz puts it, people have wants and pursue goals for *reasons*: they believe that the things that they desire, and sometimes even the pursuit of these things, is valuable. Goals and desires, then, are reason-dependent: if we did not believe that we had reasons to pursue them, we would no longer have them.

Further, we want our reasons to be *valid* ones; if our beliefs about their value are mistaken, we will not want to continue to desire them. If one desires to have a certain skill, solely because it will lead to employment in the future, one will not desire to have the skill if one's belief about its usefulness is mistaken: "The desire itself is not a reason; it is merely an endorsement of a reason independent of it."[55] And this is true both of those things that we desire for their own sake, and instrumental desires the realization of which will, we believe, serve other goals we have. And Raz puts this point strongly: "One does not wish merely not to have mistaken desires; one also does not wish to have them satisfied."[56]

It follows from these two claims that treating another with respect means treating her in accordance with sound moral principles, and that we pursue goals for reasons that we believe to be good, both in the sense of determining how best to bring the goals about, and in the sense of believing these goals to be worthwhile that we do not respect a person if we ignore the fact that her conception of the good is mistaken. In contrast to the anti-perfectionist intuition that people's choices should be respected simply in virtue of the fact that they are *their* choices, Raz argues that we have good reasons not to help others to obtain the things that they desire simply because they desire them, for their desires may be based on mistaken beliefs and if their beliefs are, indeed, mistaken, the sooner this becomes clear to them, the better. In short, not only do we desire to become autonomous, we want to know that the choices we make will genuinely help us to become so, and they cannot do this, Raz thinks, unless they are *actually* valuable, actually a means of bringing us to this goal.

The simple point that Raz is making here is that some goals are genuinely valuable while others are not, and that some methods for achieving them will work, while others won't. Just as perfectionism does not necessarily mean the coercive imposition of a way of life by one group upon another, so "perfectionist ideals may enter politics not because people believe in them but because they are valid; they are supported by true reasons, they correctly identify a valuable form of life."[57] As Mullhall and Swift point out, even an anti-perfectionist liberal "cannot coherently regard all moral judgments as mere expressions of subjective opinion. She must at least regard the judgment that people should be free to make up their own minds about how they should live as objectively valid."[58] Why, then, do they seem to believe that the lifestyle choices people make about themselves and their own lives lack the same sort of objective foundation?

Raz is suspicious of the claim that a distinction can be made "between two kinds of moral judgment: judgments about the good life, which are subjective and should be kept out of politics, and judgments about the rights and duties people have and that should govern their relations with one another, which are objective and are properly protected and enforced by the coercive apparatus of the liberal state."[59] And the same question might be asked of bioethicists: if they are so certain that the principles they employ are correct, that rights are important, that freedom is a genuine good, then why are they so reluctant to believe that the choices individuals make within a bioethical context cannot be examined, questioned, or justified in much the same way that these bioethical values can be examined and defended? How can bioethicists whose arguments depend on the presence of the Choosing Self simultaneously be so certain that autonomy is so fundamentally important, morally speaking, that it ought almost always to be respected, and so skeptical about the possibility of making justified moral judgments about the value of the things autonomous individuals choose?

And if Raz is right to think that certain ways of living our lives are objectively better than others—that it is better, say, to be a farmer than a sweat shop owner, a physician than a porn star, a journalist than a mercenary—and that we can be as sure about this as we can be that a free press is a good thing, "then he removes a major motivation for anti-perfectionism."[60] And a parallel argument can be given in the case of bioethics: can't we make the objectively justifiable judgment that there is something troubling about the desire of parents to control not only the environment in which their children are raised, but who are also willing to use genetic technologies not simply to reduce the likelihood that they will be afflicted by conditions that cause suffering, but to shape them in a fashion that conforms with their particular conceptions of the good? Can't we legitimately restrict the number of embryos that are implanted in patients undergoing IVF, even if individuals want to exceed this limit in the hope that it will increase their chance of getting pregnant, when the result may be the birth of seriously impaired newborns? If we believe that lives lived autonomously are objectively better than lives lived non-autonomously, then the same pattern of reasoning allows us to distinguish between autonomous lives that are characterized by virtuous choices, and autonomous lives that demonstrate viciousness, moral weakness, and moral failure. Moreover, we can assert that it is only in the former case that full human flourishing is achieved.

The second main aspect of Raz's view of autonomy is his claim that agents must have a plurality of valuable options to choose from. One of the fears liberals have traditionally had about perfectionist politics is that they involve the imposition of one form of life and the suppression of other forms. Raz, however, firmly believes that "there are many morally valuable forms of life which are incompatible with one another."[61] To use our earlier example, we can know that it's better for someone to spend his life as a farmer than as a sweat shop owner, without asserting that farming constitutes the *only* morally valuable form of life there is.

As Mullhall and Swift point out, Raz's argument is an interesting and unusual one. It's not simply that he deflects anti-perfectionist criticism by asserting that perfectionism is *compatible* with moral pluralism; rather, his claim is much stronger, for "his conception of autonomy seems to presuppose the truth of moral pluralism."[62] That is to say, his view of autonomy connects two quite different claims; first, that a life is valuable only if it involves the autonomous pursuit of a morally valid ideal, and, second, the claim that there are many morally valid ideals, some of which are in conflict with one another. His argument here is simple: autonomy clearly involves having the freedom to make choices, and if it also requires that the pursuits one engages in be morally valuable, then individuals must have a variety of morally valuable options from which to choose.

This means that we have to focus some attention on the question of what options are, in fact, valuable, and the considerations to which Raz is sensitive here have an important impact on the role he thinks societies and governments must play in the promotion of autonomy. If we hold the autonomous life to be of ultimate value, it must be lived in circumstances in which acceptable alternatives are present, and some of these alternatives clearly require the existence of collective goods.

The claim that an autonomous life is of ultimate value entails, Raz thinks, that "having a range of acceptable options is of intrinsic value, for it is constitutive of an autonomous life that it is lived in circumstances where acceptable options are present."[63] For Raz, the choice between good and evil is not really a choice at all: "Someone with the choice of becoming an electrician and having to murder someone is not choosing autonomously if he chooses to become an electrician, for his choice is forced. If he is to be moral, he has no choice."[64] Just as one cannot be autonomous if all of one's major decisions are coerced, or if one is constantly struggling for the bare necessities of life, one cannot be fully autonomous unless the options open to one are acceptable. We must, in short, have a variety of *goods* to choose from, if we are to be able to act autonomously. Autonomy, then, is ultimately connected with other moral values, as we can see when we ask the question whether a morally questionable choice is valuable because it was made autonomously. Is someone who autonomously does wrong morally better than the person who does wrong non-autonomously? Surely, the reverse: the more autonomous a wrongdoer is, the more evil he seems to be. Virtue and autonomy, then, can be understood not as opposed concepts, but, instead, as complementary aspects of human flourishing.

Acceptable options are dependent on the existence of certain social conditions. Even our professional roles—whether we are, for instance, lawyers, teachers, engineers, nurses, physicians, or bioethicists—depend on these professions, and the institutions they require, being recognized in certain ways in our society. And the same is true of other options, such as the option to be married. Being a husband or wife depends on being part of a socially recognized union, not merely on cohabitation with another person, as the legalization of same sex marriage in many jurisdictions demonstrates.

Clearly, then, "some of the social conditions which constitute such options are collective goods."[65] They cannot exist without a society that recognizes and supports them in certain ways. Furthermore, the existence of such goods is intrinsically valuable if they provide individuals with at least some of the options that are necessary if they are to live an autonomous life. Not only is the existence of such goods intrinsically valuable, but so, Raz believes, are some of the goods themselves: "At the very least living in a society, which is a collective good, is on this view intrinsically good."[66] The most important conclusion Raz draws from this is that moral individualism and the ideal of personal autonomy are incompatible.

The third component of Raz's conception of autonomy, and the one that most mainstream bioethicists will find easiest to agree with, involves the claim that one's valuable choices only enhance one's own sense of autonomy if they are consciously endorsed. However, Raz fleshes this claim out in a unique way, by tying it to a notion of well-being which straddles the middle ground between the claim that all that matters is that one believes that one's choices are valuable, and the claim that all that matters is, in fact, that the goals one pursues are valuable, whether or not one pursues them freely. By tying well-being to the pursuit and achievement of what Raz calls "comprehensive goals," he is able to tie the intuition that what is crucially important about a person's life is the way that life *feels* to her to the perfectionist claim that belief in the value of a goal or project adds nothing to the actual worth of that goal or project.

As we have already seen, Raz argues that we have certain wants and pursue certain goals for what seem to us to be good reasons, and if we are mistaken about the value of what we desire or pursue, it would be best if we did not have these desires or that we fail in our pursuit of these goals. But there are other sorts of goals or projects that we pursue for reasons related to the value of the pursuit itself. Some reasons for action take their value (instrumental or intrinsic) from the performance of the action itself. For instance, we want to enjoy the books we read and the films we watch, rather than merely being in a state of contentment; we want to have fulfilling careers, not simply make lots of money; we want, in short, to engage in various endeavors, not merely enjoy their rewards if they are successful. Indeed, it might even be said that there is value in a worthwhile endeavor, even if it ends in failure.

Raz notes that "I will assume that pervasive and unshakeable features of human practical thought need no justification, though they call for an explanation."[67] One of these unshakeable features is the fact that we all have certain projects that are central to our lives. Personal well-being, he goes on to say, is concerned with the question of how good or successful a person's life is from *his* point of view. We can compare the way someone's life actually is with the ways in which it might have developed, or judge certain periods of a person's life to have been more successful than others, or look at various options open to him in the present; and these are all judgments that we can make about a person's life in much the same way, perhaps, as a biographer might do. However, while we are sometimes well placed for the making of these judgments, we cannot get inside someone else's skin, and discover how much he values his life. This is because "the value of various situations for a particular person depends to a large extent on his actual goals, as they are or will be throughout his life."[68] If his life seems to us to be successful, but his goals were actually very different from his achievements, his life may feel, to him, to be a failure.

The source of these goals, Raz thinks, makes no difference to our discussion. What is important is that they are *his* goals (Raz understands "goals" in a broad sense, as meaning "his projects, plans, relationships, ambitions, commitments, and the like"[69]), and that these goals play a conscious role in his life. Consequently, if we want to improve someone's well-being, we can best do this through his goals: by encouraging him to change them if they are bad, and by helping to meet them if they are good.

Goals are nested in hierarchical structures, which means that they are quite complex; I want to complete this book because engaging in scholarship of this sort is an expected part of academic work *and* because I am interested in the topics I am reading and thinking about and want to reach some conclusions regarding them, *and* because I believe that, once I have done so, I will be better able to fill my role on the various ethics committees of which I am a member. The main exceptions to this interconnectedness are goals that are biologically determined, such as the need to eat, drink, and sleep. The consequence of all this is that an action is important, not simply because it enables one to reach a goal, but in virtue of its contribution to one's highest goals. And the more central to a person's life a particular goal is, generally speaking, the more important its achievement is to a person's well-being. Comprehensive goals are, in short, the ones which provide our lives with their "overall shape and orientation,"[70] the ones within which less important goals are nested, and, if our comprehensive goals are actually valuable, success in their achievement will constitute much of our well-being. Well-being, then, is a component of flourishing.

Raz contrasts the notion of well-being with the notion of self-interest. In simple terms, self-interest is primarily a biological concept. And there are at least four differences between these two concepts. First, while both are affected by biological needs and desires, a frustration of these needs and desires always has an adverse effect on self-interest, while a "person's well-being is not reduced by the shortening of his life, nor by the frustrating of his biological needs, when this is the means of or the accepted by product of the pursuit of a valuable goal."[71] The tragic hero, who sacrifices himself for a worthy cause, may sacrifice his self-interest, but not his well-being.

Second, the two notions are differently related to our goals. The success or failure of our goals usually has less effect on our self-interest than on our well-being. For instance, I might make a great deal of money as a commercial artist (something which is in my self-interest), but if my goal was to become a great artist (rather than simply to become rich), my lack of distinctive talent has a detrimental effect on my well-being.

Third, a failure to achieve our goals adversely affects our well-being, even if this failure remains, for some reason, unrecognized. Self-interest, on the other hand, "is unaffected by such factors. It is sensitive to a person's satisfactions with his own life. But not to whether that satisfaction or its absence is justified."[72]

Fourth, a person's well-being depends on the value of her pursuits and goals. Someone who is addicted to gambling has, all things being equal, a less successful life than a hard-working farmer does. This is not the case with self-interest, however, for her self-interest may be equally served by a number of activities, some valuable and some not. If we mistakenly engage in activities which we (falsely) believe to be valuable, our lives will be less successful than they would have been had our beliefs about what was in fact, valuable, been correct.

This distinction between well-being and self-interest is important because it allows us to articulate a conception of autonomy that, while responsive to the idea that it is important that individuals consciously endorse the choices they make, nonetheless enables us to distinguish between subjective beliefs about what is valuable (which may be incorrect), and objective criteria that determine which particular goals are worth pursuing, and which activities that contribute to their achievement are not only efficacious but, also, morally sound. It would allow us to say, for example, with respect to reproductive choice that, while the goal of becoming a parent is connected to well-being (it is a goal that, in itself, can be considered objectively valuable), not all methods for achieving this goal, even if they meet the requirements of self-interest, can be morally defended.

That is to say, even though it may sometimes be difficult to determine which goals are worthwhile and which methods for their achievement morally sound, the distinction between well-being and self-interest opens up a space in which we can ask ethical questions and make moral judgments that simply cannot be asked or made when we take the Choosing Self as our template for what autonomy comes to, without either negating the importance of respect for autonomy or imposing our views upon those who don't share them. All autonomous persons, Raz's account makes clear, should want to aim for goals that enhance their well-being, even if, at times, those goals and what is required for their achievement conflict with self-interested desires and choices. Further, while it may, on occasion at least, be a moral requirement on others that they help particular individuals enhance their well-being, and important to structure social, political, and economic arrangements in such a way that everyone is provided with the resources and freedoms necessary to identify and pursue genuinely valuable goals in morally sound ways, no such moral requirements exist when it comes to facilitating self-interested choices or goals.

The final component of Raz's conception of autonomy is captured in his claim that our autonomy consists in our being the (partial) authors of our own lives. This means that the life of an autonomous person is a work in progress it is defined not only by what it is, but also by how it got to be that way, what it might have been, and by what it might still become. And this requires that the autonomous person must have a range of adequate options open to him, and that "his life became what it is through his choice of some of these options."[73]

Autonomy, then, can be understood as both a capacity and an achievement. The reason for making this distinction is quite straightforward. If autonomy is of necessity something that we can only achieve for ourselves, societies that give autonomy a central place can only arrange their institutions in ways that are likely to produce in their citizens the critical and self-aware capacities upon which autonomy can be based. The capacity to become autonomous (which is a necessary precondition for the eventual achievement of autonomy) depends, Raz again asserts, on having a *valuable* range of options available.

The autonomy of any particular individual can be seen as resulting from a collaborative effort, one that requires the participation of others in the creation of social structures, relationships, institutions, practices, and communities, and this, in turn, requires that we have at least some substantive shared conceptions of what sorts of things are genuinely valuable. The achievement of autonomy, however, remains up to each of us: just as *you* cannot achieve *my* autonomy for *me*, so *I* cannot achieve *your* autonomy for *you*.

Raz's account can be very helpful component of a neo-Aristotelian form of bioethics, because by detaching autonomy from individualism, it allows us to consider the way in which social expectations, structures, and institutions can not only hinder someone's achievement of autonomy, but are actually necessary for that achievement. Second, by attaching the value we place on autonomy to the achievement of genuinely and objectively valuable goals, Raz opens up a space in which bioethicists can engage in substantive discussions about the worth of certain choices *without* thereby opening the door to paternalism *or* imposing their personal, subjective views about what is valuable upon others.

In this regard, it is important to remember that Raz does not tell us what the autonomous life should contain in specific detail, and neither does he claim that there is only one good way for human beings to live. Instead, he makes it clear that we can only understand why we consider autonomy to be valuable in the first place when it is connected to the achievement of valuable things, that the identification of valuable things is, in large part, a social rather than individualistic activity, and that we cannot be autonomous unless we have a range of valuable things to choose among.

Finally, as we shall see, the idea that autonomy is easily connected to the idea of authorship, with our lives having the form of an ongoing and unfolding story, introduces the possibility that we can both explore narrative dimensions of the moral life that are considered either invisible or unimportant within mainstream bioethics, and that we can come to understand what it is to be a virtuous self as a capacity that is constructed and maintained through the stories each of us tells ourselves about who we are, and how others respond to those stories; we also learn about what it means to be human, what it means to behave well and to behave badly, through narratives as much as we do through moral theories.

Further, there is a clear parallel between the development of autonomy and the development of virtue: just as we can become autonomous only over time and as a result of our own efforts, and only achieve autonomy when the social, educational, economic, and political circumstances in which we live encourage its development and exercise, so we learn to be virtuous over time, with practice, and only when the circumstances are right. Moreover, on this account, the development of autonomy and the development of virtue come together: the virtuous self must be autonomous (we are not virtuous unless we have the capacity to make judgments about what virtue requires in the particular situations in which we find ourselves, and the freedom to act on those judgments), and we cannot achieve well-being unless we make choices that are virtuous.

I believe that the case Raz makes is a strong one, and that accepting it will allow us to avoid many of the difficulties we have been exploring, including the fact that the concept of autonomy currently used within bioethics fits poorly with the experience of illness and undermines the bioethicist's claim to possess a particular kind of ethical expertise. The question becomes (and this will, in one way or another, be the focus of the rest of the book) what sorts of moral considerations we should bring to bear in our consideration of bioethical questions and issues, and what conception of the self can best capture what it might mean to be committed both to the belief that autonomy, properly understood, does capture something important about the nature of individual and human flourishing *and* that some autonomously chosen things can be misguided, wasteful, and morally wrong.

The task of the bioethicist, on this view, is, at least in part, to help individuals whom they encounter in the context of health care distinguish between choices that enhance well-being and those that do not, and policy makers come up with approaches that actually produce a wide-range of valuable options for individuals to choose from. What bioethicists cannot do, however, if they wish both to make a claim to possess professional expertise and to be able to help those in whose name they purport to direct their activities, is simply to assert, in the name of autonomy, that all choices that do not violate the Harm Principle need to be respected.

CONCLUSION: VIRTUE OR MANIPULATION?

The reason why theorists working within the liberal self-moral-political framework, and why bioethicists who derive the Choosing Self from this approach, are so reluctant to make judgments about the value of people's choices is the fear that values will be imposed on those who do not accept them. However, while the neo-Aristotelian virtue ethicist will emphasize the fact that particular social arrangements and political structures embody values, and shape both the possibilities open to us and our self-understandings, it does not follow from this that any *particular* state or set of social arrangements actually promote human flourishing. Bartlett and Collins argue that Aristotle makes it clear in the *Nichomachean Ethics* that "we too must investigate the human good so that we may know, with the greatest possible independence [of any particular conception of the human good as presented to us by any particular political community], the truth of the matter."[74]

What virtue ethics provides for us is a framework within which questions about the human good can be asked and considered, and what it means to be virtuous in any given time and place will not be answered in advance (just as what being virtuous requires of each of us cannot be known in advance of the specific situations in which we find ourselves), in any definitive and timeless way: we have to keep on working on our conceptual boat.

We need to note, however, that if we refuse to engage in a discussion of the nature of the human good, out of the belief that this question cannot be answered in shared objective terms, but only in personal ones, and because we fear that, by doing so, we will open the door to the imposition of values on individuals by other individuals or by the state, instead of defending the freedom to choose, we may be rendering persons vulnerable to manipulation and exploitation. Unless people have access to moral resources and a rich moral language that helps them make sense of their condition (such as those provided by some version of neo-Aristotelian virtue ethics), and unless we are willing to engage in substantive ethical discussions about what it might mean to flourish as individuals and as human beings, then individuals will have nothing to base their choices and conceptions of the good on but their own beliefs and desires. Beliefs, we all know, can be mistaken, and desires can be manipulated.

I want to argue not only that autonomy, as a concept, is *compatible* with neo-Aristotelian virtue ethics, but also make the stronger claim that, without the moral framework provided by some form of virtue ethics, we are less, not more, likely to actually be able to achieve autonomy because we will have no clear basis for judging whether the things we desire and believe to be valuable are genuinely so, and whether or not their achievement will contribute to our flourishing, or whether they have been given to us by marketers, advertisers, politicians, and preachers, and whether our pursuit of them furthers their interests rather than our own.

Moreover, I will argue in the final chapter that, because mainstream bioethics has come to be increasingly dominated by the figure of the Choosing Self, rather than bioethicists working to supplement the range of valuable options open to individuals, they are themselves increasingly unable to distinguish choices which are ethically sound from those that are ethically questionable, and, consequently, they increasingly defend a form of bioethics that supports manipulative and exploitative practices, rather than one that challenges and critiques them. That this is often done in the name of demonstrating respect for autonomy is an irony that would be amusing if its consequences were not so serious.

Viewing bioethics through the lens provided by virtue ethics has other implications as well. Since the roles we inhabit help determine what virtues we ought to internalize and demonstrate, being a nurse, physician, personal support worker, or bioethicist is more than a job description, it is to name professional roles which carry with them disciplinary goals and standards of practice. Consequently, bioethicists need to consider not only what virtues would be demonstrated by the good or excellent nurse, physician, or personal support worker and what practices these persons ought to engage in, but also which virtues the good or excellent bioethicist would demonstrate, what practices would shape her activities, and what teleological purpose bioethics is intended to serve. What is it that the philosopher who makes the journey from the ivory tower to the bedside of the patient—becoming, in the course of that process, a person who can legitimately be called a bioethicist—is hoping to accomplish? What, that is to say, is the purpose of bioethics, and what commitments does a bioethicist need to make in order to fulfill that purpose?

While there may be no uncontroversial way in which this question can be answered, one way of getting at the teleological purpose of bioethics is to ask what it is that the bioethicist brings to the medical context that would be lacking if the bioethicist were not there. That is to say, from the perspective provided by virtue ethics, there must be some unique contribution made by the bioethicist to the care that patients receive, to the workings of the medical institutions in which they receive it, and to the larger cultural conversation about the ethical implications of developments in medical technology and research, something which is not a duplication of what is offered by other participants in these places and spaces, or a rubber-stamping, with a kind of ethical seal of approval, of what they do. It is also important to note that, when the role played by the bioethicist is viewed through the lens provided by virtue ethics, and the activities that bioethicists currently engage in are evaluated within this framework, it may turn out that bioethicists need to understand themselves differently than they presently do, and that at least some of the activities they engage in need to be either reformed or transformed.

I will argue that a central purpose of bioethics is to provide guidance and resources for those who must make difficult bioethical choices in their own lives, to protect the interests of those who are weak and vulnerable when they find themselves in the places in which medicine is practiced and medical research performed, to work to ensure that the experiences of patients and research subjects are better than they would have been had the bioethicist not been there, and to provide a counterbalance to the forces within health care and research that push for medical efficiency, the protection of institutional reputations, and financial expediency. In order to fulfill this role, the bioethicist is required to make two distinct sorts of commitments. On one hand, the bioethicist needs to make a set of epistemic commitments that are similar to those made by the philosopher; these include a willingness to question received opinion, to work to clarify what is really at issue when conflicts arise, to try to get at the (frequently unrecognized) metaphysical, epistemological, ethical and political assumptions and commitments that underpin particular positions, and to try to get others to do so as well. On the other hand, the bioethicist needs to make a set of ethical commitments as well: to take the suffering of the sick seriously, to identify particular instances of injustice and moral failure in the institutions in which he works, and to fight against his own tendency to be co-opted by the powerful for the sake of professional recognition and social prestige.

NOTES

1. In a book about taking care of her husband as he suffered a brain injury as a result of a boating accident, Cathy Crimmins describes her encounter with a physician of this sort. After her husband undergoes brain surgery, she asks to speak with the physician who performed the operation. "The neurosurgeon never comes towards me. He's tall and craggy, with an annoyed, wooden expression on his face. You know the type: Dr. Asshole. Still, I think, maybe we have just gotten off on the wrong foot. I put out my hand and begin introducing myself. He backs away. I feel ridiculous, my hand extended to the air, still in the dirty dress over my bathing suit and reef shoes. . . . No wonder people accuse doctors of acting God-like. I waited eight hours to hear what a specialist would say about Alan's condition, and my encounter with Dr. Asshole lasted less than two minutes. I won't be told anything more specific about Alan's brain injury until well into tomorrow, when another neurosurgeon will detail it for me. The first doctor simply swooped down from the great Neurosurgery in the Sky to tell me he had nothing to tell me." Cathy Crimmins, *Where Is The Mango Princess? A Journey Back From Brain Injury* (New York: Vintage Books, 2001), 25.

2. Robert J. Fitterer, *Love and Objectivity In Virtue Ethics: Aristotle, Lonergan, and Nussbaum on Emotions and Moral Insight* (Toronto: University of Toronto Press, 2008), 26.

3. One possible exception to this claim is the application of casuistry to bioethics. Casuistry is an approach that draws on virtue ethics, and applies a form of reasoning that is rooted in this approach. However, casuistry, as presented by Stephen Toulmin and Albert R. Jonsen, places virtue ethics in the origins of the approach, and focuses primarily on its medieval and early modern practitioners, not on its ancient ones. It is then, I believe, an approach that owes parts of its conceptual framework to virtue ethics, but is not, itself, a moral approach that

encompasses a virtue-based conceptual scheme. In addition, it is better understood as an ethical method, rather than as an entire ethical theory. For more on this method, see Jonsen and Toulmin's *The Abuse of Casuitry: A History of Moral Reasoning* (Berkeley: University of California Press, 1988).

4. Aristotle, *Aristotle's Nichomachean Ethics*, trans. Robert C. Bartlett and Susan D. Collins (Chicago: Chicago University Press, 2011), 34.

5. Fitterer, *Love and Objectivity*, 26.

6. Fitterer, *Love and Objectivity*, 27.

7. Rosalind Hursthouse, *On Virtue Ethics* (Oxford: Oxford University Press, 1999), 8.

8. Hurthouse, *On Virtue Ethics*, 2.

9. Arthur Kleinman, *What Really Matters: Living A Moral Life Amidst Uncertainty and Danger* (Oxford: Oxford University Press, 2006), 18.

10. Kleinman, *What Really Matters*, 18.

11. Kleinman, *What Really Matters*, 18.

12. Kleinman, *What Really Matters*, 10.

13. Aristotle, *Nichomachean Ethics*, 1.

14. Robert B. Talisse, *On Rawls* (Belmont, CA: Wadsworth Publishing, 2001), 7.

15. Aristotle, *Nichomachean Ethics*, 33.

16. Aristotle, *Nichomachean Ethics*, 33.

17. Aristotle, *Nichomachean Ethics*, 13.

18. Jonathan Lear, *Happiness, Death, and The Remainder Of Life* (Cambridge, Massachusetts: Harvard University Press, 2000), 2.

19. Lear, *Happiness, Death*, 2.

20. Aristotle, *Nichomachean Ethics*, 13.

21. Fitterer, *Love and Objectivity*, 4.

22. Fitterer, *Love and Objectivity*, 4.

23. Aristotle, *Nichomachean Ethics*, 14.

24. Fitterer, *Love and Objectivity*, 4.

25. Hursthouse, *Virtue Ethics*, 179.

26. Hursthouse, *Virtue Ethics*, 166.

27. Hursthouse, *Virtue Ethics*, 165–166.

28. Robert C. Bartlett and Susan D. Collins, "Introduction," in Aristotle, *Aristotle's Nichomachean Ethics*, trans. Robert C. Bartlett and Susan D. Collins (Chicago: Chicago University Press, 2011), x.

29. Bartlett and Collins, "Introduction," x.

30. Bartlett and Collins, "Introduction," x.

31. Bartlett and Collins, "Introduction," x.

32. Hursthouse, *Virtue Ethics*, 218.

33. Hursthouse, *Virtue Ethics*, 218.

34. Hursthouse, *Virtue Ethics*, 218.

35. Hursthouse, *Virtue Ethics*, 223.

36. Lisa Tessman, *Burdened Virtues: Virtue Ethics For Liberatory Struggles* (Oxford: Oxford University Press, 2005), 3.

37. Tessman, *Liberatory*, 3.

38. Bartlett and Collins, "Introduction," x.

39. Bartlett and Collins, "Introduction," x.

40. Will Kymlicka, *Liberalism, Community, and Culture* (Oxford: Clarendon Press, 1989), 10.

41. Kymlicka, *Liberalism*, 10.

42. Kymlicka, *Liberalism*, 11.

43. Kymlicka, *Liberalism*, 12.

44. Kymlicka, *Liberalism*, 12.

45. Kymlicka, *Liberalism*, 13.

46. Kymlicka, *Liberalism*, 13.

47. Cheryl Misak, "ICU Psychosis and Patient Autonomy: Some Thoughts From The Inside," *Journal of Medicine and Philosophy* 30 (2005): 411–430.

48. Stephen Mulhall and Adam Swift, *Liberals and Communitarians* (Oxford: Blackwell, 1992), 255.
49. Raz, *Morality Of Freedom*, 17.
50. Raz, *Morality Of Freedom*, 18.
51. Raz, *Morality Of Freedom*, 18.
52. Raz, *Morality Of Freedom*, 161.
53. Raz, *Morality Of Freedom*, 161.
54. Mullhall and Swift, *Liberals and Communitarians*, 254.
55. Raz, *Morality Of Freedom*, 141.
56. Raz, *Morality Of Freedom*, 142.
57. Mullhall and Swift, *Liberals and Communitarians*, 256.
58. Mullhall and Swift, *Liberals and Communitarians*, 257.
59. Mullhall and Swift, *Liberals and Communitarians*, 257.
60. Mullhall and Swift, *Liberals and Communitarians*, 257.
61. Raz, *Morality Of Freedom*, 161.
62. Mullhall and Swift, *Liberals and Communitarians*, 265.
63. Raz, *Morality Of Freedom*, 205.
64. Mullhall and Swift, *Liberals and Communitarians*, 266.
65. Raz, *Morality Of Freedom*, 206.
66. Raz, *Morality Of Freedom*, 206.
67. Raz, *Morality Of Freedom*, 288–289.
68. Raz, *Morality Of Freedom*, 290.
69. Raz, *Morality Of Freedom*, 291.
70. Mullhall and Swift, *Liberals and Communitarians*, 268.
71. Raz, *Morality Of Freedom*, 296.
72. Raz, *Morality Of Freedom*, 298.
73. Raz, *Morality Of Freedom*, 204.
74. Bartlett and Collins, "Introduction," xii–xiii.

Chapter Seven

The Third Component of the Situated Self

Narratives

INTRODUCTION: A VISIT TO THE ORACLE

Bioethics is a field that revolves around case studies, short narratives of a sort largely unknown in other areas of philosophy. In bioethics, case studies serve a dual purpose: they make vivid and real the implications of the issues that bioethics grapples with, and they provide an educational tool that bioethicists use to teach students and health care workers how to apply the theoretical principles and concepts they work with to "real life" situations. While we shall see below that this use of narratives in bioethics is not usually accompanied by a consideration of why it is that bioethics makes such extensive use of this kind of tool, the work case studies do in shaping bioethical discourse is significant, and an analysis of their place in the discipline reveals interesting evidence of the important role played by narratives in descriptions of the moral life.

Case studies are a kind of fiction that paradoxically enough lies at the heart of what can be a very dry and procedurally focused subject. A number of philosophers working within a broad approach often called narrative ethics have begun to draw attention to case studies as examples of philosophical writing in and of themselves, and have raised questions about how much ethical work these case studies are actually doing. Scholars applying the tools of narrative ethics to bioethics argue that, in addition to considering ethical theories and applying moral principles to cases, bioethicists also need to consider the role played in their ethical analysis by the case studies they use to generate the ethical questions they consider, to contextualize the analysis they present, and to support the conclusions they reach.

Further, since it is precisely the features of the moral life that are best revealed in narratives and largely excluded or ignored in other forms of philosophical writing, that lie at the heart of neo-Aristotelian virtue ethics—virtues, vices, the wicked and the good, the development of moral character over time—any form of bioethics that is built on the foundation provided by virtue ethics must take stories seriously, both because of what they *reveal* to us as well as what they *do* to us.

The version of virtue ethics I present here, then, encompasses narrative ethics, and asserts that autonomy itself can be understood, at least in part, as a kind of narrative we tell about ourselves and our choices, and how these fit in with our lives considered as a whole. It is this narrative, that is to say, which makes us one person over time, morally responsible for the choices we make, and capable of giving an account of ourselves. We can see the important role played by narratives in accounts of the moral life if we turn to one of the foundational texts of philosophy, *The Apology of Socrates*, and consider not only the specific arguments that are made, but also the way in which they are placed in the context of a narrative about a particular human life which exemplifies a particular set of virtues, and the literary elements of that account which make it such a powerful and memorable piece of philosophical writing. It is to these literary elements that we now turn.

Once upon a time, a man who was on trial for his life told the jurors a strange story. The reason, he says, that he lived as he did, and performed the actions that led to his being put on trial, was that one of his friends had visited an oracle. The oracle was a Sybil, a priestess, who, when in a trance state, would be entered by the spirit of the god Apollo. When possessed by the god, she could make predictions and prophecies, and provide cryptic answers to specific questions. "Who is the wisest one of all?" his friend Charephon asked, and was told that no one was wiser than Socrates. When Charephon reported to Socrates what the Sybil had said, Socrates was puzzled, and he states that, "When I heard these things, I pondered them like this: 'What ever is the god saying, and what riddle is he posing? For I am conscious that I am not at all wise, either much or little. So what ever is he saying when he claims that I am wisest? Surely he is not saying something false at least; for that is not sanctioned for him."[1] And so, he says, he found himself at a loss to make sense of the oracle's words.

Anyone who has studied philosophy knows how the story goes: Socrates did not believe that he was the wisest man at all, and so he went around asking questions of those who appeared to be wiser than he. It turned out, of course, that none of those he questioned were able to tell him, in any conclusive or persuasive way, what it was that they knew, or explain how they knew it. Nonetheless, many persisted in believing that they were experts in their chosen occupations, and they became annoyed by Socrates' questioning. Indeed, he said, although he felt compelled to understand what the words of the god conveyed by the oracle really meant and so continued his interrogations, he did so "all the while perceiving with pain and fear that I was becoming hated."[2] The conversations lead Socrates to conclude that perhaps, after all, the oracle was right: unlike those he questions, at least he knows what he does not know.

This story is important to philosophers for a number of reasons. Of particular significance for our discussion is that it provides a model for the epistemic and moral commitments a philosopher must make, at least if we consider being a philosopher as a role in the sense that virtue ethics asserts we should. These commitments are bound up in the image Socrates presents of himself as the gadfly, and the image is startlingly unflattering: the gadfly is an annoying insect, whose buzzing is irritating and whose bite is painful. No one really likes having the gadfly around, and yet, Socrates claims, the gadfly serves a vitally important social purpose: it wakes individuals up when they are in danger of sleepwalking through their lives, and, in so doing, helps them realize what is most important, and, ultimately, forces them to begin to think about how they ought to live.

The task of the gadfly is precisely to ask questions about the things that almost everyone takes for granted, to make "normal" ways of thinking and doing appear strange, as things that need to be examined and evaluated afresh, and to challenge the beliefs that others have about themselves. The image of the gadfly, and the way in which it is presented in the form of a narrative account of a particular human life, does three things that are important for the conception of autonomy I am presenting, and for the role it might play in bioethics. First, the image of the gadfly gives us a model of the virtuous philosopher as a kind of courageous irritant, as someone who is willing to challenge others and take personal risks in order to ask questions that no one else thinks (or wants) to ask, even when this is personally costly: the gadfly is likely to be swatted when his questions become too probing and painful.

Second, this image of the gadfly sets out a set of epistemic commitments that must be made by the philosopher: a willingness to pursue truth (even if one never fully captures it), to see where the argument might take us even if this conflicts with our present beliefs, and to be suspicious of our own certainties, particularly when they are widely shared with others. Third, because the image of the gadfly is presented in the context of a narrative, it reveals the power that stories have to serve as sources of moral knowledge, to provide evidence that is morally significant, and makes the case, by example, that stories are things that moral philosophers ought to take seriously.

With respect to the third point, think about the utter strangeness of the story that lies at the heart of this account, Charephon's visit to the oracle.

This story is as strange as any story about turning water into wine or wine into blood, or a goose laying golden eggs. Booth uses the story of the goose that lays the golden eggs to illustrate the process by which stories become part of our selves, and influence those selves as we take them in. He asks, "What happens to us when we follow such a simple story?"[3] He observes that this is not an easy question to answer: "Whatever it is, it happens so frequently and with such seeming simplicity that we find it difficult even to recognize what a strange and wonderful process we undergo as we use a sequence of words like this [the words which compose the story] to create, not so much in our heads as in our souls, a narrative laden with the *kind* of significance that stories about our own life might have."[4] Stories, he argues, affect us in fundamental ways. "When a story 'works,' when we like it well enough to listen to it again and to tell it over and over to ourselves and friends . . . it occupies us in a curiously intense way. The pun in 'occupy' is useful here. We are occupied in the sense of filling our time with the story: its time takes our time. And we are occupied in the sense of being taken over, colonized: occupied by a foreign imaginary world."[5]

Consider, again, the story that Socrates tells about the oracle. It contains elements so fantastical that it could almost be a fairy tale: the consultation with the mysterious oracle, the cryptic answer to the question asked by Charephon, the hero's quest to find out the meaning of the riddle, and the way in which his life was transformed as a result. How does a story about a consultation with an oracle fit with the model of the examined life that philosophy professors present to students when they teach this dialogue, and how is our understanding of the philosophical points made in this dialogue colored by this narrative? What standards of evidence are in play when reference to such a consultation can constitute an important part of Socrates' defense strategy? Indeed, what might it be like to live in a world in which the space occupied by the gods is so close to the human world that an oracle can see through the veil that separates the two, and give serious advice to politicians and military men? To use Booth's terminology, when we are colonized by a story like the story about Charephon's visit to the oracle, we are "occupied by a foreign imaginary world."[6]

This story, moreover, is a story-within-a-story. As Nehamas observes, the characters in Platonic dialogues are themselves fictional creations. We seldom notice this fact, but instead view them as "real" people about whom accurate reports are being made because "the exceptional verisimilitude of Plato's writing overcomes our staunchest precautions and seduces us into taking his dialogues not as works of literature and imagination but, instead, as transcriptions of actual conversations."[7] This means that our analysis of these dialogues must go beyond a philosophical examination of the explicit arguments that are presented, but must also consider their literary features: the role of character and plot, the use of irony, the relationship between author and reader, and, of course, the interplay between philosophical argument and literary imagination. We cannot, that is to say, pay attention only to the words the characters use; we must also ask why Plato created characters with those particular features, and what it is that we, as readers, are meant to learn from them. Nehamas suggests that one of the things we are meant to learn is that *we* are like the people Socrates questions, rather than (as many readers would like to believe) like Socrates, and that intellectual arrogance is a philosophical and moral failing.

If we follow this line of thinking, it is reasonable to suggest that one of the things Plato is trying to teach us is that ethics is not simply concerned with how we resolve moral problems or answer ethical questions, as though these things are simply intellectual puzzles, but about orienting our lives around particular values, so that both our reasoning and our choices are shaped by this orientation. The moral life is full of emotions, surprises, triumphs, and failures, composed of moments of grace and, sometimes, threatened by fierce conflicts. The moral life, in short, is more like a novel than an instruction manual, and descriptions of what it is to think, feel, and act ethically are often difficult to convey, except through the telling of a story. As Elliot observes, "The moral life involves the unexpected. . . . It involves events that happen by surprise, which we can't predict or control: a dismissal letter from the Dean; a fishtailing car on the ice; an inheritance from a long-lost uncle; the birth of a child with cystic fibrosis."[8] And, he asks, "How would you convey these things, and the way they can turn your life upside down, in a philosophical essay? You can *write* in a sentence that surprise is a part of the moral life, as I did earlier . . . but you can't actually express this sense of the unexpected or surprise in the absence of narrative. Surprise happens in stories. It is hard to surprise your reader in an essay without resorting to profanity."[9] In short, the moral life encounters, and requires us to engage with, the *peripeteia*.

This is one of the reasons why the Platonic dialogues are so powerful and memorable; they present philosophical arguments that are written in such a way that features usually thought to belong only in narratives are also present. They show us heroes and villains, as well as characters who are self-deluded, manipulative, courageous, and loyal; they embody plots; they contain elements of the supernatural, and present us with personality conflicts; and they allow us to be surprised, puzzled, engaged, and moved, just as we are when we read a good novel. Consider the *Apology* again. It encases an intriguing story told by Socrates about Charephon's visit to the oracle within a narrative written by Plato about Socrates on trial (both literally and metaphorically) for *his life*: defending himself, that is to say, in the face of charges that might result in his execution *and* defending the way in which that life was spent and the values around which his activities revolved. And when we read it, we respond to it in the way we respond to all good stories, emotionally and physiologically: it is one of the few pieces of philosophical writing which can bring a lump to the throat of clever and sometimes jaded philosophy professors, and students who have appeared indifferent and even bored when exposed to other philosophical material will sometimes report that they were in tears by the end. To use Booth's language, it is a story that can colonize us, if we let it, and in so doing, it allows us to imagine a richer and more complete moral universe than we might otherwise have been able to.

The story of Socrates, then, is one that we remember long after we have read it, and it is the kind of story that can change our lives, if we are willing to let it. "The truth about stories," Thomas King writes, "is that that's all we are."[10] King examines two creation stories, one an indigenous North American story about a woman (whom King names "Charm") who fell from the sky, and created the world with the help of the animals, and the other the more familiar story of Adam and Eve. The first story imagines a creative and cooperative universe, while the second imagines a created and hierarchical one; the second posits a harmonious world that moves towards chaos, while the first posits a chaotic world that moves towards harmony. Each story, therefore, encourages us to understand the world in a particular way. Moreover, King argues, the two stories are mutually exclusive: to accept the world imagined in one story requires us to be blind to the world imagined in the other. Because stories imagine and create worlds, they shape our understanding of what is real and what is important, of how things connect to one another, and where everything belongs. Consequently, King believes, everything is composed of stories: "It was Sir Isaac Newton who said, 'To every action there is always opposed an equal reaction.' Had he been a writer, he might have simply said, 'To every action, there is a story.'"[11] And, he continues, "Take Charm's story, for instance. It's yours. Do with it what you will. Turn it into a television movie. Forget it. But don't say in years to come that you would have lived your life differently if only you had heard this story. You've heard it now."[12]

The same is true of the story that Plato has Socrates tell about his life in the *Apology*: it is, quite literally, a story that asks us to live our lives differently; and, after reading it, whatever else we do with it—dismiss it, forget it, write a paper on it—we can't say that we've never heard it. As Nehamas notes, what the Platonic dialogues teach us is that the "logical examination of beliefs is a part but only a part of the examined life . . . philosophy is not only a matter of reading books: it is a whole way of life, even if . . . it does not dictate a single manner of living that all should follow."[13] And, while Nehamas does not quite say this, many of the central elements of the moral life the role of character, the place of emotions, the nature of our connections to others can only be conveyed with any degree of realism in narrative form.

CASE STUDIES: THE ROLE OF STORIES IN BIOETHICS

The connection between stories (or narratives as they are also commonly called) and other forms of philosophical writing is not always clear and uncontroversial. While many philosophers are suspicious about using narratives in their work (with the exception, perhaps, of thought experiments— might we not see Rawls's concepts of the original position and the veil of ignorance as a kind of story that Rawls tells to us?[14]), or of presenting philosophical ideas in story form, the example of Plato's dialogues, which are considered by many to be among the finest works of philosophy ever written, demonstrates that narratives and philosophical writing need not be considered distinct and mutually exclusive.

Indeed, many moral philosophers have begun to challenge the assumption that fictions and philosophy are entirely separate by drawing attention precisely to the way in which central features of the moral life can be best illuminated through an exercise of the imagination which takes the form of narrative presentations. Martha Nussbaum argues that fiction can help us understand what it is to be fully human in ways that standard philosophical writing is unable to.[15] The place to find the complex, allusive, and particularized features which are essential to fully understanding the nature of the moral life is primarily in fictional narratives, Nussbaum asserts, and an important way to grasp what is required of us as moral agents "is to live as good characters in a good story do, caring about what happens, resourcefully confronting each new thing."[16] Richard Rorty believes that philosophers should become "liberal ironists," who connect fiction and poetry to works of philosophy, because it is only through works of literature that we have access to the inner lives of other people, can begin to imagine what it might be like to be them, and, in particular, to understand what it is that humiliates them. The liberal ironist, as Rorty understands him, will not distinguish between writing that is "philosophical," and writing that is not; instead, he will draw on the moral resources available in a wide variety of literary sources.[17] Susan Neiman argues that we can find solutions to the moral and political problems facing us by returning to Enlightenment values, which, she argues, are illuminated as much by the moral imagination as they are underpinned by the claims of reason. In the process of making her case, Neiman employs the stories of Sodom and Gemorrah, Abraham and Isaac, Job, and Odysseus, not only to *illustrate* her philosophical claims, but, more importantly, to *ground* them.[18] Colin McGinn makes the case that, unless moral philosophy takes questions of character seriously and considers what fiction might reveal about different kinds of characters, "moral philosophy is still not living up to what we have a right to expect of it. . . . The aim of the moral philosopher is to do justice to the varieties of moral experience, to the entire range of the ethical life, and this . . . requires us to go beyond the usual assumptions and methods."[19] In order to do justice to the ethical life, he argues, we must turn to fiction: "There is more to the moral life than what ethical words mean and what we should do about this and that."[20] Finally, Richard Kearney suggests that stories, quite literally, make us human: "It is . . . only when haphazard happenings are transformed into story . . . that we become full agents of our history."[21] And, he continues, "This becoming historical involves a transition from the flux of events into a meaningful social or political community what Aristotle and the Greeks called a *polis*. Without this transition from nature to narrative, from time suffered to time enacted and enunciated, it is debatable whether a merely biological life (*zoe*) could ever be considered a truly human one (*bios*)."[22]

While bioethics revolves around case studies, it often does so in a remarkably unselfconscious, and even strikingly oblivious, way. Thomas May, for instance, presents a series of case studies to underpin his defense of autonomy in the context of medical treatment. He uses the case to illustrate the philosophical points that he is making—for example, that health care professionals should not override the desires of patients, or that patients ought to have adequate information provided to them when they are asked to make a decision about their care. But the cases themselves are not presented as anything more than straightforward descriptions of the facts—indeed, some cases are presented with additional evidence of verisimilitude, such as the claim that they are "based on an actual case history."[23]

Similarly, in their introduction to a set of beautifully detailed and extensive case studies, John Freeman and Kevin McDonnell are careful to note that, while the cases they present are fictional creations, they are based on real events: "This book is about the difficult moral decisions that arise ever more frequently in the course of medical practice. . . . Although we have presented them as fictional cases in order to explore their many nuances, they all originate from first-hand experience. They represent amalgams of true cases we have seen, discussed in depth, and sometimes personally managed."[24]

Case studies, in short, are often presented as though they are simply objective descriptions of the issues that arise in bioethics, and many authors also add that they are based on *real* events and, indeed, events that the authors themselves have sometimes been part of. This claim is intended to make the cases appear more real, more factual and simply descriptive and, hence, more legitimate than they might be seen to be if they were only fictional creations based on nothing more than an exercise of the author's imagination. Many bioethics textbooks include cases for analysis, but few say much about the place of cases in the theoretical structure of bioethics, or spend much time considering the ethical work that these cases do as examples of philosophical writing presented in narrative form.[25]

However, as Tod Chambers argues, a "concern with the nature of narrative should be of pivotal concern to bioethics because the ethics case is central to the discipline. . . . In the present state of the art, bioethics... is entrenched in stories."[26] Bioethics cases encompass everything from the seemingly straightforward descriptions of the facts of "real" cases to fictional, but still apparently "factually-grounded" case presentations, to the more cryptic and mysterious cases peopled by characters called "Dr. Z." and "Ms. C," to short works of science fiction set in some imagined but possible future in which, for instance, parents have the power to determine the genetic make-up of their children, and can control their interests, talents, and experience.[27]

NARRATIVE ETHICS AND THE CONSTRUCTION OF ISSUES IN BIOETHICS

One of the most difficult challenges for moral philosophers is to capture the disparate elements that go into living a moral life, and doing justice to the most important elements of that life, even if we are able to identify what those elements are. As Elliot observes, there seems to be an intractable gap between moral description and moral experience: "It is extraordinarily difficult, if not impossible, to capture the countless subtleties which go into the perceptions and judgments of each person involved: the hopes, fears, prayers, guilt, pride and remorse, the conflicting emotions which accompany any irrevocable decisions, the self-imposed pressure to carry through with an action once a decision has been made."[28] Every decision we make depends as much on beliefs, commitments, and assumptions as it does on the rational deliberations that we employ to resolve the problem. And, Elliot notes, to "express these things, even to perceive them consciously, requires a talent possessed by few of us other than novelists or poets."[29]

Those who critique mainstream bioethics from the perspective of a (broadly understood) narrative ethics approach assert a number of things. First, that in addition to employing standard ethical theories and principles, we need to use the images of novelists and literary critics to make sense of our moral predicaments. Second, that we need to spend as much time thinking about the way in which we construct and articulate moral problems as we do in trying to decide what decision we should make. Principled bioethics focuses much attention on helping us to reach a decision, but tends to ignore the possibility that the way in which the moral problem is articulated or presented makes certain decisions appear reasonable or unreasonable, and renders other possible solutions entirely invisible. Finally, narrative ethics, in its strongest form, offers the hope that narrative approaches will allow us to see and to map new moral landscapes, to view precisely the things that novelists and poets (to use Elliot's terms) explore, in the expectation that by so doing, we will be able to narrow the gap between moral descriptions and moral experience.

In his analysis of the literary characteristics of bioethics cases, Chambers observes that cases are "framed": "Framing encloses something and thereby sets it off from other forms of communication and interaction. Frames act as signals that what is inside should be attended to differently from everything else."[30] In bioethics texts, cases are framed in a number of ways: they appear at the end of a chapter, they are "indented, italicized, or printed in a different type."[31] Framing is used to suggest the fact/value distinction, and, consequently, set bioethicists, who deal with "real" issues and have a legitimate place at the bedside of the patient or on the ethics committee, apart from moral philosophers, who like to play with hypothetical thought experiments, and who belong only in the classroom or at philosophy conferences. In short, "the act of framing presents the case as separate data and not in any way influenced by the philosophy."[32]

In addition, "factual" or "true" cases are often framed differently from "fictional" or "made up" ones. They may be distinguished by where they are placed in the text and by how they are named. Munson, for instance, includes factual Case Presentations at the beginning of his chapters, and Decision Scenarios, composed primarily of fictional or fictionalized ones at the end[33]; Vaughn includes a "Classic Case File" in his chapters[34]; Pence has written a book, *Classic Cases In Medical Ethics*, which gains much of its validity from the claim that the cases included are, indeed, *classic*, not only because they have become part of the data of bioethics, but because they are *true*. As he puts it, "I believe that knowing about real cases and how they were resolved is a real education in ethics for people who will one day make ethical decisions."[35] "Real" cases support a particular kind of ethical analysis in part, of course, because we already know what happened, but also because all bioethicists are familiar with the "Dax" case, and who Louise Brown and Marybeth Whitehead are. And, because bioethicists know who *they* are, they tend to view the way in which these cases have been used to frame and shape the issues as though they are simply factual as well. "Fictional" cases, in contrast, are designed precisely to let us, those who read them, make the decision: we cannot know, nor do we need to know, how any decision we might make "works out"; instead, we only need to know whether it is a decision we can rationally defend through the application of bioethical principles or arguments.

However, it is arguably the case that even "factual" cases contain "fictional" elements, and that any sharp distinction made between "real" cases and "imaginary" ones is as deceptive as some critics believe is the framing of cases to suggest that they are uncontaminated by the philosophical assumptions and commitments that occur elsewhere in the text.[36] Like fictional cases, they too are stories. We can, therefore, identify three categories of cases: "classic" cases, which have already occurred, and have had a role in shaping bioethics; fictional or imaginary cases which may, nonetheless, be based on real events; and "live," or ongoing ones. It is this last category, that is usually considered by ethics committees.

When working through or trying to resolve a case that is occurring in "real life," as ethics committees are required to do, there is also a mix of fictional and factual elements. Committee members are provided with information that is usually presented or written up in the form of a case, and such descriptions always involve a degree of authorship: someone made a decision about what to include and what to exclude, from what (or whose) perspective the story should be told, and how the characters are presented. In the absence of these narrative underpinnings, a simple statement of the "facts" would be nothing more than the "dislocated sequence which Dr. Johnson offers us in his notes of his travels in France: 'There we waited on the ladies—Morvilles—Spain. Country towns all beggers. At Dijon he could not find the way to Orleans—Cross roads of France very bad—Five soldiers—Women—Soldiers escaped—The Colonel would not lose five men for the sake of one woman—The magistrate cannot seize a soldier but by the Colonel's permission, etc."[37] While all of these points may be factually true, they are nonsensical, unless we place them in a coherent narrative. What working through these live cases reveals, according to some narrative ethicists, is that the line between fact and fiction is not always easy to draw. All case presentations—indeed, all descriptions of actual moral problems—require emplotment: "To emplot is to propose a plot that transforms what still are incoherent things-that-are-happening into experience that has meaning."[38]

When we deal with live cases, they are like fictional ones, in that we don't yet know how they will work out; as in classic cases, however, we know that "how they turn out" is importantly connected to the decisions and recommendations made by the ethics committee and these decisions and recommendations, in turn, are shaped by the way in which the ethical issue is revealed through the way in which the case was presented.

What this demonstrates is that narratives are no less legitimate sources for bioethics to draw on than are medical descriptions, moral theories, or ethical principles. Booth is correct when he asserts that "every presentation of a time-ordered or time related experience that in any way supplements, reorders, enhances, or interprets unnarrated life"[39] is a narrative, and so any adequate ethical analysis of human experience must encompass "all narratives, not only novels, short stories, epics, plays, films, and TV dramas, but all histories, all satires, all documentaries, all gossip and personal anecdote, all biography, all 'storied' ballets and operas, all mimes and puppet shows, all chronicles"[40]—and, we can add, all bioethical case studies, whether classic, fictional, or live, and all narratives documenting the experience of illness. Booth argues, further, that even if there are those who are suspicious of narratives, who wish to live entirely in a world of "facts" (if, indeed, any such persons exist), they cannot escape: "We all live a great proportion of our lives in a surrender to stories about our lives, and about other possible lives; we live more or less *in* stories, depending on how strongly we resist surrendering to what is 'only' imagined."[41] Indeed, we might say that fictional narratives are sometimes ethically truer than factual reports, and that all reporting of events involves the work of the imagination, in terms of how these events are described and ordered, what elements are included and excluded, and from what (or whose) perspective the story is told.

The challenge that narrative ethics offers to mainstream bioethics is acute: those who draw our attention to the literary features of case studies, and make explicit what they both reveal and conceal about what might be the morally justifiable choice to make suggest that we need to think as much about the stories we tell as we do about the principles and theories we apply; and illness narratives (which we will consider in more detail in the next chapter) pose an even greater challenge because they suggest that bioethics is not performing one of its most important tasks, namely, helping to make the experiences of those who find themselves in need of medical attention better than they would otherwise have been. The first challenge suggests that bioethics needs to be supplemented by the insights of narrative ethics; the second suggests that mainstream bioethics is largely a failure, that a whole new paradigm for medicine's encounter with patients, and bioethics' mediation of that encounter, is needed.

Both of these challenges revolve around a conception of the virtuous self as storyteller, as constructed out of stories and functioning through them, and of social institutions and practices—such as hospitals and medicine, universities and bioethics, and the roles that these institutions and practices create and support, like doctors and bioethicists—as likewise narratively constructed, composed as much by the stories they tell about who they are and what they do and the acceptance by others of those stories, as they are by their knowledge and actions. And, most importantly, what narrative ethics offers, and allows bioethics to access, is a richer and more satisfying description of the moral life: richer, because it encompasses more, more satisfying, because it opens us up to new possibilities and deeper understandings than mainstream bioethics currently provides. It is through these stories that virtues and vices are revealed, the effects of oppressive and exploitative arrangements demonstrated, and possible ways of living well or living badly are articulated. Stories provide our initial access to the moral life, and serve as the basic building blocks for the development of moral character. Application of the Neurathian procedure in bioethics will require stories to be told, to be contrasted and compared to one another, and to be accepted or rejected.

CASE STUDIES AS LITERATURE: THINKING ABOUT STORIES

Case studies, like all stories, invite us to suspend our disbelief and to enter imaginatively into the world inhabited by the characters who populate them, and to engage with them on their own terms. Consider the following case study that is reproduced in full, which provides a variation on two stock bioethical characters, the Non-Compliant Client and the Dedicated Doctor. (In an act of framing, the book from which this case is taken presents the case studies in italics, while the accompanying commentaries are presented in non-italicized text).

Patients We Love To Hate: The Non-Compliant
Ms. C is a 45-year-old with adult-onset diabetes (AOD). She has a good understanding of the disease and its complications, gained from watching her mother, aunt, and sister manage their AOD and its complications, and from having attended several diabetes education courses. When diagnosed five years ago, Ms. C was 20 percent over her ideal body weight. She was advised to lose weight, exercise at least twenty minutes three times a week, follow a 1500-calorie American Diabetic Association diet, and take an oral medication (Diabeta) twice daily to control blood sugar levels.

Ms. C has complied poorly with this regimen. As sales director for a major corporation, she travels frequently. Her job requires that she wine and dine clients. When traveling, she often skips lunch, drinks more wine than is advisable, and exceeds 1500 calories a day. She reports, with a grin, "Wine and desserts! Those are the things I really enjoy! You could call them my hobbies." She rarely exercises because she "hates to sweat" and occasionally misses one of her daily doses of Diabeta because she is "rushed." She has steadily gained weight and is now forty percent over her ideal body weight. Her self-monitored daily blood sugar levels reflect huge swings between striking elevations (when she overeats or forgets her medicine) and life-threatening hypoglycemia (when she remembers her drug but fails to eat at regularly scheduled intervals).

As a result of her poorly managed diabetes, Ms. C is a regular visitor at various emergency rooms (ERs). In the last six months she has been admitted seven times with depressed or elevated blood sugars. On three occasions, the police brought her in because she was driving erratically. She has begun to experience visual blurring and numbness in her feet.

Ms. C claims to understand both the short-and-long-term risks of her disease, but has no apparent interest in altering her behavior to avoid complications. Her physician, Dr. Z, one of only three internists in her hometown of 12,000, has repeatedly spent lengthly sessions counseling Ms. C in an attempt to motivate changes in her behavior. He has also referred her to a diabetic nurse educator to identify techniques to control her diabetes, techniques Ms. C might find more "user friendly"; to a dietician to educate her about dietary control when she is working; and to a psychologist to help her understand her (in his opinion) obstructive behavior, all to no avail. Ms. C has refused to see any of these providers more than once or twice. She reported that the nurse specialist was "so thin he couldn't appreciate what I go through"; that the dietician "needed to lose twenty pounds herself, so how much could she know?" and that the psychologist's staff rudely refused to accommodate her schedule. Most recently Dr. Z recommended that she begin insulin injections to better manage her blood sugar levels. Ms. C refused, stating that she fears her hypoglycemic episodes would be even worse with insulin. When Dr. Z insisted that her health requires behavior modification and change in medication, Ms. C yelled, "How many times do I have to tell you I am not interested in giving up the few things I enjoy? It's your job to get rid of these problems, not mine!"

It is at this point in the story that the ethical dilemma reveals itself:

Dr. Z finally reached his limit. Six weeks ago he told Ms. C that he could no longer care for her, that she should find another doctor because, two months hence, he would refuse to see her. Today Ms. C showed up at his office and reported that none of the other internists or primary care physicians (most of whom have cared for her during one or more of her ER visits) would agree to take her as a patient. Dr. Z replies that he will only continue as her physician if she agrees to the previous behavioral changes they have discussed. Ms. C insists her life will be devoid of any pleasure if she follows Dr. Z's instructions, adding, "Look, I just want to minimize my symptoms. My mother took drugs to improve her circulation. Why can't you just give me those and quit trying to make me someone I'm not? If I'm willing to put up with the aggravation, why aren't you?"
Dr. Z really does not want to care for Ms. C. He is tired of arguing with her and believes that he is fighting a losing battle in terms of managing her disease. Still, since none of his colleagues will assume medical responsibility for her, his termination of their relationship will mean her only care will be through the ER. This will mean that no single physician is coordinating her care, that her "normal" status is never checked, and that no proactive approach is taken. Still, he is not convinced she will be worse off; after all, his coordinated care and proactive approach have not made any apparent difference to her health status.
Is Dr. Z morally obligated to continue to care for Ms. C? [42]

This is a fairly typical (if slightly longer than most) example of the sorts of cases that provide the basis for an important part of bioethical analysis. It is taken from a book of case studies, and each case is accompanied by ethical analyses presented from a number of perspectives such as the perspective of a nurse, an ethicist, a psychologist, and a physician. The analyses provided fall firmly within the framework provided by principled bioethics. Indeed, the introduction to the cases asserts that "these principles . . . are completely uncontroversial, in the sense that everyone grants their relevance to the practice of medicine."[43] These analyses provide a useful way of examining the ethical issues raised by the cases, but treat the cases themselves as though they are straightforward and transparent descriptions of a particular set of circumstances that give rise to an ethical dilemma that must be resolved by the bioethicist. It is this ethical dilemma, that is to say, which is the appropriate subject of bioethical analysis, while the case presentation itself is presumed to be morally and theoretically neutral.

Bioethicists who employ the tools of narrative ethics, however, remind us that cases are stories not only those that appear as fictional creations in bioethics textbooks, but also renditions of "Classic" cases, and even ongoing "live" cases that are presented to ethics committees for practical resolutions. Chambers, who has done much insightful work in this area, argues that bioethicists need to be more self-aware about the possibility that their ethical analyses may be shaped by the way in which the case is presented. He observes that, when "ethicists write cases, they are rhetorically imposing a world upon us, a world that excludes as well as includes those particularities that allow us to make the best possible moral decisions."[44] Because cases "impose a world on us," Chambers argues that there is no such thing as a completely neutral or entirely objective case study. Rather, case studies are a highly structured form of philosophical writing, and they encourage us to view ethical issues in particular ways, and discourage us from noticing other ethical possibilities. Chambers observes, for example, that cases always present the situation they describe from someone's perspective, even when they appear to be presented in the neutral terms of the unbiased observer: "It is important to note that the passive voice, which hides the agent of action and is so much a part of the standard form of the medical case history, exists primarily to suggest that the narrative is apersonal, that is, the narrative is objective and 'scientific.'"[45] In order to demonstrate that this is not the case, Chambers suggests a simple test: simply shift the pronouns around, and see whether the story still flows coherently. This will allow us to "determine whose narrative it is . . . [to] situate the narrator."[46]

If we try this exercise with the case of Ms. C and Dr. Z, and replace Dr. Z with "I," the narrative flow remains intact: "I recommended that she begin insulin injections. . . . I finally reached my limit. . . . I really don't want to care for Ms. C. I am tired of arguing with her and believe I am fighting a losing battle. . . ." In contrast, if we replace Ms. C with "I," the narrative flow is lost, and the story becomes jarring and even peculiar: "I claim to understand both the short and long-term risks of my disease, but have no apparent interest in altering my behavior to avoid complications . . . I insist that my life will be devoid of any pleasure if I follow Dr. Z's instructions. . . . Dr. Z really does not want to care for me. He is tired of fighting with me and believes he is fighting a losing battle in terms of managing my disease." What this switching of the pronouns around reveals, then, is that the case is presented, not from a neutral, objective perspective, but is, rather, Dr. Z's own story. Narrative ethics asks us to think about why the authors chose to write this case in the third person: why does presenting a case in this way make it a more legitimate tool for bioethical analysis than if it were presented as Dr. Z's personal take on his frustration with trying to deal with Ms. C? Narrative ethics also asks us to consider whether the authors themselves are even aware that the way in which they have told the story of the encounters between Dr. Z and Ms. C encourages us to see the situation from the doctor's perspective, rather than the patient's.

It is important to note that this privileging of a particular perspective when case studies are constructed is usually done unconsciously rather than deliberately: authors genuinely believe that they have presented their cases fairly and objectively, that they are straightforward descriptions of the sorts of ethical issues which arise in the context of medicine.[47] However, it is equally important that we be aware of authorial perspectives because our analysis of a case will be shaped, also in unconscious ways, by the perspective from which a case is written and from whose perspective the story is told. While we will sincerely believe that we have engaged in an objective analysis of the issue, that we have taken on the persona of what might be called (borrowing from Mill) a disinterested rational spectator, our analysis is likely nonetheless to be contaminated by the way in which the author has imposed a world on us, and which of the characters we identify as central to the story, and which we identify as peripheral.

Consider, again, the conflict between Dr. Z and Ms. C. The case appears, on an initial reading, to be a straightforward account of an irresponsible patient who is largely to blame for her own health problems, and a dedicated physician, who desires nothing more than to take care of her health care needs, and who becomes understandably frustrated by her refusal to follow his advice. We are immediately predisposed to take the physician's side, to sympathize with his frustration, and to wonder whether a patient like Ms. C is worth wasting any more time on. In short, we are encouraged to take a side in the dispute between them and it's pretty clear which side we ought to take. Moreover, as soon as Ms. C is labeled as "non-compliant," she becomes a stock bioethical character: the kind of patient who as the title given to the case makes explicit "we love to hate." When we apply principles to this case, our analysis of it falls into a familiar pattern: we must weigh Ms. C's right to exercise her autonomy, even if her choices are misguided, against her physician's obligation to act beneficently toward his patient, as well as his right to act on his professional judgment.

In the case of Dr. Z and Ms. C, there is little contest: Dr. Z is the hero, and Ms. C is the problem: indeed, if he is the hero, then she is the villain. In two out of the three commentaries that accompany this case, the commentators side with Dr. Z and view Ms. C with a marked degree of hostility. One states that "Ms. C relinquished her role as a responsible partner in the patient-physician relationship when she chose to direct her health care in irrational ways,"[48] and Dr. Z has no more moral obligations towards her. Indeed, the commentator adds, "Ms. C's behavior makes her a medical saboteur. Her omissions and commissions are instances of subversion and are very likely to defeat the efforts of the most dedicated health care professional."[49] Another notes that, "one can easily see why Dr. Z and his colleagues have such a negative reaction to Ms. C. She can be presumptuous, demanding, and disrespectful. . . . Ms. C's profligate approach to medical care monopolizes resources that could be better used to treat more acute, emergency cases."[50] Only one of the commentators considers why it is that Ms. C is acting in these self-destructive ways. Perhaps she is depressed about her medical problems, and perhaps "the discrepancy between the reality of her condition and what she would like her life to be is so painful that Ms. C immediately self-medicates through wine and food in an attempt to dull the pain."[51]

As long as we view this case as a neutral account of an encounter between a dedicated physician who is struggling to help a non-compliant patient—one who, moreover, is irrational, irresponsible, presumptuous, demanding, and disrespectful—it is easy to give an ethical analysis of the case that sympathizes with the physician's frustrations and places the responsibility for her condition squarely on Ms. C's shoulders: who, indeed, would want to treat a patient like that? And if she is so profligate in her use of health care resources, who can argue against the claim that the physician has a moral obligation to make good use of health care resources (including his time), and that this fact, combined with his personal frustrations, suggest that Dr. Z no longer has a moral obligation to treat Ms. C? However, after performing the test of switching the pronouns around and seeing that the case presentation is not at all a neutral account, but rather tells the story from Dr. Z's perspective, we can no longer be so confident that the analysis provided by the commentators is not shaped by their unconscious acceptance of the physician's point of view; the comments they make about Ms. C, with her "irresponsible" attitude, "profligate" use of medical resources, and the "presumptuous disrespect" (who does she think she is, anyway?) she displays towards her caring physician, suggest an emotional identification with Dr. Z, and that their apparently objective ethical analysis has been colored by this identification.

Bioethics case studies constitute a particular form of philosophical writing, and, as Chambers notes, they bring with them certain genre expectations as a result. Just as something labeled a romance novel must contain a love affair to satisfy its readers' expectations, and just as a book described as a murder mystery will disappoint its reader if no one gets killed (even if it, nonetheless, tells an entertaining tale), so too not every description of events that take place in a medical setting meets the genre requirements of a bioethics case study. Chambers identifies the following features as essential parts of the genre.

The first feature is the right kind of reportability. In a narrative, something happens, usually when some kind of transgression occurs. What counts as reportability depends on the genre: in the bioethics case, the transgression consists of a series of events which lead to the creation of an ethical dilemma, a situation in which, ethically-speaking, we are not sure what should be done: is Dr. Z morally obligated to treat Ms. C? If this case were presented as a medical case study, rather than as a bioethical one, the kind of transgression, and the expectations of reportability, would be different: are insulin injections the most appropriate treatment for Ms. C's diabetes?

Second, bioethics cases are usually plot-driven: they "focus on action rather than setting and character development."[52] The settings are usually neutral: as Chambers puts it, these cases could occur "anywhere in which allopathic medicine is practiced."[53] In the case of Dr. Z and Ms. C, it doesn't really matter what state these events took place in, or even what country. In terms of character development, bioethics cases are apsychological: the characters are subservient to the action, and character traits are only mentioned "when they directly relate to the cause of actions."[54] Ms. C's character traits are only relevant because they contribute to her physician's frustration, and his frustration is only relevant because it is what gives rise to his threat to fire Ms. C as his patient. Even features like race, gender, and religious belief are only mentioned if they are deemed relevant to the action; we are not asked to consider, for example, whether there is any significance to the fact that Dr. Z is male and Ms. C is female, let alone whether there are any other differences between them that might be contributing to the judgment that she is nothing more than a non-compliant patient. (If the gender roles were reversed, would a male version of Ms. C be considered "presumptuous"? Would we read the case differently, if there was some indication that Dr. Z and Ms. C were of different racial or cultural backgrounds?)

Finally, with the exception of "classic" cases, bioethics cases invite us, the reader, to end the story. *We* decide how the conflict should be resolved: it is up to *us*, not *Dr. Z*, to decide whether or not Ms. C should continue as his patient and if the story were ended *after* he had made a decision (whatever it was) there would be no ethical problem for us to address.

Chambers argues that these features not only turn the bioethics case into a particular kind of narrative, he also claims that, for all their usefulness, the genre-expectations built into case studies can be tyrannical: they push us in some ethical directions, and minimize the importance of, or even exclude, others. Most importantly for this discussion, they provide little space for the voices of those who are ill to be heard, and, because they are apsychological, they focus our attention on what actions should be performed, rather than on the characters of those who make the decisions and those who will be affected by them. Consequently, bioethics cases typically "do not provide the kind of information that virtue ethicists deem as essential" to considering questions about the nature of the moral life.[55] This, in turn, encourages us to think that the central, if not the only, concern of ethics is to determine what actions should be undertaken.

The bioethics case that meets the genre expectations, arguably, fits nicely with the principled approach to bioethics; indeed, principles and cases become mutually self-supporting. The bioethics case is constructed so that it asks us to think only about what should be done, what action should be performed, and the principles help us both choose that action and defend that choice to others. Furthermore, we don't need to know anything about characters and motivations because the principled approach suggests that anyone who is sufficiently rational would, in similar circumstances, apply the same principles in similar ways. We do not need to ask about the moral characters of Dr. Z and Ms. C (indeed, while we see the case through Dr. Z's eyes, we know almost nothing about him beyond his role as a physician, and that he is frustrated), we need only to decide whether he or any doctor in his position has a moral obligation to keep on treating her, and whether she has a right, rooted in her autonomy, to make her own choices even if they appear to be misguided and self-destructive.

One way to resist "the tyranny of genre expectations" is to think more carefully and self-consciously about the stories we tell in bioethics, and about how we tell them. Bioethicists, Chambers and Montgomery argue, need to recognize that all case studies—not only fictional creations like the narrative about Dr. Z and Ms. C, but also when they come in the form of a presentation to an ethics committee about a current "live" dilemma—are essentially short stories, and any attempt to tell them no matter how hard the teller strives to present an objective account, "in the very act of telling, is persuading listeners to take a particular position by shaping the telling of events in a particular way."[56] This encourages the listener or reader to understand the story in the way that the teller sees it.

This is important because, as we just seen, the point of using cases in bioethics is to reach a decision: there are *consequences* to the way in which the story is told. And, Chambers and Montgomery note, because case studies are plot-driven, there can be a temptation to reduce cases to simple plots, because we can't include everything, and, anyway, not everything is equally important. But this temptation, they argue, should be resisted because we can be ethically misled by the way in which the story is told. The plot will determine whether for instance we are telling a story about an irresponsible and presumptuous non-compliant patient, a story about an unsympathetic and bullying physician who is unwilling to take the time to learn about the issues his patient is grappling with, or even a story about the ethical challenges generated by a scarcity of medical resources. "Ethical deliberations, as every hospital administrator understands, is an exercise of power, and it takes place where some might least expect it: in decisions about how a story will be told,"[57] because the way in which the story is told fundamentally shapes what decision will be made.

Cases, like other kinds of stories, need closure, and closure occurs at the point at which nothing further can be added. Closure, in case studies, takes two forms: first, the conclusion of the interpretive process; and, second, the literal end of the story. The first form interpretive closure is reached when there are no further questions to be answered. This kind of closure is not structural, it is epistemological, and it is reached when we have worked through all the ethical possibilities raised by the narrative until there is nothing more to say. (This kind of closure, however, does not preclude the possibility that, in the future, new evidence might not cause the case to be revisited.) The second form—structural closure—is achieved when the story ends, and a decision is made. The task of the bioethicist, Chambers and Montgomery argue, "is not so much to end the story. . . . It is rather to envision an ending or more than one to the unfolding story."[58] What *could* be done is, through this process, transformed into what *should* be done.

These types of closures and the possibilities they open up and the ones they close off are shaped by the way in which the case is told or written. Consequently, they note, "When considering a case, it is instructive to ask how its plot ('What is going on there?') is influencing the decision being made ('What is going on here?')"[59] They assert that much can be learned by replotting a story from the perspectives of other participants. This is at once an exercise in empathy, a way of revealing the rhetorical status of the preliminary account, and a means of widening perspective in search of a durable understanding of the case."[60]

If we apply this proposal to the case of Dr. Z and Ms. C, and tell the story from what we imagine might be *her* perspective, rather than *his*, it looks very different:

> *Ms. C is forty-five years old, and suffering from adult onset diabetes. She comes from a family with a history of the illness: her mother, aunt, and sister all have diabetes, have struggled to manage the disease, and suffered from its complications. Her aunt recently had to have a foot removed and is now in a wheelchair, and her mother and sister have also experienced serious health issues as a result of their diabetes. Getting the disease as well was one of Ms. C's worst fears, and she felt overwhelmed and depressed when she was diagnosed five years ago. Those feelings are still present today. She knows that she weighs more than she should, but has struggled with weight issues all her life, and, while she has embarked on a number of diets over the years, sometimes managing to lose weight as a result, she has inevitably gained it back, and more. Each time this happens, she feels even more depressed and unable to cope.*
> *Ms. C has a demanding job that requires that she travel frequently, and wine and dine clients. She has found it difficult to stick to the 1500 calorie diet her doctor has put her on, given the fact that she is often in airports and moving*

between time zones; moreover, when she is required to take clients out to dinner, she has found that she is more likely to "make the sale" if she joins them in a glass of wine and lingers for conversation over desert. When she tried to stick to her diet during these business meals, clients became uncomfortable. Despite her best efforts, she has had a difficult time maintaining an appropriate blood-sugar level, although she faithfully monitors it closely.

Ms. C is becoming profoundly depressed about her inability to manage her weight and maintain normal blood sugar levels. After seeing her mother and sister experience severe and life-threatening hypoglycemic episodes after being placed on insulin, she is terrified that the same thing will happen to her if she starts taking insulin injections. She has tried to convey her concerns and fears to her physician, Dr. Z, but he has been very unsympathetic and critical: when she tried to explain that very few things give her pleasure in life, and joked that wine and desert were her "hobbies," instead of picking up on her depression and anxiety, he made it clear that he believed that all her health problems were entirely her fault, and he dismissed her request to be put on the same drugs that so helped her mother when she developed circulatory problems. Ms. C now feels so intimidated by Dr. Z and his barely disguised dislike, that she sees him as little as possible, especially since at her last visit he threatened to dismiss her as a patient if she didn't lose some weight. This has resulted in her having to make more trips to the ER than she would like, but she feels that she has no other choice when her symptoms become too severe.

She would really like to find someone else to be her primary care physician, but the town she lives in is small, and all the other physicians already have full patient lists. She has recently begun to experience blurred vision again, but she is scared that if she makes another appointment with Dr. Z, he will tell her that he is no longer willing to treat her. While the ER provides excellent care when she finds herself in a medical crisis, it is not a good place to turn to for ongoing help in managing her condition. What should Ms. C do?

What rewriting cases in this way reveals is that the complexities of bioethical issues are more clearly seen when cases are retold from more than one perspective. Narrative ethics, when applied to case studies, reminds bioethicists to be self-conscious and self-reflective about the way in which they "tell their stories," and encourages them to explore case studies from multiple perspectives. We need, that is to say, to see not only *through* the story to the ethical question that lies beneath, but also to think *about* the story itself, and how it may be influencing what we see to be at issue and understand to be at stake.

CONCLUSION: FROM CASE STUDIES TO ILLNESS NARRATIVES

If central and important elements of the ethical life can only be revealed in narrative form, as many moral philosophers have persuasively argued, bioethicists need to take narratives seriously as well. Of particular importance to a form of bioethics that approaches issues through the framework provided

by virtue ethics is the way in which stories demonstrate the connection between actions and moral character, the interplay between the protagonists
that generates the moral dilemma and whose mutual participation is required
to implement any proposed resolution, and the way in which ethical issues
are placed in a temporal context: ethical dilemmas have a history, and solutions to them have consequences. In addition, bioethics itself is steeped in
stories, a fact that all bioethicists need to pay more attention to: it is striking
that bioethicists spend so much time considering the field's myths of origin,
and anchor much of their bioethical deliberations in case studies, but tend,
with a few notable exceptions, not to spend much time thinking about the
narrative dimensions of the work they do, or to consider the philosophical
implications of working with an approach to ethical questions that revolves
around case studies. Arguably, bioethicists ought to pay a significant degree
of attention to the way in which they tell their stories, and how they employ
them in their ethical analyses. At the very least, they ought to rewrite cases in
various ways, recount the events from the perspectives of various characters,
and consider the way in which the ethical judgments they draw might be
shaped by the way in which the ethical dilemma was presented.

But this is not all that stories do. As we shall see, while bodies are
constructed out of DNA, flesh, and bone, selves are substantially constructed
out of narratives, out of the stories we tell ourselves about who we are, the
stories we tell others about who we are and the stories they tell to us about
themselves, and the stories we tell each other about who we are together.
Indeed, giving an answer to the questions we earlier identified as crucial to
the concept of selfhood—who am I? who are you? who do you say I am? and
who should I say you are?—can only be answered through the telling of a
story which provides our answers with context, content, and temporal order.
Any satisfactory conception of autonomy, then, will have to pay a significant
degree of attention to the place of narratives in our individual articulations of
our conception of the good, and to our mutual deliberations about what might
be required if we are to live well together, and it is through illness narratives
that bioethicists can best acquaint themselves with the inner lives and experiences of those whose interests and concerns provide the moral foundation
upon which bioethics is built, and who are most affected by the recommendations bioethicists make.

In the next chapter, we will consider what it means to be a self in the face
of illness and suffering, and why bioethicists need to take illness narratives
seriously. Bioethicists, we shall see, need to consider not only the place of
stories in their ethical deliberations, but also the role that they ought to play
in ensuring that patients are provided with the space in which to tell their
own stories, and given the attention necessary for those stories to be taken
seriously.

NOTES

1. Plato, *Apology* in *Four Texts On Socrates*, trans. Thomas G. West and Grace Starry West (Ithaca: Cornell University Press, 1984), 69.

2. Plato, *Apology*, 70.

3. Wayne C. Booth, *The Company We Keep: An Ethics of Fiction* (Berkeley: University of California Press, 1988), 138.

4. Booth, *The Company We Keep*, 138–139.

5. Booth, *The Company We Keep*, 138–139.

6. Booth, *The Company We Keep*, 139.

7. Alexander Nehamas, *The Art of Living: Socratic Reflections From Plato To Foucault* (Berkeley: University of California Press, 1988), 38.

8. Carl Elliot, *A Philosophical Disease: Bioethics, Culture, and Identity* (New York: Routledge, 1999), 126.

9. Elliot, *A Philosophical Disease*, 126.

10. Thomas King, *The Truth About Stories* (Toronto: House of Anansi Press, 2003), 2.

11. King, *About Stories*, 28–29.

12. King, *About Stories*, 28–29.

13. Nehamas, *The Art of Living*, 42–43.

14. In a novel entitled *The Witch of Exmoor*, Margaret Drabble explores some of the implications of Rawls's thought experiment, and encourages the reader to consider what it might mean to treat Rawls's proposals practically rather than imaginatively, and, in so doing, she demonstrates that Rawls's proposals are as much a work of the moral imagination as they are a rational exercise of the intellect. How would it work?, her characters ask. Would a button have to be pressed? " 'And would you wake up,' asks Simon… 'with all the memories of a person who had been brought up in the new society? Would they have been implanted, like in that robot movie? So that you could remember nothing else?' 'You would wake up,' says David, teasingly, impressively, 'with the memories of a person who has been born into and lived in a society run on the principles of fairness and justice.''Wow!' says Emily. 'That is science fiction.'" Margaret Drabble, *The Witch of Exmoor* (San Diego: Harcourt Brace & Company, 1998), 7.

15. As she puts it, "How should one write, what words should one select, what forms and structure and organization, if one is pursuing understanding? (Which is to say, if one is, in that sense, a moral philosopher?) Sometimes this is taken to be a trivial and uninteresting question. I shall claim that it is not. Style itself makes claims, expresses its own sense of what matters. Literary form is not separable from philosophical content, but is, itself, a part of content an integral part, then, of the search for and the statement of truth. But this suggests, too, that there may be some views of the world and how one should live in it—views, especially, that emphasize the world's surprising variety, its complexity and mysteriousness, its flawed and imperfect beauty that cannot be fully and adequately stated in the language of conventional philosophical prose, a style remarkably flat and lacking in wonder but only in a language and in forms themselves more complex, more allusive, more attentive to particulars." Martha C. Nussbaum, *Love's Knowledge: Essays On Philosophy and Literature* (New York: Oxford University Press, 1990), 3.

16. Nussbaum, *Love's Knowledge*, 3–4.

17. As Rorty puts it, "We would like to be able to admire both Blake and Arnold, both Nietzsche and Mill, both Marx and Baudelaire, both Trotsky and Eliot, both Nabokov and Orwell… The task of enlarging the canon takes the place, for the ironist, of the attempt by moral philosophers to bring commonly accepted moral intuitions about particular cases into equilibrium with commonly accepted general moral principles." Richard Rorty, *Contingency, irony, and solidarity* (Cambridge: Cambridge University Press, 1989), 81.

18. "Values," Neiman argues, "become real when they become embodied, and we are touched by the forms in which they appear. Not even our minds are moved by argument alone, to say nothing of our hearts and our hands and all the other things that keep us going. If the Enlightenment has a body, it's never portrayed as seductive. This is one reason why historical argument hasn't succeeded in undermining suspicion of the Enlightenment. Here philosophy

and history need the help of literature, which moves us more because it moves more of us. Tone and emphasis and nuance are literary notions demanding literary means..." Susan Neiman, *Moral Clarity: A Guide For Grown-Up Idealists* (Orlando: Harcourt, Inc., 2008), 121.

19. Colin McGinn, *Ethics, Evil, and Fiction* (Oxford: Clarendon Press, 1997), 2.

20. McGinn, *Ethics, Evil, and Fiction*, 2.

21. Richard Kearney, *On Stories* (London: Routledge, 2002), 3.

22. Kearney, *On Stories*, 3.

23. Thomas May, *Bioethics In a Liberal Society: The Political Framework of Bioethics Decision Making* (Baltimore: The Johns Hopkins University Press, 2002), 14.

24. John M. Freeman and Kevin McDonnell, *Tough Decisions: Cases In Medical Ethics*, 2nd ed. (New York: Oxford University Press, 2001), vii.

25. Lewis Vaughn, for example, includes both a "Classic Case File" in each chapter of his textbook, as well as "Cases for Evaluation": the former are presented as descriptions of "famous" bioethics cases, while the latter are described as "recent news stories followed by discussion questions." Their purpose is to "give students the chance to test their moral reasoning on challenging new scenarios that range across a broad spectrum of current topics." Lewis Vaughn, *Bioethics: Principles, Issues, and Cases* (Oxford: Oxford University Press, 2010), x. Nowhere is it suggested that these descriptions or scenarios might, themselves, be doing ethical work; rather, they are presented as neutral descriptions of moral issues which can be the subject of philosophical analysis. Likewise, while Ronald Munson notes that "In the Case Presentations, I sketch out the most important cases in bioethics in narrative accounts," the reason for doing so is not to explore, in philosophical terms, what ethical work these "narrative accounts" are doing, it is to help readers connect abstract moral thinking with "real life" concerns: "The most important aspect of Case Presentations, in my view, is that they remind us that in dealing with bioethical questions, we are not engaged in some purely intellectual abstract game. Real lives are often at stake, and real people may suffer or die." Ronald Munson, *Intervention and Reflection: Basic Issues In Medical Ethics*, 8th ed. (Belmont, CA: Thomson-Wadsworth, 2008), xx. While this reminder is an important one, Munson does not address the question of why this goal is accomplished better through a narrative presentation, rather than, say, through and abstract argument. In his view, Case Presentations simply require us to look *through* the narrative to see the "real life" events the narrative describes, and he says nothing about the possibility that the narrative itself might require philosophical analysis, or consider whether the narrative form might allow us to access elements of the moral life that other forms of ethical writing might be unable to. Of the Decision Scenarios presented for student analysis and class discussion, they are described as "brief, dramatic presentations of situations in which ethical or social policy decisions have to be made," and their purpose is to get "the reader to decide what the problems are and how they might be dealt with by a particular moral theory or by principles argued for in the readings." (Munson, *Intervention and Reflection*, xx). Again, their role is to provide a context for analysis of particular ethical questions, but not, themselves, to serve as narratives which can also be subject to philosophical exploration.

26. Tod Chambers, *The Fiction of Bioethics: Cases as Literary Texts* (New York: Routledge, 1999), 3.

27. As a character in one of these cases signs to her husband, "I made the appointment for next Thursday at the Genomic Center. Can you make it? You have to be there to help make the final decisions about the proper combination of genes. Brad, this is so exciting. I can't imagine how mom and dad just left everything to chance and then prayed for the best . . . if we're only going to have one child, she ought to be perfect." Freeman and McDonnell, *Tough Decisions*, 163.

28. Elliot, *A Philosophical Disease*, 144.

29. Elliot, *A Philosophical Disease*, 144.

30. Chambers, *The Fiction Of Bioethics*, 17.

31. Chambers, *The Fiction Of Bioethics*, 18.

32. Chambers, *The Fiction Of Bioethics*, 18.

33. Munson, *Intervention And Reflection*, xx.

34. Vaughn, *Bioethics*, x.

35. Gregory E. Pence, *Classic Cases In Medical Ethics: Accounts Of The Cases And Issues That Define Medical Ethics*, 5th ed. (Boston: McGraw-Hill, 2008), v.

36. Chambers, *The Fiction Of Bioethics*, xv.

37. Quoted in Alasdair MacIntyre, *After Virtue* (Notre Dame, Indiana: University of Notre Dame Press, 1984), 214–215.

38. Arthur W. Frank, *Letting Stories Breathe: A Socio-Narratology* (Chicago: University of Chicago Press, 2010), 136–137.

39. Booth, *The Company We Keep*, 14.

40. Booth, *The Company We Keep*, 14.

41. Booth, *The Company We Keep*, 14–15.

42. Becky Cox White and Joel A. Zimbelman, *Moral Dilemmas In Community Health Care: Cases And Commentaries* (New York: Pearson-Longman, 2005), 80-82.

43. White and Zimbelman, *Moral Dilemmas*, 5.

44. Chambers, *The Fiction Of Bioethics*, 177–178.

45. Chambers, *The Fiction Of Bioethics*, 27.

46. Chambers, *The Fiction Of Bioethics*, 28.

47. This has become evident to me when case studies are written up and presented for discussion in ethics committees. The authors of the cases (including me, on occasion) genuinely believe that they are presenting a straightforward and factual account of a situation that has generated an ethical dilemma. However, what the discussion often quickly reveals is that important "characters" have been left out, or that the case presentation has been shaped by the particular professional competencies of the author—who is often surprised when his working assumptions are challenged by those who come to the table with a different professional background.

48. White and Zimbelman, *Moral Dilemmas*, 87.

49. White and Zimbelman, *Moral Dilemmas*, 87.

50. White and Zimbelman, *Moral Dilemmas*, 91.

51. White and Zimbelman, *Moral Dilemmas*, 90.

52. Tod Chambers, "What To Expect From An Ethics Case (And What It Expects Of You)," in *Stories And Their Limits: Narrative Approaches To Bioethics*, ed. Hilde Lindemann Nelson (New York: Routledge, 1997), 175.

53. Chambers, "What To Expect From An Ethics Case," 175.

54. Chambers, "What To Expect From An Ethics Case," 175.

55. Chambers, "What To Expect From An Ethics Case," 182.

56. Tod Chambers and Kathryn Montgomery, "Plot: Framing Contingency And Choice In Bioethics," in *Stories Matter: The Role Of Narrative In Medical Ethics*, ed. Rita Charon and Martha Montello (New York: Routledge, 2002), 79–80.

57. Chambers and Montgomery, "Plot," 82.

58. Chambers and Montgomery, "Plot," 83.

59. Chambers and Montgomery, "Plot," 81.

60. Chambers and Montgomery, "Plot," 81. In an interesting essay entitled "Context: Backward, Sideways, and Forward," Hilde Lindemann Nelson engages in this exercise. She takes a case that originally appeared in the *Hastings Center Report*, and which seems to be a straightforward story about an HIV-positive gang member recovering from a gunshot wound who is being sent home from the hospital to be nursed by his sister. He does not want his family to know about his HIV-status, or that he is gay. The ethical question attached to the case is: does the physician have a duty to warn the sister? Nelson rewrites this case several times and notes that these re-writings do not exhaust all the available possibilities and each re-writing suggests that very different ethical questions are actually central to the narrative. For example, one re-writing suggests that the central issue concerns Medicaid rules and the distribution of health care resources, as these rules are the reason why it was decided that this patient should be sent home, rather than remaining at the hospital to be treated. Interestingly, in the original case, it states that "It was felt that he could safely complete his recovery at home" (40), which makes it appear that the decision was not made by anyone in particular, and, therefore, no particular person's responsibility. These re-writings also bring the issue of gender to the fore: why does everyone, from the physician to the family, simply think it appropriate for the sister to put her

own life on hold, and take on the task of nursing her brother? Hilde Lindemann Nelson, "Context: Backwards, Sideways, and Forward," in *Stories Matter: The Role Of Narrative In Medical Ethics*, ed. Rita Charon and Martha Montello (New York: Routledge, 2002), 39–47.

Chapter Eight

The Fourth Component of the Situated Self

Suffering

INTRODUCTION: WHERE IS THE BIOETHICIST?

One of the most appealing, if deceptive, features of the conception of autonomy that is embodied in the figure of the Choosing Self is that it suggests that we have control over the way in which our lives go. It tells us that, in order to live well, we simply need to have some conception of the good, some idea of what values follow from that conception, and then choose, out of the possibilities open to us, the one that will best accord with those beliefs. It suggests, in short, that what we make of our lives is entirely up to us; even when faced with illness, we can still act autonomously, still express our deepest values through the choices we make. The self that underpins this model, then, is essentially disembodied (or, perhaps, encased within a body, but not significantly affected by this placement). We have already seen, in the discussion of feminist approaches to bioethics, that autonomy so conceived is poorly equipped to deal with (or even notice) the ethical significance of the fact that we are gendered beings. In this chapter, I want to draw attention to another feature of our embodiment, namely, our frailty and mortality. We will all experience illness, some of us will suffer greatly as a result, and all of us will die.

Since bioethics is a field that exists precisely because human beings have these features, and so, at various stages in their lives, must seek medical attention, and, in so doing, move into the spaces in which bioethicists work, it is both interesting and ironic that mainstream bioethics works with a model of autonomy that fits so poorly with the realities of human embodiment. Another genre of stories, namely *illness narratives*, also offers a critique of mainstream bioethics, but from a very different perspective than those we have already considered. A form of virtue ethics that is committed to a model of autonomy that can help us make sense of the predicaments and possibilities generated by the fact of embodiment, and that understands narratives to be important sources of bioethical knowledge, must pay attention to these stories as well.

What these illness narratives reveal, with striking consistency, is that the model of autonomy personified in the Choosing Self is utterly inadequate to capture the nature of the sorts of choices individuals must make when confronted with serious illness. In such situations, the issue is often not so much to ascertain what treatment, out of the possibilities available, ought to be chosen; it is, far more fundamentally, how to maintain one's sense of selfhood in the face of illness and suffering, and how to confront the inescapable reality that one will die, and not at some unknown point in the distant future, but in days, weeks, or months.

The conception of autonomy I am proposing, then, is one which takes the implications of our embodiment as being of deep ethical significance, and seeks to provide a context in which the confrontation with the *peripeteia* generated by illness and suffering can be made sense of. As autonomous beings who are inescapably embodied and consequently mortal, any choices we make, and any conceptions of the good we endorse, must always take the ethical significance of our physical reality into account. The challenge, from the perspective of virtue ethics that takes as its ethical frame of reference the concept of a whole human life, is how we can live well not in spite of our frailty and inevitable death, but in light of these inescapable features of our humanity.

Illness narratives serve as a salutary reminder of the ethical implications of our embodiment, of the most fundamental purposes of medicine, and they raise questions about the role that bioethicists ought to play in the encounter between patients, physicians, and other health care workers. The sick and vulnerable, who turn to medicine for treatment and care, need to be able to trust that those into whose hands they place themselves and their bodies will not only provide the treatment they need, but will also recognize them as *persons* who are suffering, and whose voices need to be heard.

Medicine, that is to say, ought not to be concerned only with what medical treatments are appropriate and whether they succeed or fail, but also with the selves who suffer illness and on whose bodies the treatments are performed. However, illness narratives often reveal what Eric Cassell identifies as a central paradox of modern medicine, namely, that "even in the best settings and with the best physicians it is not uncommon for suffering to occur not only during the course of disease but as a result of its treatment."[1]

This paradox is generated by the fact that, Cassell argues, modern medicine provides "no basis for an understanding of suffering,"[2] because while it has a place for diseases, organs, and "objective" tests to determine what is taking place in the sick body, it has no place for the subjective sufferings of the person who experiences the illness. As Cassell succinctly puts it, "bodies do not suffer, persons suffer."[3]

Frank articulates this subjective experience of suffering as he was treated for two serious and life-threatening illnesses, and, as he does so, he makes his experiences "objective," in the sense that his suffering is made (partially) accessible to others: "Critical illness takes its travellers to the margins of human experience. One step further and someone so ill would not return. I want that journey to be recognized."[4] Although his diseases were successfully treated, Frank articulates a profound and lasting experience of suffering despite his survival. "I always assumed that if I became seriously ill, physicians, no matter how overworked, would somehow recognize what I was going through. I did not know what form this recognition would take, but I assumed it would happen," he writes. "What I experienced was the opposite. The more critical my diagnosis became, the more reluctant physicians were to talk to me. I had trouble getting them to make eye contact; most came only to see my disease. This 'it' within the body was their field of investigation; 'I' seemed to exist beyond the horizon of their interest."[5] Richard Cohen, who suffers from MS, as well as enduring two bouts of colon cancer, writes about the "loneliness of illness": "The feeling of emotional abandonment by physicians, the very people who should be counselors as well as care providers, can be devastating. When that happens, a rapidly increasing sense of isolation is inevitable."[6]

From a bioethical perspective, what is particularly striking in these illness narratives is how absent bioethics appears to be in the face of the suffering experienced by patients. Like the story of the dog that did not bark in the night, this absence seems to require an explanation. One possible reason for this invisibility is that mainstream bioethics approximates the remoteness of scientific medicine, with the focus placed on ethical issues detached from the particularities of the situation and the idiosyncrasies of the people involved. When an ethical crisis occurs, bioethicists tend to try to identify what kind of problem it is in the same way that physicians try to make a diagnosis (Is this a case of non-compliance? An end of life issue? Is the patient competent?), and then to determine the appropriate decision-making procedure. (Should autonomy take precedence here, or beneficence? Is there a substitute decision-maker who needs to be consulted?) And then, finally, to arrive at the correct or at least ethically defensible solution. (The patient is competent, and can make her own treatment decisions; the legal documents identify the son as the substitute decision-maker, so we should ask him what he wants for his mother; the feeding tube can be removed.)

The ethical issues raised, the appropriate principles and procedures to apply, and a determination of what should be done are detached from the person in mainstream bioethics in much the same way that Cassell argues scientific medicine detaches diseases from their manifestations in particular patients. The person who is the object of medical treatment is both there and not there: he is both *anyone* in this kind of circumstance, and, consequently, *no one* in particular. Like the disease, the ethical issue appears, and must be attended to; and the point of bioethical analysis is primarily to reach a decision about what action should be performed, in much the same way that the task of the physician is to treat the disease process. Both can be detached from the persons who are experiencing them: they could be *any* patient suffering from colon cancer or heart disease, not this particular person, with her hopes, fears, desires, goals, character, personality, and relationships.

To put this point another way: it's not clear that mainstream bioethics, any more than modern medicine, provides a framework within which suffering can be acknowledged and assuaged. Bioethicists are consequently confronted with another paradox: how is it possible for a bioethics that gives autonomy a central place, which is oriented around facilitating patient choice, to pay so little attention to the actual experiences of suffering persons? Illness narratives demonstrate both the limits of autonomy as it is usually understood, as well as the limitations of mainstream bioethics when faced with sick and dying patients.

BIOETHICS AND ILLNESS NARRATIVES

The goal of medicine, Cassell argues, is the relief of suffering; moreover, he asserts, suffering "is an affliction of the *person*, not the body."[7] For the bioethicist, as well as the physician, reading illness narratives can be a sobering experience because many of them describe intense suffering, not only as a result of the disease process but also and sometimes primarily because of the way the narrators were treated by physicians and other health care professionals. By "illness narrative," I mean any account of the experience of illness written from the perspective of the sufferer. While many illness narratives are written in the first person, one individual's experience can also be reported by someone else. Frank, for example, in his discussion of the nature of illness in *The Wounded Storyteller* recounts his own experiences, but also reports the experiences of others, many of which are expressed in the first person: they are, we might say, first-person accounts of illness, encased in a first-person account of illness. Frank's account, then, is more than simply his *own* story about his *own* experience; it is also an exploration of the experience of illness more generally. Cohen's reporting on the lives of five people suffering from illness describes what he is told by them and reflects on their experiences in light of his own struggles with serious and chronic disease.[8] I am using "illness narratives" as an all-encompassing term, one that covers both first-person accounts and accounts reported by others.

Not only do illness narratives support Cassell's observation that, paradoxically, far from relieving suffering, medical treatment can often increase it (even if it cures patients of their disease), but the suffering described in these accounts appears utterly untouched by the presence of the bioethicist, and the institutional context within which patients encounter health care providers seems only superficially shaped by more than forty years of contemporary bioethics. Sure, these patients may have given informed consent to their medical treatments and their autonomy may have been respected (and these things are, indeed, important), but they express various degrees of rage, disbelief, and despair about their experiences as ill persons. These emotions are engendered not simply, or even primarily, by the disease, but by the way in which health care professionals treated them.

As Havi Carel notes, in an exploration of illness that is at once a first-person illness narrative that describes her experiences after being diagnosed, at thirty-five, with a progressive, untreatable, and ultimately fatal lung condition, and a thought-provoking philosophical discussion of illness, that many of her interactions with health care professionals were alienating, isolating, and dehumanizing. "These kinds of encounters with doctors and nurses have repeatedly surprised me; no one ignored my questions or requests. But few cared to make the encounter more comfortable and less frightening for me. No one asked me how I felt about my illness," she writes. And, she goes on to say, "I quickly learned that when doctor's ask 'How are you?' they mean 'How is your body?' That when an X-ray of my lungs is up on the screen and several doctors stand around addressing my 'case,' they will not include me in their discussion. That they will not want to know how my life has changed because of my illness, how they could make it easier for me."[9] Her description of her experiences (as is the case with many illness narratives) echoes Frank's observation that "it" (the disease) is what is of interest to health care providers, not the "I," the person who experiences illness.

The absence of any sign of bioethics in these narratives is not only striking, it is something that needs explanation. Ethics is concerned with questions about how we ought to treat one another and what it means to live well, not only when things are easy, but also in the face of adversity: that is why the image of Socrates at his trial, both articulating a vision of what he understands to be the nature of the ethical life, and choosing to conduct himself in a way that reflects this understanding, is such a powerful one. The example of Socrates also reminds us that questions of ethics are practical and that the ethical life is an active one, concerned as much with what we do as with what we think. Finally, it reminds us that ethics is inescapably social, bound up not only with how we see ourselves and with the justifications we provide for our actions, but also with how others view us, and with whether they find those justifications meaningful and convincing. If any branch of philosophy should take the "I" and its suffering seriously, surely it is this one. As Cassell succinctly puts it, "Central to any moral understanding is the concept of the person. Ethical standards; rules about good and bad, right and wrong; rights and their corollary obligations; matters of custom and conscience that guide the moral aspects of life are always in terms of persons. . . ."[10] Moreover, he goes on to say, in a phrase which echoes the central thesis of this book, it "follows that all understandings are based on some idea of the nature of persons, whether manifest or latent."[11]

Consequently, he argues, how physicians treat patients is largely driven by their theoretical understanding of what medicine is and what it treats—namely, a scientifically grounded and objective enterprise that identifies and treats diseases which are located in bodies. He argues that the reason why physicians continue to fail to treat patients as persons[12] and, consequently, increase their suffering "is that in the intellectual basis of modern medicine, sick persons and their diseases are not *logically* a part of disease oriented medicine."[13] He goes on to say that to think of things as logically related means that they "are connected in the mind—to think of one leads to thinking about the other. Disease theory has no relation to person—in disease theory it does not matter what person has the disease—and therefore, the common complaint that patients are overlooked in the treatment of their diseases is another way of stating that, in the intellectual basis of modern medicine, patients and their diseases are not logically related."[14]

The claim that there is no logical place for persons in disease-oriented medicine, only their medical conditions, is of fundamental importance when it comes to assessing illness narratives because it suggests that the failures of particular physicians to treat their patients as persons should not simply be seen as individual failings, but, rather, as something which results from their training, and from the intellectual paradigm that structures the theory and practice of scientific medicine. (Indeed, in support of this contention, I have heard patients being referred to as though their identity were synonymous with their disease: "The heart attack" or "The stroke." At a public forum on issues in long-term care, I once heard a woman speak, with great frustration, about the difficulty she was having trying to get workers and health care providers to stop referring to her mother as "The Alzheimer's in room 104." Her point, of course, was that while her mother *had* Alzheimer's, this disease was not the sum total of her identity.)

Cassell's analysis also helps explain why the observations and complaints made by those who write illness narratives are so similar: their diseases, genders, personalities, and situations may vary, but their description of their experiences with medical treatments and by health care professionals articulate the same kinds of insults and reveal similar resulting traumas. Their most consistent complaint is that they were treated as a disease rather than as a person, that their voices were not heard (even though their choices were respected), that they were given no opportunity to tell their stories, and that their suffering was dismissed or went unacknowledged. Moreover, these similar complaints occur in response to treatment in very differently structured medical systems: Cohen's, and those whose stories he tells, took place in the United States; Frank's in Canada; and Carel's primarily in the United Kingdom. While these health care systems, as noted, are structured very differently, what they have in common is that their medical practitioners all work within the same disease-based theoretical framework, which employs what Cassell labels "An anachronistic division of the human condition into what is medical (having to do with the body) and what is nonmedical (the remainder) [which] has given medicine too narrow a conception of its calling."[15]

Arguably, it is not only medicine that ought to have as its goal the relief of suffering but bioethics as well. Indeed, the moral issues that bioethics focuses on, the lessons learned from the Classic Cases, and the application of moral theories and principles to medical practice are difficult to explain without assuming a recognition on the part of bioethicists of the importance of suffering, and a desire to minimize it wherever possible. Moreover, as we have already seen, bioethicists gain much of their professional credibility from the claim that they have made a legitimate move from the ivory tower to the bedside of the patient because they have something important to contribute to the way in which medicine is practiced and medical institutions run, something which is unique, and which would otherwise be lacking without their presence. Why else would they be able to offer guidance to physicians, lead ethics workshops for hospital staff, and advise administrators on hospital policy?

What bioethicists have to add, given the nature of ethics, it seems not unreasonable to argue, is precisely a perspective which balances the deficiencies of disease-based medicine, namely, a reminder that patients are more than bodies and diseases, they are persons, and that the "I" is as important as the "it," if not more so; and, moreover, that ethical questions are not answered by deciding what ought to be done about "it," but by ensuring that actions are not disconnected from the persons who perform them, or from those upon whom they are performed. The suffering articulated in illness narratives, then, not only provides a critique of the theoretical basis of current medical practice, but also poses an implicit indictment of mainstream bioethics: whatever its accomplishments, it is failing to provide a sufficient reminder that patients are persons, and, therefore, it also has a role to play in their ongoing suffering. As Howard Brody observes, "Just as modern medicine has developed many ploys for dismissing stories it would rather not hear ('The patient is uninformed; the patient is depressed'), bioethics has developed quite an extensive list of its own ploys ('The patient lacks decisional capacity; the decision, while rationally deliberated, is inauthentic; the surrogate's evidence is not clear and convincing')."[16]

The absence of bioethicists from illness narratives could be explained in a number of ways. First, and most simply, it might be asserted that, despite the suffering reported in illness narratives, these stories are reports of subjective experiences which need to be taken with a large grain of salt—indeed, John Hardwig, in a critique of narrative ethics which will be considered more extensively below, expresses this point sharply: "Exclusive reliance upon patient autobiographies [which Hardwig takes to be the primary concern of narrative ethics in bioethics] . . . would weaken the practice of medicine. . . . Wherever accuracy is important, there are serious questions about whether we ought to attend exclusively or even primarily to autobiography," he argues. We need to be careful when it comes to judging the truth of the stories we are told: "Consider, first, small things. Medical students are taught to double the amount of alcohol I say I consume and perhaps also the number of cigarettes I say I smoke. The veracity of the sexual history I give is suspect, as is the story I tell about what I eat or why I am seeking pain medication. Users of illegal substances often deny drug use. Child abuse, spouse abuse, and elder abuse invite cover stories."[17] If patients lie about all *these* things, what reason do we have to trust their accounts of how they were treated by physicians and other health care providers? At best, their interpretations are suspect; at worst, their stories are untrue.

This sort of objection demonstrates a distrust of patients and a dismissal of the role that subjective experiences might play in bioethics; interestingly, it is mirrored in the framework of scientific medicine, in which symptoms reported by patients are viewed as suspect unless and until objective tests reveal a cause. "Sickness," Cassell asserts, "has to be validated by doctors."[18] I will say more below about this distrust of subjective accounts in bioethics, and explain why I believe an adequate bioethics needs to find a way to encompass such narratives. For now, I will simply note that both the *experience* of suffering and the *experience* of illness are both *necessarily* subjective: none of us has access to anyone else's experience of these things. However, we all know that we have been sick and that we have suffered (and that if we are not currently experiencing these things, we inevitably will at some point in the future), so these experiences are not *only* personal to each of us and completely inaccessible to others. As Carel observes, "We are all ill at some point or another. The vast majority of us will die from some kind of illness. Illness and decay are universal features of life . . . so why is the illness, as a woman with cancer wrote to me, 'a dirty little secret that sick people share?'"[19] She argues that philosophers interested in questions of illness—a category that surely ought to include bioethicists—need to take phenomenological approaches seriously. Such approaches treat subjective, first-person experiential reports as legitimate material for philosophical exploration, "thus challenging the medical world's objective third-person account of disease"[20] or the bioethicist's attempt to duplicate this objective approach as much as possible. In short, it is one thing to say that physicians or bioethicists should employ judgment when assessing experiential accounts of illness; it is quite another to view patients with suspicion, and the stories they tell about themselves with distrust.

Second, and in a related defense, it might be said that the subjective experiences reported in illness narratives, however they were viewed by the persons who experienced them, do not necessarily describe activities which involved ethical transgressions, or situations which were ethically complex enough to require the attention of the bioethicist. They never, that is to say, became "cases" in which bioethical expertise was needed or sought, or which needed to be referred to an ethics committee. In other words, it might be argued, while these stories may provide provocative insights into how a person felt about his medical treatment, and even provide some sense of his suffering, it does not follow that illness narratives are ethically interesting, or that the suffering reported is ethically problematic: perhaps the diagnosis of disease and the experience of illness almost inevitably produce suffering.

While this may, perhaps, be technically true, since I have yet to come across an illness narrative, no matter how dire and painful, which makes reference to a referral to a bioethicist or to a bioethical consult (hence, my observation that the absence of bioethics and bioethicists from such narratives is striking), it does not necessarily follow that no ethical issues were present, or ethical transgressions did not occur. Carel, for instance, reports that one of her physicians grabbed her without warning, and yanked up her sweater so violently that the seams ripped, in order to see whether she had marks on her back.[21] One of the patients whose story Cohen recounts was told nothing about what he was being tested for until the moment before he was to undergo a painful needle biopsy in his stomach.[22] Most fundamentally, however, the suffering reported in these illness narratives is itself an ethical issue; if bioethicists are doing little to relieve suffering, then something is missing from the theoretical framework bioethicists are employing, and from their professional practices.

Third, in response to this last claim, it might be asserted that the insights bioethics offers are still being ignored by the medical establishment, that bioethics still needs to carve out a fully recognized place for itself, and that once it has done so it will be better placed to address the issue of patient suffering. This claim is unconvincing, however, because a strong case can be made that bioethicists have, indeed, achieved an important place for themselves, both within health care institutions and as advisors who help shape health policy: most hospitals now have an ethicist, an ethics committee, and a research ethics board, all of which are supposed to ensure that the treatments provided and the research conducted meets ethical standards and that care is offered in a way that meets patient needs. Bioethicists, moreover, advise politicians and lawmakers on how they should respond when issues of bio-ethical significance appear. Bioethics, that is to say, is marked not by failure in terms of its institutional placement, but by remarkable success. Conse-quently, as Brody notes, when we critique modernist or scientific medicine, there is evidence that bioethics deserves some of the criticism, "as it is shown to have become an integral part of the postmodernist medical enterprise and not, as it may proudly and naively assumed during its recent renaissance, a critical attack upon and corrective of that medical system."[23]

Finally, and most plausibly (given the weakness of the previous explana-tions), we must consider the possibility that mainstream bioethics is itself structured in such a way that makes it difficult for the voices of patients to be heard and provides little space for their stories to be told, and that bioethics as currently formulated has been so successful in integrating itself into health care in large part because it has carved out a place for itself which supports and even mirrors the structures of institutionalized medicine, and works within an intellectual framework which, as a result of its claim to provide expert and specialized ethical guidance, must minimize the importance of, or even exclude, the perspectives of non-experts, including patients. Although bioethicists will, of course, fight to ensure that the right of patients to make autonomous choices is respected, this does not require them to do more than ascertain what their choices are. Although respect for autonomy is arguably the most important principle in mainstream bioethics, illness narratives dem-onstrate that its presence has not translated into "listening to patients" in the way that such narratives suggests is necessary if they are to feel that they have been treated as persons. In other words, mainstream bioethics paradoxi-cally simultaneously upholds the importance of autonomy and resists taking the stories of patients seriously.

Consider, for instance, an objection Hardwig makes to narrative ethics and the inordinate weight which, he argues, narrative ethicists pay to auto-biographical accounts of illness which are both epistemically weak—they may be untrue, self-deluded, biased—and morally suspect: oppressive to other people because such stories only tell one side of what occurred and because they wrong other characters who are molded so that they fit into the story in the right way: "Blindness to the *moral* weakness of autobiography is, I believe, rooted in the much too simple patient-centered ethics that was traditional in medicine and has been taken over by contemporary bioeth-ics."[24]

The solution Hardwig offers to what he considers to be an inappropriate focus on patients in bioethics is that, if we choose to consider illness narra-tives at all, we (meaning physicians and bioethicists) should function as biographers: we should listen to what patients say about themselves, listen to what others say about them, apply our own understandings of what has shaped them and what is important in the context in which their stories are presented, and then offer a reliable biography that pulls all these strands together. While Hardwig claims that he recognizes that there is no one true story, that the physician or bioethicist who tells the story will bring her own authorship to it, his account nonetheless seems to privilege the perspectives of the bioethicist and the physician over that of the patient. It is bioethicists and clinicians who must become biographers, and they must treat first-person illness narratives with suspicion because the stories told by patients are so untrustworthy: not only do patients lie, they can be self-deceived, trying to present a favorable image of themselves to the listener or reader, and if, as he appears to believe, "illness makes most people more self-absorbed, self-centered, or inconsiderate, more regressed into a primitive or immature self,"[25] then the stories they tell will be morally suspect as well. We should, in short, "be especially wary of relying on a sick person's story."[26]

Hardwig's argument seems to suggest that illness itself transforms people into unreliable narrators, and that the *last* thing physicians or bioethicists should do is take illness narratives seriously. This claim comes perilously close to Walker's description of the way in which "necessary identities" are imputed and solidified, particularly between identities that are dominant (in this case, those of physicians and bioethicists) and ones that are subordinate: the experiences of the subordinates can be ignored because "what they are in a position to know better than everyone else what it is like to be in their place is one of the things they are presumptively disqualified from accurately reporting."[27] Moreover, she goes on to say, "It is not just that their views don't count; given whom these people are, their views can't count. Women only manipulate and complain. Slaves lie and run. Servants loaf and steal. Laborers are stupid. Natives are childish. No identity is so necessary as one that successfully precludes its bearer confuting it."[28] The imputation of necessary identities, then, works to maintain existing power structures and to support dominant theoretical frameworks. Any model of bioethics that does not make a place for the narratives of patients to be told and heard, especially if this exclusion is based on a belief that patients are untrustworthy and that their stories are both epistemically and morally suspect, is a model which will find it difficult to take seriously the issue of patient suffering, let alone work out methods to address it. It is, moreover, a bioethics that will privilege the perspectives of experts (physicians and bioethicists) over those they seek to help, and, by doing so, will undermine its ability to achieve its own goals.

Carel tells an interesting story of this process of necessary identification, and describes the way in which it privileges certain kinds of professional expertise by delegitimizing subjective experiences. She notes that both her parents are medical doctors, and that she remembers them "complaining about families of patients becoming irrational. I . . . [remember] the awe and humiliation with which people knocked on our door, asking to see the Doctor."[29] When she became ill, everything changed: "Suddenly they [her parents] were sitting on the other side of the desk. They were the ones seeking answers, begging at the doctor's door, saying 'but surely . . .' and 'there must be *something*.' Watching them turn from confident figures of authority to emotionally defeated parents seeing their sick child become sicker, made it clear to me that there is some unspoken severance, some invisible but clear dividing line, separating 'us' from 'them.'"[30]

Hardwig's arguments seem to defend a bioethics that places bioethicists and physicians on one side of the line, and patients on the other. How can you have your story listened to by other people who view autobiographical narratives with suspicion? Why is their ability to create a "reliable" biography privileged over the patient's telling of her own story? Carel revealingly observes that when, as a professor of philosophy, she began to give presentations about the nature of illness, other participants wanted to know more about her identity: "Is she a patient or an academic? It somehow seemed to make a difference."[31] As a (presumably) healthy academic, her claims about illness were deemed to be more credible than they would have been if they were expressed by an ill person making observations informed by her own experiences. In short, the claim that illness makes sick persons a *less* reliable source of information *even about themselves and their own experiences* defends a view of bioethics, which, indeed, provides very little space for the voices of patients to be heard.

The very success that bioethicists have had in being recognized as professionals who do, indeed, have a legitimate place at the bedside of those who are ill means that bioethicists have, almost of necessity, allied themselves with physicians, hospital administrators, and policy makers: bioethicists, like them, are professionals, not patient advocates. Brody suggests that many people are drawn to bioethics "for the same reasons our colleagues were attracted to medicine: we can observe human suffering at close range, allow ourselves to feel good about our desire to help, but remain invulnerable behind the armor of our professional expertise, claiming all along that we cannot allow emotional engagement to interfere with the detachment and objectivity demanded by our craft."[32] As long as physicians cling to the dream that they can provide effective scientifically based treatment and bioethicists to the belief that they can provide objective and theoretically sound moral advice without being personally touched by the patient's suffering, Brody concludes, "then no one is *listening to the patient's story, the suffering remains without meaning, and healing has been rendered impossible.*"[33] Illness narratives remind us of the importance of listening to patients' stories, the consequences when these stories go unheard, and the suggestion that a bioethics that does not take stories seriously, no matter how technically efficient, and theoretically straightforward, is utterly unsatisfactory.

CROSSING THE POSTMODERN DIVIDE: THINKING WITH STORIES

The most radical challenge to mainstream bioethics offered from the perspective of narrative is arguably Frank's assertion that we should cross the postmodern divide and think with stories. While the approaches to narratives that we have already examined—that we should consider the literary elements of case studies, and that we should expand the framework of mainstream bioethics in such a way that it can allow illness narratives to be told and heard—imply that bioethics can be adapted to encompass narrative concerns, Frank's challenge suggests that the underlying assumptions of bioethics need to be reconsidered. That is to say, if the first approach suggests that bioethics needs a makeover, and the second implies that it needs an addition, Frank's approach suggests that it needs to be torn down and then rebuilt on an entirely new foundation.

Illness narratives, in Frank's view, are the cries of wounded storytellers; in order to heal, they must transform the experience of illness into a story which allows them to express who they are and what illness has done to them *on their own terms*, not on the terms that medicine (or bioethics) sets out for them. Moreover, Frank argues, illness stories are *embodied*: they, quite literally, come out of the body,[34] and so they are, simultaneously, the cry of a wounded and inarticulate body trying to express itself, and the cry of a person who must struggle to tell his own story, on his own terms, in a medical context which is designed to force him to translate what the body feels into symptoms, and the person into someone who acts in ways which a patient ought to act: bravely confronting illness, embracing the medical treatment offered, and patiently waiting for the attention of physicians. "The active roles in the drama of illness all go to physicians. Being a patient means, quite literally, being patient."[35] And, he goes on to say, "Daily life in a hospital is spent waiting for physicians. Hospitals are organized so that physicians can see a maximum number of patients, which means patients spend maximum time waiting. You have to be patient. Maybe the doctor will come this morning; if not, maybe this afternoon. . . . When the physician does arrive, he commands center stage."[36]

When Frank describes sick people as "wounded storytellers," he asserts that they need to be able to tell their illness narratives in order to make sense of what is happening to them. Serious illness, he observes, not only threatens the body, it leaves the person stranded, without a map and a destination. The only way they can resituate themselves is through the stories they tell about their illness: "The ill person who turns illness into story transforms Fate into experience; the disease that sets the body apart from others becomes, in the story, the common bond of suffering that joins bodies in their shared vulnerability."[37]

The claim that all of us, as embodied and therefore as similarly vulnerable creatures are connected, is important: stories must not only be told, they must also be heard. Every illness story, therefore, has two sides: the *personal* (what the story describes of the experiences of the person telling it) and the *social* (how the story is received and the expectations of the one hearing it, which can either allow the story to be told on its own terms or distort it, transforming it into terms which are more acceptable to the listener). Because storytelling is social in this way, it creates ethical obligations for both the one who tells the story and the one who hears it. The teller has an obligation to present a story that is as truthful as possible, and the listener has an obligation to try to understand that truth. Moreover, since all of us are highly likely, at some point in our lives, to be the ones who are ill, who need to have our own illness narratives heard, we also have a self-interested reason to ensure that such narratives are treated with respect.

In keeping with the metaphor of being on a journey, and searching for a new destination, Frank argues that we need to cross the postmodern divide. On one side of the divide lie the expectations of medical and moral certainty provided by scientific (or modernist) medicine and standard bioethics, as these are described and enacted by highly trained experts. Those on this side of the divide believe that objective answers to medical and ethical questions can be found, and they ask people to model their lives and choices on these theoretical certainties, rather than the other way round. On this side of the divide, the "experience of illness begins when popular experience is overtaken by technical expertise, including complex organizations of treatment,"[38] and it is the narrative of the physician, not the patient, that predominates: "The story told by the physician becomes the one against which others are ultimately judged true or false, useful or not."[39] This is also the side of the divide occupied by the contemporary bioethicist, who draws on a particular understanding of ethical theory to justify her moral claims, and who applies principles to resolve moral dilemmas: she must slot the experiences of patients into this framework and reconstruct them, when necessary, to ensure that they fit. And, in this modern context, what is required of the ill person who seeks medical care is what Frank labels "narrative surrender": "The ill person not only agrees to follow physical regimens that are prescribed; she also agrees tacitly . . . to tell her story in medical terms."[40]

On the other side of the divide, however—the side that Frank has moved to, and where he urges us to join him—there are no such things as "objective truths" which exist independently of particular human beings and the stories they tell about themselves and their experiences. We are, Frank claims, made up, as selves, out of stories, and so are the worlds we, as human beings, create together. Without stories, we would have no way of making sense of our sensory experiences, let alone come up with medical, ethical, or any other kind of abstract concept: "Stories inform in the sense of providing information, but more significantly, stories give form—temporal and spatial orientation, coherence, meaning, intention, and especially boundaries—to lives that inherently lack form."[41]

Because of the work that stories do, they have a significant ethical dimension not in the simplistic sense that reading stories will make us better people (a dubious proposition at the best of times) but much more fundamentally: it is only through *narratives* (which Frank understands in the same broad sense that Booth does, and that I am employing in this discussion) that we can even have a sense of moral concepts at all, of things being good or bad, better or worse, and in this sense, stories make us human. Frank asserts that we should not simply tell stories, or analyze them, but recognize that they work on us, shaping us in the process. Moreover, there is nothing beyond or beneath stories against which stories can be measured: there are just more and other stories, of different sorts, and told for various purposes. As he puts it, "human life depends on the stories we tell: the sense of self that these stories impart, the relationships constructed around shared stories, and the sense of purpose that stories both propose and foreclose."[42]

Stories, then—the ones we tell about ourselves, the ones others tell about us, and the ones we tell each other about our shared social world—are, to use King's phrase, "all there are." Reality, Frank believes, does not exist independently of the stories we tell about it; rather, "Stories enact reality: they *bring into being* what was not there before."[43] This claim has significant implications for bioethics because it suggests that even the principles we recognize as legitimate, as having the power to move us to action and of having the capacity to help us think clearly about bioethical issues do not exist independently of stories, but are, rather, rooted in them. Philosophers, Frank notes, tend to distrust stories because they are fallible, and to search for objective principles that can provide the moral decisions they make (or so they hope) with a degree of certainty. However, Frank argues, "claims based on some version of reason seems no less fallible. There is no machine that can unerringly sort good actions from bad, and if the world is a place where stories breathe and human freedom is a perpetual project, the lack of such a machine is just fine."[44]

Even more troubling for those who assume the validity of, and work with, an ethics based on principles, while it is the case that principles can tell us what is good or bad in particular instances, it is *stories*, Frank believes, not *objective reason*, which ultimately tells us which principles to endorse: when "people are pressed to account for their reasons or principles, sooner or later they fall back on stories. People's belief that an act is the right thing to do, at a minimum acceptable and at most ethical, is embedded in the stories they have learned years before, as those stories have been adapted through the narrative trajectory of repeated telling. Few of these stories may be actively recalled; they are mostly a tacit resource."[45]

Frank's account, then, presents a far-reaching challenge to modernist medicine (and, of course, to mainstream bioethics). First, Frank observes that such medicine (and such bioethics) requires patients to transform their narratives into a form that is acceptable. To use Carel's terminology, patients have to transform first-person lived experience into third-person objective narratives: "we [patients and physicians] will speak to one another in a dry, emotion-free way, patients quick to mimic the doctor's sanitized way of speaking about their illness, their body. A further decline in lung function is 'natural progression of disease.' Pain is 'a symptom.' Fear cannot be spoken about."[46] As patients do this, the story ceases to be "theirs," and becomes someone else's.

Even more fundamentally, however, Frank's claim that "stories are all there is," means that his approach, if accepted, requires us to give up the modernist beliefs we hold about where our principles come from (that they are identified solely through the exercise of reason) and how they are justified (also solely through the exercise of reason). Instead, if we not only see them as rooted in stories but also (and even more fundamentally) see our willingness to accept them *as rational*, as therefore making a claim on us, as *also* (tacitly and perhaps unconsciously) rooted in stories that we have been told and whose values we (also unconsciously) have accepted, then bioethicists must give up not only their belief that their moral framework is rationally grounded and their decisions justified, but perhaps also their claim to possess a certain kind of professional expertise *that others should pay attention to.*

In short, whereas most narrative approaches suggest that we should think *about* stories, which implies that we are able to divide descriptions of the world into categories, placing those we label narratives into one category which can then be compared with descriptions that are not narratives (for example, which are medical, scientific, or ethical), Frank's position asserts that all (and any) descriptions are either straightforward narratives or ultimately grounded in narratives. Consequently, we can't evaluate those descriptions we designate as stories using other kinds of descriptions; we can only play stories off against one another, and see what happens.

There are two important implications that follow from Frank's account that bioethicists working within a virtue-based, narratively sensitive form of bioethics need to take seriously. First, his observation that stories need to be told *to someone*, not just *by* someone, is important, because it connects the teller and listener together in a reciprocal relationship which places an ethical burden on both. The teller must construct a story that is not so idiosyncratic and disordered that it is impossible for others to make sense of; and the listener cannot pretend that she has not heard it, or that it is not important. To use King's terminology, if the illness narrative constitutes the cry of the wounded storyteller, then bioethicists can't say that they would have done things differently if only they'd heard the story: they've heard it now, heard it told in multiple illness narratives, and they ought to treat it as morally significant.

Second, to accept the centrality of narratives when it comes to providing adequate descriptions of the moral life, and of their importance in constructing selves which are capable of recognizing and responding to the world along its moral dimensions, does not compel us to say that all stories are created equal, or that we cannot find more and less satisfactory frameworks to make sense and use of them. Indeed, part of the task of the bioethicist becomes, in the model I am proposing, not only to play stories off against one another, but also to identify within particular stories the sort of evidence that the virtue ethicist must take seriously: virtues, vices, examples of what it is to live well or to live badly (and why), and, of course, what virtues ought to be displayed by those who occupy particular roles: nurses, physicians, hospital administrators, personal support workers—and bioethicists.

NARRATIVES AND THE CREATION OF INTERSUBJECTIVE MEANING IN BIOETHICS

I want to conclude this chapter with a brief discussion of the reluctance that many bioethicists show towards understanding narratives as constituting both an important source of information when they come in the form of illness narratives, and an important kind of philosophical writing (not merely as a neutral tool for analysis) when they come in the form of case studies, and why this reluctance contributes to a bioethics that finds it difficult to address patient suffering. Finally, I will make a few suggestions about which elements of the narrative critique provide important insights that should be included within an adequate bioethical framework.

First, it is a feature of narratives that they need to be both told and heard; they cannot do their work—whether their purpose is to provide a description of the world, reveal one person's inner life to others, or to entertain, among other possibilities—unless there exists both a storyteller and a listener. Consequently, narrative ethics implies relationships, and asserts that ethics is a fundamentally mutual enterprise that we engage in together, rather than a rationally based exercise that individuals can engage in on their own. Narrative ethics when understood as a form of virtue ethics, therefore, as in other expressive-collaborative approaches, requires us to recognize that "doing ethics" is, as much as anything, a social activity embedded in real lives and enacted through practices.[47] Its purpose is not, therefore, to provide a mechanism by which objective moral certainties can be identified or a set of rational principles discovered; it is, rather, to help us live together in meaningful and productive ways. The image of Socrates defending himself and his beliefs at his trial is a useful reminder that ethical beliefs must translate into claims and actions that are intelligible to others if they are to be meaningful. A bioethics that does not adequately address so basic a feature of the human condition as suffering in the face of illness which is compounded by medical treatment, whatever its other strengths, largely fails the test of intelligibility. What, then, are its goals, and what other purposes is it serving?

There are two major reasons, according to Cassell, why medicine has had a difficult time addressing patient suffering; and, I believe, the same reasons also contribute to the difficulty that bioethics has in coping with this phenomenon: "The first is a continuing failure to accord subjective knowledge and subjectivity the same status as objective knowledge and objectivity."[48] In both medicine and bioethics, objective criteria which are understood in a way appropriate to scientific investigations (or what Carel calls the "third person" perspective) are seen to carry more weight, both theoretically and practically, than first-person or subjective accounts *even when* those accounts are about something *only* patients know, namely, what it is like to be them.

Bioethicists are more comfortable determining whether what a patient says or does reveals them to be competent or incompetent, compliant or noncompliant, clear-thinking or delusional, rather than with actually listening to what they have to say about what they are experiencing, not only because of their illness, but also because of its treatment. Once we have slotted them into the appropriate category, we know what to do; actually hearing what they have to say might challenge the usefulness of the categories bioethicists are employing, and make our job more difficult. This point reveals another deficiency in the model of autonomy-as-choice that mainstream bioethics currently employs: not only does it not provide sufficient resources to help individuals decide what choice they ought to make out of the range of possibilities that are open to them, it also does not require bioethicists to take their suffering seriously. It is their decisional capacity that is important, not the nature of their subjective experiences, even when those subjective experiences might be entirely relevant to an ethical analysis of their situation.

It is important to note that to argue that bioethicists ought to think carefully about illness narratives is *not* to claim that we must endorse or applaud everything that we see and understand as a result. Some people are, indeed, confused, incompetent, or selfish, and the stories they tell about themselves can reveal them to be so, while others demonstrate that they are brave, caring, and humorous, valiantly coping with the challenges they face. However, thinking in narrative terms allows us to employ a richer vocabulary than we are able to if we only stick with principles and standard ethical theories. We can think not only about rights and autonomy, weigh the benefits of acting in accordance with a cost-benefit analysis against the claims of justice, but also about heroes and villains, the wise and the foolish, and about various forms of human strengths and weaknesses: courage, honesty, self-deception, hubris, intransigence, and so on, and not just in terms of those bioethicists make decisions for, but also in terms of themselves.

Moreover, we should notice, to use Frank's metaphor, that what is *wounded* when the voices of patients are not heard on their own terms, when subjective accounts of what it is like to experience illness and suffering are not considered to be appropriate matters for ethical analysis, is the *self*: that part of each of us which necessarily experiences things subjectively, but needs to have that experience recognized by others if it is to be fully validated as meaningful and significant (and, again, it is important to remember that recognizing someone's experiences as meaningful and significant is not synonymous with saying that we must take everything they report at face value, without employing further thought and judgment). Illness narratives, then, describe what it is to be a *wounded self* not just a sick or injured one, but one whose suffering has been compounded by the fact that those who should respond ignore its cries for help.

The second feature that prevents physicians from taking suffering seriously, Cassell argues, is "an increasing denial of the inevitable uncertainties in medicine and a quest for certainty."[49] Medical tests are understood to be a source of objective certainty about what is wrong with the patient, and the reports patients make of their symptoms are considered suspect unless validated by such tests. This quest for certainty arguably shapes bioethics as well: to understand morality as consisting in a rationally based collection of moral laws or as providing a set of objective principles which all rational and morally committed persons ought to accept, to see case studies as objectively neutral material suitable for detached ethical analysis, is all to make a commitment to the theoretical-juridical model of morality.

There is no place for subjective narratives within this theoretical-juridical model because subjective accounts are, by definition, *not* objective, *not* subject to law-like generalizations, and more concerned with what people actually do, or have done, than with what they should do. Far from being sources of moral certainty, they instead challenge the frameworks many contemporary moral philosophers impose on the world, and to take them seriously requires that we give up on the "quest for certainty" presupposed by theoretical-juridical accounts.

Rejection of narrative approaches and subjective perspectives in bioethics seems predicated on the belief that, to accept them, would require us to exchange rational and objective moral justifications that provide a certain kind of certainty with ones that are irrational, subjective, and altogether uncertain. As Hursthouse puts it, it has been commonly held that the task of normative ethics "was to come up with a set . . . of universal rules or principles which would have two significant features: (a) they would amount to a decision procedure for determining what the right action was in any particular case; (b) they would be stated in such terms that any non-virtuous person could understand and apply them correctly."[50] This model of what ethics should do fits well with mainstream principle-based approaches to bioethics: a decision-making procedure is identified, which can be used by all persons with appropriate intelligence and competence, and it will tell them with a considerable degree of certainty what action they ought to perform. Moreover, different people who apply the same procedure in identical or importantly similar circumstances should come up with the same results, regardless of whether or not they are virtuous persons (or virtuous bioethicists). Who would exchange *this* for something explicitly less certain, more nebulous, such as the character-oriented and narratively informed guidance provided by virtue ethics?

While I will address this question further in the final chapter, I want now to argue that the kind of certainty that would be lost is almost entirely illusory, connected more to the sense that bioethicists have of themselves than to their ability to make disinterested and objectively valid claims. It is common for bioethicists to disagree profoundly on important ethical issues, and to reach very different conclusions about what should be done in particular cases. It is quite astonishing that bioethicists working with principles and dominant ethical theories continue to assert that their judgments are objectively justified *despite* the persistence of particular issues (abortion, euthanasia, and the appropriate basis for the distribution of resources, to name but a few), and in the face of the disagreements demonstrated when bioethicists are asked to provide commentaries on case studies, and to propose solutions to the ethical dilemmas they generate. The frustration exhibited by students in bioethics classes or health care workers in ethics workshops when instructors or facilitators simultaneously tell them that "there is no one right answer" (which is why the topics discussed are *issues*) *and* try to teach a method (namely, some version of principled ethics, usually accompanied by an ethical framework designed to lead to a solution) which suggests that, indeed, there is a right answer which can be reached if only we choose the appropriate principles and apply them correctly (even if we can't reach agreement on what that correct answer actually is) demonstrates a recognition of a tension that lies at the heart of contemporary bioethics. How can bioethicists simultaneously claim to be providing a method that allows users to rationally justify their moral claims and conclusions regardless of their ethical commitments, personal experiences, and moral character, when bioethics focuses on a multitude of disagreements, and the field is characterized by persistent ethical issues that bioethicists seem unable to resolve?[51]

It is important to note, however, that giving up the quest for certainty in bioethics is *not* to assert that we must give up on the idea of moral justification, or of making sense and meaning out of the ethical challenges we face. I want, therefore, to distinguish the *quest for certainty* from the *quest for moral justification*. The quest to determine which of our beliefs we are justified in holding is the quest that all philosophers, in some form or other, engage in,[52] and whatever advances we have made in our philosophical understandings, we have clearly not reached the end-point of our investigations. (If we had, there would be nothing left for any of us to say.) The quest for certainty, in contrast, has as its goal the attainment of answers we feel confident about so confident about, in fact, that once we have attained them, we do not need to look any further.

However, if we move away from the theoretical-juridical template and the expectations it places on us about what morality should look like and how it should work, we can clearly see that certainty and justification are distinct, and even opposed, concepts; moreover, a desire for the kind of certainty suggested by theories which follow this template reflects a particular kind of emotional commitment we make to our beliefs—a commitment that allows us to feel confident about our assertions and to feel comfortable dismissing the views and perspectives of those with whom we disagree as simply wrong, while the concept of justification requires us to make an epistemic commitment to keep on questioning even our deepest beliefs, to listen to other people especially when they disagree with us, to make sure that we have not ignored anyone's perspective because we do not believe that they have anything significant to say, and to challenge others when we disagree with their conclusions.

The distinction that I want to draw between certainty and justification can be seen more clearly, perhaps, if we compare the claims I am making about ethics to the nature of progress in the discipline of medicine. While medicine, at any period in its history, functions on the basis of beliefs it holds to be correct and perhaps even certain, this medical certainty is nonetheless distinct from the question of whether those beliefs are justified: just as a medical textbook from one hundred or even fifty years ago is now an historical artifact rather than a guide to treatment, so, I can assert with some confidence, an up-to-date medical textbook available today will similarly reveal itself to be full of errors and misconceptions a century from now. Indeed, Duffin observes, ideas considered to be correct "at the beginning of a medical education are sometimes false by the end."[53]

The quest for certainty, then, is concerned as much with our orientation towards our beliefs and the status we wish to confer on them as it is with their validity, while the quest for justification is concerned with their objective status, independent of our beliefs about them; and we can never know for certain, in medicine or bioethics, that our beliefs are justified. The quest for certainty can be dangerous because it can encourage us to believe that our beliefs are correct and to defend them accordingly; the quest for justification, in contrast, encourages us to keep on looking, to keep searching for better, more adequate, more complete answers to the questions we ask and to keep asking ourselves, indeed, whether *those* questions are the right ones.

However, the belief that moving away from the theoretical-juridical template and giving up on the quest for certainty (which encourages us to think that *only* ethical conceptions which fall into the propositional, law-like forms expected by this model actually count) will leave us with nothing ethically significant to say seems to be a widely shared misconception about narrative ethics. For example, John D. Arras suggests that accepting illness narratives in the way that Frank and other narrative ethicists ask us to do requires us to simply endorse what the teller reports, and that, as we do so, we must suspend our capacity to make moral judgments: "So long as the narrator has suffered and claims the mantle of authenticity, that in itself justifies the story told. . . . But if all we do is strive to comprehend, if we are exclusively concerned with discerning coherence within a person's narrative, then we have no space left over for moral judgment."[54] Tom Tomlinson argues that, while narratives may serve as an interesting addition to bioethics, only principles can provide us with adequate guidance for our decisions and provide them with moral justification: "What is untenable is the idea that narrative provides a mode of justification that is independent from or superior to appeals to moral principles. Neither interpretation nor narrative coherence offers the tools needed for choosing from among all the interpretive and narrative possibilities."[55]

It is ironic that those who are skeptical about narrative approaches to bioethics on the ground that such approaches do not offer ethical certainty seem quite comfortable claiming that a principled approach is superior in this regard, even though it, too, often results in profound and deep disagreements, not only about what should be done, but, also, about what is truly at issue, ethically speaking. I have participated in educational workshops designed to familiarize health care workers with the principled approach and have observed, when the participants are divided into groups which are all given the same case study to analyze, that their construction of the ethical issue the case raises will differ, as will the conclusions they reach about what should be done and that none of the analyses they provide, or the decisions they make, is clearly "wrong," either clearly unethical, clearly involving a misinterpretation of the principles, or clearly a misapplication of them to the case. In short, they must *interpret* the case study *before* they can begin to analyze the ethical issues it raises and the ethical issue identified is not independent of that interpretation. The interpretation, that is to say, comes first, and only then can the principles be applied.

In terms of the objection that narrative ethics asks us to simply take illness narratives *as is*, to look only for coherence and authenticity, it is arguably the case that there can be no such thing as a straightforward, uninterpreted, and unmediated story: rather, as Booth demonstrates in his analysis of the short (one paragraph) story of the goose that laid the golden eggs, *all* stories ask us to call on *shared* meanings before they can be understood, and these shared meanings form a kind of web which links our individual subjectivities together, making our experiences of stories mutual as well as individual. In the case of the story of the amazing goose, we have to have shared understandings of terms like "goose," "golden," and "eggs," we need to be able to imagine a goose who both acts naturally by laying eggs, *and* supernaturally, by laying ones that are made out of gold, *and* we need to be able to understand the moral of the story which applies to all real human beings, even though this moral is transmitted through a story which we know could not actually occur. [56]

Consequently, even if we are asked to take illness narratives "on their own terms" (as the authors appear to ask us to do), this means that we must take them seriously rather than dismiss them, and that we should make an effort to understand what the storyteller is trying to say, and what the story asks of us; it does not mean (because it *cannot* mean) suspending our judgment or resisting the urge to interpret. Indeed, it can be argued that there is, ultimately, no such thing as a purely subjective narrative (with the exception, perhaps, of the internal dialogue that takes place in our own heads), because, as many accounts of the role played by narratives make clear, not only do stories need both tellers and listeners, but the meaning of the story and judgments about its significance are generated between them. Even a story told in the first-person, which recounts the subjective experience of suffering, must be presented in such a way that it is intelligible to others if it is to be understood, and it therefore takes on a kind of objectivity when it is told it is put "out here," set loose in the world, [57] and made accessible to others, who cannot simply understand it in the way that the storyteller does, but must interpret it. While stories may be told from a subjective perspective, that is to say, they can only be understood intersubjectively, and it is in this intersubjective space that they can be analyzed and evaluated.

CONCLUSION: MORALITY AND THE CREATION OF INTERSUBJECTIVE UNDERSTANDING

Morality, indeed, should also be seen as something which is created intersubjectively; what counts as a moral reason, what moves us to act, what constitutes a reasoned judgment and how such judgments differ from irrational ones, all of these things are products of shared understandings, not the result of individuals rationally identifying moral certainties that exist "somewhere else." To put this point bluntly: the only reason that principled bioethics occupies the place it does, the only reason the liberal self-moral-political framework shapes our thinking about autonomy so forcefully, or the concepts of rights and utility play the role that they do in bioethical analysis, is not that they are necessarily true in some timeless sense, but that bioethicists have reached an intersubjective understanding that these terms and concepts are meaningful, and that they should affect how they act and determine what counts, for them, as adequate moral justification.

As Walker puts it, we *can* find standards of justification for our own moral beliefs, and we *can* describe to others what those justifications are. However, "we *can't* . . . assume that our judgments ought to have authority over them, much less that it is a test of our or anybody else's moral beliefs that they achieve universal authority. And we certainly *can't* presume that the strength of our justification to us warrants our seeing to it that they believe as we do."[58] In short, what counts as a justification for *me* (say, an appeal to Kant's Categorical Imperative) can only count as a reason for *you* if we have an intersubjective understanding that, indeed, the kind of guidance offered and justification provided through the application of this test is meaningful. The failure of Socrates to persuade the jurors at his trial of the merits of his claims about the nature of the examined life and why they should treat his presence among them as a blessing (he is, after all, the gadfly whose sting prevents them from sleepwalking through their lives) and as an example (it is not only he, Socrates, who should lead an examined life but all human beings) suggests that they did not share his commitments, that no intersubjective understanding of their validity was reached. Likewise, if the principled approach to bioethics ceases to occupy the place it currently does, if there is a change in the intersubjective understanding of bioethicists about what constitutes the appropriate theory and method for bioethical deliberations, then the principles that currently shape decisions, provide justifications, and move us to action, will cease to do so.[59]

Another way to put this is to remind ourselves that, as we saw in chapter 1, moral theories create entire moral universes, and invite us to step inside and situate ourselves there; once we have done so, we will see what our fellow inhabitants also see, and will think like they do. But what counts as a reason for us, and moves us to action, will not be the same as it will be for those who inhabit different moral universes. The calculations that seem reasonable, rational, and compelling to the utilitarian will be anathema to the Kantian.

It is important to reiterate, however, that to make this claim is not, simultaneously, to assert that everything is up for grabs, morally speaking, or that "anything goes." Because moral meanings (like meanings of every other kind) must be intersubjectively agreed upon, if they are to carry authoritative weight, we can evaluate moral claims in light of arguments, provide evidence for or against particular propositions, judge which best capture central elements of the human experience, and conclude that some are more useful, more productive, richer, more reasonable to hold and defend than others, and, finally, that some may be closer to the truth than their competitors. But what constitutes valid arguments, convincing evidence, and relevant experience is something we will have to decide among ourselves: these things won't be discovered by particular individuals in some abstract place that is only reached through the exercise of a certain kind of reason, but will also have to pay attention to significant human experiences (such as the experience of suffering) as well. Whether our focus is on ethical claims, medical evidence, or scientific discoveries, what counts as the appropriate method and what is seen to provide adequate evidence, is all intersubjectively, not individually, decided.

As we saw in chapter 1, we can infer the moral worlds imagined in particular ethical theories from the framework provided by those theories; we can play them off against one another and make a reasoned choice about which one provides the best place to situate ourselves because it seems to us to better capture important elements of the moral life than its competitors. And we need to ask ourselves whether the most adequate moral world is one that is at least partially shaped by narratives or one that excludes them from its framework, and whether understanding the self as narratively structured and social life as intelligible, at least in part, because of intersubjective understandings which include a store of shared stories, provides a more comprehensive take on the nature of the moral life than accounts which do not include these features.

The image of Socrates is helpful for seeing why arguing that moral understandings are discovered together does not require us to give up on the concept of justification, while the quest for certainty can actually inhibit the quest to determine which of our beliefs we are justified in holding. If Nehamas is right to remind us that we are not, as most of us would like to think, like Socrates, but, rather like those he questions, then, if we had been at the trial, we might have been among the jurors who sentenced him to death. To accept the proposition that Socrates was right and the jurors wrong (as most philosophers have done for centuries) is to say that, while Socrates was unable to reach intersubjective agreement with the jurors who felt certain about the correctness of their beliefs, that is not the end of the story: he has (metaphorically speaking) been able to achieve it with us, not only because of the arguments he gives or the example he provides, but also because the story he tells about himself and encourages us to become a part of is one that seems truer than the position of the jurors.

Moreover, Socrates, through his conversations with others demonstrates that, if there are objective truths somewhere "out there," they must be discovered together through focused conversation, and that our moral beliefs are demonstrated not only in how we think, how vigorously we defend our positions, or in what we say, but, even more importantly, by what social activities those claims legitimate, and by what we do and how we live. The moral world, in this story, is simply inseparable from the social world. And how hard it is to remember that Socrates' wisdom lies in the recognition that he knows what he does not know! The belief that we can make any claims to moral certainty, that *our* chosen principles are rationally justified and therefore more authoritative than their competitors, and our current theoretical frameworks objectively valid, is to demonstrate the misplaced confidence of the accusers rather than the wisdom of Socrates, and to endorse a perspective which inhibits our ability to engage in the quest for justification.

In short, a bioethics which takes itself too seriously, which sees itself built on a particular set of moral certainties, as more akin to a science than to an art, as something which must abstract itself from the particulars of real people and their experiences lest it be distracted and led astray by them, a bioethics that has little place to discuss virtuous or vicious characters or what moral commitments a virtuous bioethicist needs to make, is a bioethics that will be unable to encompass important aspects of what it is to be human, what it might mean to be embodied and therefore vulnerable, and which will find it difficult to make sense of suffering, let alone develop practices which might help to minimize it. Paradoxically, by claiming to be able to do too much, mainstream bioethics ends up being able to do too little, and, as we shall see in the final chapter, can be led astray, can end up endorsing what it ought to question, and questioning what it ought to endorse.

NOTES

1. Eric J. Cassell, *The Nature of Suffering and the Goals of Medicine* (Oxford: Oxford University Press, 2004), 29.
2. Cassell, *The Nature Of Suffering*, v.
3. Cassell, *The Nature Of Suffering*, v.
4. Arthur W. Frank, *At The Will Of The Body: Reflections On Illness* (Boston: Houghton Mifflin Company, 1991, Afterword, 2002), 54.
5. Frank, *At The Will Of The Body*, 54.
6. Richard M. Cohen, *Strong At The Broken Places: Voices Of Illness, A Chorus Of Hope* (New York: Harper Collins Publishers, 2008), 77.
7. Cassell, *The Nature Of Suffering*, xii.
8. Kleinman makes an important and useful distinction between *illness* and *disease*. "Illness" refers to the "experience of symptoms and suffering" (3); "disease," in contrast, "is the problem from the practitioner's perspective. In the narrow biological terms of the biomedical model, this means that disease is reconfigured *only* as an alteration in biological structure or functioning." (5-6). My usage of these terms follows this distinction. Arthur Kleinman, *The Illness Narratives: Suffering, Healing, and the Human Condition* (New York: Basic Books, 1988).
9. Havi Carel, *Illness: The Cry Of the Flesh* (Stocksfield: Acumen, 2008), 39.
10. Cassell, *The Nature Of Suffering*, 25.
11. Cassell, *The Nature Of Suffering*, 25.
12. Cassell notes that, paradoxically, even though pain is now routinely talked about in medical circles, suffering is still undertreated. Pain and suffering, he argues, are not synonyms, and treating the former does not necessarily fully address the latter. And the situation, he believes, may be getting worse, not better. "Since the first edition of *The Nature Of Suffering and The Goals Of Medicine*, medical care has become ever more dependent on an increasingly sophisticated technology and ever more concerned with the economic aspects of medicine. At the same time, physicians are less skilled at what were once thought to be the basic skills of

doctors: discovering the history of an illness through questioning and physical examination, and working toward healing of the whole person. For too many doctors the power of their tools has made it seem (wrongly) that it does not matter *whose* disease or *whose* body it is, that all that counts is the power of the technology. Both patients and doctors seem more dissatisfied and the central problems in medicine addressed in the first edition are, if anything, worse." Cassell, *The Nature Of Suffering*, xi.

13. Cassell, *The Nature Of Suffering*, 130.

14. Cassell, *The Nature Of Suffering*, 130.

15. Cassell, *The Nature Of Suffering*, 33.

16. Howard Brody, "Who Gets To Tell The Story? Narrative In Postmodern Bioethics," in *Stories And Their Limits: Narrative Approaches To Bioethics*, ed. Hilde Lindemann Nelson (New York: Routledge, 1997), 23.

17. John Hardwig, "Autobiography, Biography, and Narrative Ethics," in *Stories And Their Limits: Narrative Approaches To Bioethics*, ed. Hilde Lindemann Nelson (New York: Routledge, 1997), 57.

18. Cassell, *The Nature Of Suffering*, 258.

19. Carel, *Illness*, 9.

20. Carel, *Illness*, 8.

21. Carel, *Illness*, 4–5.

22. Cohen, *Strong at The Broken Places*, 77-79.

23. Brody, "Who Gets To Tell The Story?," 22.

24. Hardwig, "Autobiography and Narrative Ethics," 50–51.

25. Hardwig, "Autobiography and Narrative Ethics," 60.

26. Hardwig, "Autobiography and Narrative Ethics," 60.

27. Margaret Urban Walker, *Moral Understandings: A Feminist Study In Ethics*, 2nd ed. (Oxford: Oxford University Press, 2007), 83.

28. Walker, *Moral Understandings*, 83.

29. Carel, *Illness*, 40.

30. Carel, *Illness*, 40.

31. Carel, *Illness*, 42.

32. Brody, "Who Gets To Tell The Story?," 29.

33. Brody, "Who Gets To Tell The Story?," 28.

34. Arthur W. Frank, *The Wounded Storyteller: Body, Illness, and Ethics* (Chicago: The University of Chicago Press, 1995), 2.

35. Frank, *At The Will Of The Body*, 56.

36. Frank, *At The Will Of The Body*, 56.

37. Frank, *The Wounded Storyteller*, xi.

38. Frank, *The Wounded Storyteller*, 5.

39. Frank, *The Wounded Storyteller*, 5.

40. Frank, *The Wounded Storyteller*, 6.

41. Frank, *Letting Stories Breathe*, 2.

42. Frank, *Letting Stories Breathe*, 3.

43. Frank, *Letting Stories Breathe*, 75.

44. Frank, *Letting Stories Breathe*, 156–157.

45. Frank, *Letting Stories Breathe*, 157.

46. Carel, *Illness*, 41.

47. Beauchamp and Childress's claim, considered in chapter 1, that the principles of bioethics are embedded in, and drawn from, the "common morality" can be seen as a recognition of the social nature of ethics. However, their assertion that persons who don't agree with the principles they identify are, by definition, people not committed to morality, suggests that their defense of, and belief in these principles is grounded in something *other* than shared social recognition. That is to say, "rational commitment" to these principles appears to come first, and then the opinions of those who share those commitments are deemed to provide support for the claim that their origin lies in the common morality. An ethics truly grounded in the "common morality" (should such an ethics be deemed desirable) would have to take seriously the pos-

sibility that those who don't agree, rather than simply being persons who are not committed to morality, are actually individuals who have different moral beliefs.

48. Cassell, *The Nature Of Suffering*, xii.

49. Cassell, *The Nature Of Suffering*, xii.

50. Rosalind Hursthouse, *On Virtue Ethics* (Oxford: Oxford University Press, 1999), 39–40.

51. Of course, someone might respond to this claim by saying that *no* bioethicist actually asserts that ethical certainty exists, and this might be technically true; however, the claims bioethicists make about the place of principles in the field, the assertion that Beauchamp and Childress make that these principles are distillation of *the* common morality rather than expressions of *a* moral approach, the advice bioethicists offer to physicians and politicians, the statements bioethicists make to the media, and the tone of many of the books and journal articles written by bioethicists, all suggest that bioethicists possess a particular kind of professional expertise and that what they offer is not opinion, but, rather, sound moral judgment, all suggest that bioethics makes a claim to possess a degree of ethical certainty. Consider, for example, the tone and content of the following quote from John Harris, who is defending the right of individuals to make use of technologies of enhancement and dismissing worries that the use of such enhancements would be unfair or unjust because they might benefit some individuals more than others: "I favor and defend enhancements as absolute rather than as positional goods. I defend them because they are good for people not because they confer advantages on some but not on others. I am therefore uninterested in any collective action problems that result from their use for positional advantages rather than for the betterment of individuals or of humankind. The morally justifiable enhancements owe their moral justification to the fact that they make lives better, not to the fact that they make some lives better than others. Therefore, the collective action problem that results from the fact that people invest in enhancements either to get an edge or to protect themselves from being made worse-off by others having them when I do not in a way that leaves everyone poorer and no one better off than anyone else is a problem for them and not for me, or the enhancing technology. 'Serves them right,' you might say, and you'd be right!'" John Harris, *Enhancing Evolution: The Ethical Case For Making Better People* (Princeton: Princeton University Press, 2007), 29.

52. Even those who challenge the concept of truth itself, paradoxically, suggest that the claim that there is no such thing as truth is truer than the proposition that there is such a thing as truth. In *Contingency, irony, and solidarity*, for example, Richard Rorty argues that we should give up the quest for Truth and settle for truths. However, the reasons he gives for this change suggest that we will have a truer (if not Truer) understanding of politics and ethics if we do so.

53. Jackalyn Duffin, *History of Medicine* (Toronto: University Of Toronto Press, 2004), 126.

54. John D. Arras, "Nice Story, But So What? Narrative and Justification In Ethics," in *Stories And Their Limits: Narrative Approaches To Bioethics*, ed. Hilde Lindemann Nelson (New York: Routledge, 1997), 2–3.

55. Tom Tomlinson, "Perplexed About Narrative Ethics," in *Stories And Their Limits: Narrative Approaches To Bioethics*, ed. Hilde Lindemann Nelson (New York: Routledge, 1997), 132.

56. Booth, *The Company We Keep*, 125–155.

57. For more on the concept of stories being "set loose in the world," see Arthur W. Frank, *Letting Stories Breathe*. 35.

58. Walker, *Moral Understandings*, 242.

59. The concept of intersubjectivity, and its implications for ethical theory, will be considered again in the final chapter.

Chapter Nine

The Fifth Component of the Situated Self

Practices

INTRODUCTION: TWO MODELS OF BIOETHICS

It is the movement from the comfortable and theoretically focused world of the ivory tower, through the more practically oriented spaces of the ethics committee and the institutional research board, a journey that culminates at the emotionally charged place at the bedside of the patient, that transforms the philosopher into a bioethicist. This journey has dimensions that are both metaphorical and spatial. It requires a shift of academic focus, from abstract topics to applied ones, and it is initiated by an invitation to enter new places and spaces: the hospital, the hospice, the long term care home, and the ethics committee. What justifies this journey, and legitimates this transformation, is the claim that the bioethicist has an important and unique contribution to make to these medical settings, that his presence makes these spaces morally better than they would be if he were not there, and that what he has to offer in the way of professional ethical guidance could not be provided by anyone else.

Moreover, there is something seductive and appealing in this transformation. As a result of the journey, individuals gain professional recognition that they would otherwise lack, being converted in the public perception from slightly odd and largely useless academics who have little comprehension of the problems faced by those who do "real" work, to respected professionals, whose views are sought by journalists, who can give important educational workshops to health care organizations, and whose judgments are respected by hospital administrators when expressed in ethics committee meetings, by researchers when presented to institutional research ethics boards, and by physicians and nurses when difficult decisions need to be made about what should be done for particular patients.

But what is it that bioethicists should say, do, and be? What is it that justifies the invitation to leave the ivory tower, the transformation that occurs as a result, and what is the nature of the contribution bioethicists make to these medical settings? What I want to consider, as I put in place the final characteristics of the Situated Self and describe the moral universe through which that self moves, is what follows if we conceive of bioethics as a practice, rather than as a set of technical skills and a job description, what sort of practice it might be, and what sort of internal goods it might confer on its practitioners. We now have two clear models before us of what it is that the bioethicist brings, the one offered by mainstream bioethics, and the virtue-based approach that I have been developing. These models are strikingly different, and the assumptions and features of one are largely incompatible with the characteristics of the other.

Mainstream bioethics employs a model of ethical reasoning that falls within the theoretical-juridical framework; consequently, it is largely procedurally focused, and concerned with determining the appropriate method for resolving moral dilemmas. On a practical level, once the appropriate principles and values have been identified and a procedure for applying them developed, any specific question or issue can be analyzed, and perhaps even resolved, as long as the method is followed correctly; on an abstract level, once the appropriate theoretical approach is identified, it can be applied to questions as diverse as the morality of genetic enhancement to the appropriate distribution of health care resources. In this model, ethical reasoning functions as a kind of sorting and organizing mechanism: issues are placed into appropriate categories (for example, informed consent, duty to warn, or maternal-fetal conflict), analyzed in accordance with the relevant principles and values, and, finally, reduced to a small, manageable number of possible responses, which themselves can then be further analyzed according to the same methods so that, through this process, one clearly reveals itself to be superior to its rivals.

This form of bioethics, as we have seen, is oriented around a conception of autonomy that consists primarily in the capacity to choose; what is morally relevant is that choices be facilitated, as long as the Harm Principle is not violated in some clear and uncontroversial way. If resources permit, then substantive questions about the morality of particular choices are largely irrelevant, as long as the constraint on choice imposed by the Harm Principle is respected. Consequently, bioethicists are often concerned with limiting the scope of governmental regulation, since regulations have the effect of limiting choice; as a corollary, the market has been viewed as a facilitator of choice, and many bioethicists have been quick to support the sale of goods as varied as reproductive materials and services, organs, and health care.

In this model, in addition, the moral character of the bioethicist is irrelevant, as are the substantive ethical views of the particular persons who occupy this role. Indeed, it is fair to say not simply that these views are *irrelevant*; even more fundamentally, they are *unacceptable*: given the model of autonomy that is employed, the moral commitments and resulting judgments of particular bioethicists are little more—and can be little more—than personal opinions. Their commitments, therefore, must be to ethical theories (particularly Kantianism and utilitarianism), to autonomy understood as choice, to the Harm Principle, and to the principles and procedures that follow from them. Their role, then, is to ensure that the proper policies are developed and the correct procedures followed. An appropriate place for bioethicists to do their work, therefore, is at the level of policy development, and their role is to translate those policies into a set of procedures that can be employed in the relevant institutions, and to ensure that they are followed.

The bioethicist, in this model, can legitimately be a trusted advisor to those who are powerful—whether they are politicians, hospital administrators, or medical researchers—because it is only at this level that one can have a say about which policies are created and how they might be instantiated in the form of practical procedures. The bioethicist, then, functions as a kind of bureaucrat; as we saw Thomas May nicely sum up the role, the bioethicist is concerned with ethics education (which largely consists in teaching the principles of mainstream bioethics and presenting a method for applying them); case consultation (in which the bioethicist facilitates the application of those principles and methods to particular cases); and policy development (which reflects those principles and makes a place for those procedures to be applied). The task of the bioethicist, then, is essentially to ensure that the correct procedures are followed, that autonomy is respected and its exercise facilitated, to refrain from expressing his own moral views, and to prevent other decision makers from expressing theirs.[1]

Individual bioethicists, consequently, are interchangeable with one another: it is policies, procedures, principles, and respect for autonomy as choice that is important, not the ethical commitments of the particular persons who inhabit this role. In this perspective, asking questions about the moral character of the bioethicist is not only inappropriate, but is actually offensive, suggesting that the questioner misunderstands the nature of bioethics, is judgmental, and is willing to impose his private moral views upon others who do not share them. In short, a bioethicist who wants to make substantive moral judgments and ask questions about moral character is simultaneously incompetent and dangerous.

The virtue-based model I have proposed, and which I have been developing over the last few chapters, is quite different along all these dimensions. It works within the template provided by expressive-collaborative approaches, those that understand ethics as consisting not in a set of policies or procedures, but, rather, in a set of practices; extends the scope of morality to include narratives of all kinds because it is often through narratives that human beings articulate and explore dimensions of the moral life that are invisible when we think only in terms of principles, policies, and theories; and a conception of autonomy that situates the self in the space between well-being (a concept that is connected to the idea of human flourishing) and self-interest (which is responsive to personal desires and individual choice).

In this conception of autonomy, facilitating particular choices is not sufficient to ensure that the capacity for autonomy will develop, or that those choices allow autonomy to be exercised. Three additional things are required: first, that the person choosing have an adequate range of morally valuable options from which to choose; second, that the choice made contributes to her flourishing, as an individual and as a human being; and, third, that the choices individuals want to make not be the result of manipulation, exploitation, or deception. Moreover, it is through making choices that virtues or vices are inculcated and demonstrated. Consequently, choices are never discrete episodes in an individual's life; rather, they contribute to, or detract from, the development of an adequate moral character. In this model, the concept of human flourishing (perhaps never fully worked out, but always there as a backdrop to moral deliberations—deliberations, in part, about what human flourishing consists in) provides a measure against which choices can be evaluated, institutional policies examined, and practices critiqued.

In this model, it makes no sense to see the personal moral commitments of the bioethicist as irrelevant or inappropriate, or to consider his moral character unimportant; indeed, it is these commitments and the kind of moral character he demonstrates that determine, in large part, whether particular individuals who inhabit the role are adequate or inadequate bioethicists. The excellent bioethicist, like the excellent physician or excellent nurse, will demonstrate particular virtues that are intrinsically connected to the role he occupies; and just as a physician who lacks compassion or a nurse who is callous cannot be considered virtuous, so, too, a bioethicist who cares more about procedures than persons, or who, in order to protect his status as trusted advisor, is unwilling to challenge authority, cannot be considered virtuous. In order to determine in more detail what the virtues of a bioethicist might consist in, and what form their expression might take, it is necessary to think about the *telos* of bioethics: what is the purpose of bioethics, and, consequently, what is the purpose of the bioethicist?

The origin myth of bioethics tells us that bioethics was originally conceived of as providing a necessary corrective to the exercise of medical power in order to protect the interests of patients and research subjects, and the role of the bioethicist was to challenge authority when necessary in order to protect the weak and vulnerable, to think critically about developments in medical technology and about their social implications, and to critique widely accepted patterns of thinking and doing when they fell short of philosophical credibility and could not be ethically justified. These still seem to me to be worthy goals, and something which should serve as the unique contribution made by bioethicists to medical practice, research, and technological development; it is, therefore, in light of these goals that contemporary bioethics should be viewed, and the role played by the bioethicist evaluated. What these goals immediately reveal is that we should be suspicious of the desire to be a "trusted advisor" because the role played by a trusted advisor is largely incompatible with the role of a critical observer who is willing to challenge power and authority for the sake of the weak and vulnerable. Trusted advisors, whether in industry, politics, or medicine are an important and powerful part of the system, and their job is not to critique the institutions that provide them with this elevated and important role, but, rather, to ensure that those institutions function efficiently and are favorably viewed by those on the outside.

The great strengths of the model that currently dominates mainstream bioethics are obvious: the principles and procedures it employs are widely accepted, they provide an efficient and concise method for working through difficult ethical issues, they have found a respected place within the workings of health care institutions and in the culture at large, and they ask nothing more of the bioethicist than that he respect autonomy, have a knowledge of principles, procedures, and ethical theory, and the intellectual capacity to apply them in particular contexts; who would trade these things for something different, more nebulous, less exact? Who would choose to trade the pristine and clear language of principles for the language of moral virtue and human flourishing, with all the baggage that, for many ethicists, this terminology carries with it? Who would want to have to consider not only the ethical judgments they make, but also the way in which those judgments shape, and are shaped by, their own moral character? Why should anyone, that is to say, trade the first model for the second one? I want to argue that, despite these strengths, the mainstream model is deeply unsatisfactory, and that it needs to be replaced with a model that contains the resources virtue ethics can provide.

The strengths of mainstream bioethics as currently practiced are largely undercut by the weaknesses of this approach, and both its efficiency and success come at a high cost. In terms of offering specialized expertise that only the bioethicist can provide, the fact that the model of autonomy around which mainstream bioethics revolves largely precludes the possibility of making justified substantive moral judgments makes it unclear what sort of expertise the bioethicist has to offer that is unique and indispensable; moreover, the persistence of patient suffering, despite both the presence of the bioethicist in the world of health care, and the emphasis on autonomy as choice that he endorses, raises questions about the extent to which health care institutions have been reshaped by the incorporation of bioethics. The argument so far, then, asserts that bioethicists have not (yet) made the kind of contribution it was hoped they would when the field was created and as the role of the bioethicist was professionalized.

I now want to make, in this chapter, the stronger claim that bioethics (and bioethicists) have had a significant impact on health care, medical and pharmaceutical research, and on cultural discussions of bioethical issues, but that that impact is very different from what most bioethicists purport (and perhaps believe) it to be. Far from playing a significant role in helping to ensure that these spaces and the practices that take place within them become ever-increasingly more ethical, bioethicists now frequently endorse activities they ought to question and sometimes even reject, and the role played by bioethicists is often to provide a particular sort of legitimation to activities that would occur regardless of whether or not they were included in making decisions about them.

I want to argue, in addition, that this situation should not be understood as resulting from a failure on the part of particular bioethicists, but should be seen, rather, as a structural and theoretical failure: for individual bioethicists, it can be difficult to critique the policies and practices of the health care institutions in which they find themselves because, as feminist bioethicists observe, bioethicists who ask hard questions, who are difficult to manage, will have their invitation to enter into health care spaces rescinded, and will quickly be replaced by others who are more agreeable. In addition, and even more importantly, the theoretical structure provided by mainstream bioethics makes it difficult to find grounds for the ethical challenges bioethicists might want to make, even when they are personally willing to make them.

The focus of this chapter, then, is on the way in which institutions and social structures function to enhance or inhibit human flourishing, how bioethicists might find ways to act as a virtuous bioethicist should, despite the resistance they are likely to face, and what sorts of theoretical foundation virtue ethics can provide to address these institutional and professional concerns. I will make the case that a fundamentally important role of the bioethicist (indeed, the role that legitimates the journey from the ivory tower and the transformation that occurs over the course of that journey) is to work to reshape institutions and activities that demonstrate manipulation, exploitation, or injustice, that cause or exacerbate the suffering of those who are ill, into places and practices that can create the conditions necessary for human flourishing. To more fully understand the state of contemporary bioethics, and the sorts of activities it currently legitimates, I will begin with an exploration of Carl Elliot's examination of the pharmaceutical industry.

THE TRUSTED ADVISOR, THE GADFLY, AND THE WATCHDOG

In *White Coat, Black Hat*, Elliot tells a dramatic tale about current practices in the pharmaceutical industry, its effects on health care, and the role played by the bioethicist in providing an ethical justification for them. The bioethicist occupies a central place because it is the bioethicist who must approve particular research proposals when they are presented to institutional research boards, and the bioethicist whose arguments lend moral credibility to risky medical research in the first place. Elliot's account is fascinating, not only because of the light it sheds on aspects of research on human subjects that are usually hidden, but also because, when it comes to the place of bioethics and the important role played by bioethicists in legitimating this research, it can simultaneously be read in two very different and, indeed, incompatible ways.

On one reading, the reading that corresponds to the first model set out above, it is an account of the phenomenal triumph of bioethics, of its move from the margins of the world of medicine and medical research to the very center, and of the transformation of the bioethicist from external critic of the medical system to powerful insider. On the other reading, the one that reflects the perspective of a virtue-based approach to bioethics, it is a narrative of utter failure, of a bioethics rendered ethically impotent and morally suspect, and of bioethicists so co-opted by their desire for professional recognition and personal prestige that they can no longer question what they ought to question, reject what they ought not to accept, or challenge activities that they ought to view as ethically unacceptable. In the first reading, the appropriate role for the bioethicist to play is that of trusted advisor, someone to whom the rich and powerful can turn to for advice and validation; in the second, the appropriate role is that of the gadfly or watchdog. Indeed, the gadfly and the watchdog can be seen as two parts of the character of the virtuous bioethicist: the gadfly represents the epistemic commitments to question, to challenge, to irritate, to take nothing for granted that are borrowed from the discipline of philosophy, while the watchdog represents the moral commitments the bioethicist must make to do what he can to protect the weak and vulnerable, to address exploitation, manipulation, and injustice, and to promote the conditions necessary for human flourishing.

These two readings are as incompatible with one another as is the creation story of Charm and the one centered on Adam and Eve, and acceptance of one largely precludes acceptance of the other. Moreover, while the models of the bioethicist as gadfly and watchdog can be understood as complementary aspects of a single person, neither is compatible with the goal of being a trusted advisor: Gadflies sting and watchdogs bark and bite, while trusted advisors smooth out difficulties and make life easier for the rich and powerful. I will argue that it is the second reading—the one of failure—that more fairly represents the state of mainstream bioethics today than the first one does; to see why this might be the case, we need to explore Elliot's description of the pharmaceutical industry and its effect on the practice of medicine and medical research in some detail.

The world that Elliot describes is a world in which the accumulation of wealth and the exercise of power masquerade as scientific research designed to benefit the sick and vulnerable members of society; a world in which doctors are transformed into businessmen, and PR companies create diseases for which already existing drugs can be marketed as treatments; and a world in which pharmaceutical companies test drugs on homeless alcoholics and professional "guinea pigs," and continue to market lethal drugs even after they become aware that they are dangerous. As Elliot forcefully puts it, "We have constructed a system in which deception is often not just tolerated but rewarded"[2]; introduced social and legislative changes [which] have transformed medicine into a business. . . . [That] because of medicine's history as a self-regulating profession, no one is really policing"[3]; and these choices have led to a decline in the scientific credibility of medical research, contributed to the corporatization of the university, and allowed the scope and power of the pharmaceutical industry to increase exponentially: in 2009, it was the third most lucrative industry in the world, and during the 1990s the first, ahead of big oil.

This is a world in which professional paid "guinea pigs" serve as research subjects, taking personal risks for money; their participation in medical research, given the number of trials they are part of, raises questions not only about the ethics of paying individuals to be research subjects, but also about the validity of the results which emerge from these drug trials. It is a world in which fake medical journals that look indistinguishable from genuine ones are created as part of a marketing strategy, and academic physicians paid to put their names on articles they did not write, in which the results of drug studies they did not conduct are reported in favorable terms. It is a world in which diseases are created and branded, so that whole new categories of patients are identified as having conditions that need to be treated with pharmaceuticals. Finally, it is a world in which physicians are transformed into drug advertisers and public relations reps, dangerous medications are aggressively marketed, and research proposals are expeditiously approved by for profit institutional research boards.

And where, we might reasonably ask, are the criticisms of these activities in the bioethical literature, and by ethicists working in the field? Astonishingly, bioethicists, rather than being critics of the processes whereby drug companies have transformed medicine and medical research into marketing and commercial enterprises, have themselves become part of the system. They, too, take money from pharmaceutical companies, sit on for-profit institutional research boards (IRBs), and some of the research money that supports university ethics centers is provided by these corporations. Like the doctors whose involvement adds credibility to the activities they participate in and the corporations they speak for, bioethicists, too, provide credibility through their ethical approval of these processes. Indeed, since bioethicists use ethical arguments to justify and socially legitimate the activities of all these other individuals, they are arguably the most compromised actors of all. Elliot reports that, after a young man named Jesse Gelsinger died in a poorly designed gene therapy trial that had no chance of providing personal benefits to him and from which the state of his health should have excluded him, two bioethicists wrote an op-ed piece lamenting the possibility that Gelsinger's death might lead to tighter regulation of such trials, and, consequently, slow the pace of medical research. "We do a disservice to Jesse Gelsinger and others who have been hurt or killed in medical research by simply adding layers of bureaucracy in the path of clinical research,"[4] they stated.

Surprisingly (particularly in light of the fact that the origin myths of bioethics often see the field as emerging in heroic response to the abuses suffered by research subjects in unethical experiments), far from asking whether future deaths and injuries of research subjects could be reduced or even prevented by stricter regulation, the goal of clinical research itself was seen to be beyond question and any costs incurred in the achievement of this goal, therefore, justified. In this drama, the role of the bioethicist is understood to consist not in asking ethical questions and challenging the imperatives of powerful corporations—to ask, for example, whether the research in question is really done to benefit humanity, or whether it is performed for the sake of the profits it will produce, and whether, even if it is demonstrably the former, whether this end is so valuable that it justifies the death of research subjects—but to ensure that research continues as efficiently and expeditiously as possible.

In a similar vein, Elliot reports that when it came out that Lilly had used homeless alcoholics as research subjects, and the company went into damage control, it hired a team of bioethics consultants. Far from asking questions about whether "poverty, illness, and addiction render subjects vulnerable to exploitation by powerful corporations, the bioethicists concluded that 'It is not unethical or exploitative to use homeless people in Phase 1 studies if the system of subject selection is fair, consents are well-informed, and the risks are not exceptional for the pharmaceutical industry.'"[5] Again, this response is striking because it ignores all the questions a bioethicist might be expected to ask, and assumes the values of an industry that a bioethicist might be expected to critique.

At his conclusion of his discussion of the ethicist, Elliot wonders whether, in contemporary bioethics, there is any longer a distinction between serving the corporate machine and personal honor. "Once the very discipline of bioethics is itself part of the machine," he observes, "service is an honor.

Laurie Zoloth, the former president of the American Society for Bioethics and Humanities, has written that the real temptations of industry associations are not financial but the honor and status of corporate consultancies." And, Elliot concludes, if "she is right and advising a corporation is an honor, then bioethicists have already made the shift from outsider to insider, from critic of the machine to loyal servant."[6] Again, from within the perspective of the bioethical mainstream, this shift is hard to analyze, let alone declare to be ethically problematic or even unethical: the important place now held by the bioethicist simply indicates that bioethical expertise has been recognized by the powerful, that it should be paid for like every other kind of professional skill, and that the role of the bioethicist is, moreover, an honorable one, something that philosophy or medical students might aspire to.

The bioethicists' particular contribution is to provide moral legitimacy to pharmaceutical research and to the companies themselves. One way for companies to limit potential questions about their research protocols or their advertising activities is to note that they ran these things by an ethicist first, who gave approval for what they are doing. Indeed, some bioethicists have even provided advice on how potentially controversial drugs (like Viagra) might be marketed, so that possible customers respond with enthusiasm, rather than embarrassment or disgust. Some ethicists, then, essentially function as a specialized kind of PR expert, and, Elliot asks, "What does it say about bioethics when the ethicist is indistinguishable from the public relations counsel?"[7] While critics often suggest that the primary concern here is one of conflict of interest can the ethicist, for example, advise a pharmaceutical company, for a fee, on how to market a drug, *and* provide unbiased advice on the (for profit) IRB that approves the research protocol for testing that drug? Elliot thinks that there is a much deeper concern here, and that is a question about the future of bioethics itself. Bioethicists have gained professional recognition by claiming to possess a specialized kind of ethical expertise, and it is this purported expertise that allows them to become trusted advisors to corporations. But, Elliot observes, "embracing the role of trusted advisor means foregoing other potential roles, such as that of critics. It means giving up on pressuring institutions from the outside, in the manner of investigative reporters."[8] Moreover, he notes, "As bioethicists seek to become trusted advisors, rather than gadflies or watchdogs, it will not be surprising if they slowly come to resemble the people they are trusted to advise. And when that happens, moral compromise will be unnecessary, because there will be little left to compromise."[9] And, I would add, little of ethical interest or significance is left to say.

But suppose at least some ethicists working in the field of bioethics want to be both more (and less) than trusted advisors, do, indeed, want to be gadflies or watchdogs (or, to paraphrase Rorty, would like to be both in alternative moments), on what basis could they take on one or the other of those roles? They are not only incompatible with the role of trusted advisor (the client will get as irritated with the gadfly who asks difficult questions as the Athenians became with Socrates, will worry about being bitten by the watchdog, and both will hinder the efficient achievement of the goals the client wants to accomplish), but the framework of mainstream bioethics itself incorporates many of the values that might be challenged by the gadfly or watchdog.

As we saw in the first part of the book, contemporary mainstream bioethics is dominated by the figure of the Choosing Self. While the Choosing Self draws on elements of the other selves and approaches that we considered (for example, the procedural orientation of principlism, the willingness to engage in a cost-benefit analysis from utilitarianism, and an emphasis on the importance of rights, a concept that partially corresponds to the means-ends formulation of Kant's Categorical Imperative), the central place it currently occupies is largely a result of their collective failures. The model of autonomy it employs is drawn primarily from liberal political theory, and then largely detached from the political framework in which the impetus for its creation arose out of a search to find a mechanism to ensure democratic peace, and in which autonomous choices must be constrained by liberal principles of justice.

Because the Choosing Self embraces a conception of autonomy in which the value of autonomous choice can be utterly detached from a substantive discussion of the value of the ends towards which choice is directed, it becomes a self that is very comfortable in the world of commerce. The Choosing Self, indeed, often equates autonomous choice with the freedom to buy and sell. In addition, because it includes no measure (except the Harm Principle, narrowly construed) against which choices can be substantively evaluated, it is also ill equipped to consider questions of social justice, and of the way in which some people may be deprived of the resources not only to *act* autonomously (because they have few, if any, good options open to them), but even to *imagine* different possible futures for themselves.

As a result, many bioethicists who work with this conception of the self end up justifying and defending activities and policies that are ethically questionable: the lucrative market in the buying and selling of human reproductive materials is justified on the ground that it supports the right of desperate infertile couples to become parents through the generous "donations" of paid egg and sperm "donors"; the purchasing of kidneys by wealthy North Americans from impoverished persons in the Third World is defended as a freely entered into and autonomously chosen transaction which benefits both parties[10]; and genetic enhancements (should they ever be possible) are applauded by bioethicists who dismiss the objection that such enhancements will only be available to the few and the wealthy, and, therefore, treat issues of social justice with indifference or even scorn. As Harris puts it, to those who object to such enhancements on this basis, "Just as it is not wrong to save some lives when all cannot be saved, it is not wrong to advantage some in ways that also confer a positional advantage when all cannot be bettered in those ways."[11] Harris makes it clear that he expects to be one of the people who would be able to take advantage of any enhancements that become available, and so is untroubled by questions about justice or fairness. "Suppose that further depletion of the ozone layer made humans very vulnerable to melanoma and it was discovered that green skin afforded complete perfection. Suppose further that a safe intervention would change skin pigmentation to the required shade of green. I am sure that I would go green, and if I had to make the intervention in newborns I would do it for my children. Others might prefer their children normal and cancerous . . ."[12] Moreover, he continues, with a certain degree of callousness, "My kids might have a hard time until all their friends were dead, but I imagine that there would be enough caring greens like me to provide them with more durable companions—and they would have the last laugh."[13]

The issue here, however, is not the specific arguments made by particular bioethicists, or even whether or not they themselves believe in the positions they advance; it is, rather, the theoretical structure that both underpins their claims and makes only certain kinds of justifications plausible, while rendering alternative perspectives untenable or invisible. The framework employed by mainstream bioethics encourages us to think in individualistic and capitalist terms, even within spheres where such thinking would once have been thought inappropriate, such as medicine, academia, and the family. How can one make the case that there is something ethically questionable about a bioethicist being paid to sit on a for-profit IRB, when the ethical model one is using allows one to easily justify this type of ethical entrepreneurship as a contribution one is making to protect research subjects (wouldn't it be worse if the bioethicist were not there to ensure that adequate informed consent forms are written and signed?), and forces one's critics to try to make the opposing case using language and concepts that are ill-suited to the articulation of a different ethical perspective? How can one argue against a bioethicist's right to exercise her autonomy in this way, and to have her professional expertise recognized and compensated for in the same way in which the expertise of other professionals is recognized and paid for, without raising questions about that person's integrity which are perhaps unfair, and, in any case, could be solved by replacing *that* ethicist with another one whose integrity is unimpeachable?

The critique of bioethics which I have been offering, which culminates in this chapter, is premised on the belief that bioethics is *important*, that it *can* and *should* have a central role to play in helping to articulate values in the context of medicine and medical research, and in shaping societal responses to technological and social developments which have an impact on people's lives and health; but it is also premised on the belief that bioethicists can't fulfill this role if what they want to be is trusted advisor, rather than gadfly or watchdog, and that being a gadfly or watchdog is difficult within mainstream bioethics which, increasingly, often appears to do little more than justify exactly the sorts of activities (like defending the right of pharmaceutical companies to test drugs on homeless alcoholics as long as they signed a consent form[14]) that bioethicists ought to ask hard questions about.

However, in order to make this case, given the assumptions of mainstream bioethics and the way in which they set the terms of the debate, we need to find a moral standpoint which is both external and comprehensive: an ethical perspective, that is to say, which is sufficiently different in its description of the nature of morality that it does not assume what it ought to question, and comprehensive enough not only to cover the scope of the issues examined in bioethics, but, even more fundamentally, allows bioethics to critique itself. I have argued that virtue ethics can provide us with just such an external and comprehensive approach; I now want to consider more specifically how it might be applied to health care institutions, to the activities that take place within them, and to the practices engaged in by bioethicists. If mainstream bioethics has developed a theoretical framework that is able to justify the activities that Elliot describes, and if ethicists working within this framework have found an important place for themselves within the corporate structure of pharmaceutical companies and help to facilitate their activities, mainstream bioethics may have achieved enormous institutional and social success, but must, nonetheless, be considered largely a moral failure.

PRACTICES, WELL-BEING, AND SITUATED AUTONOMY

Among Aristotle's great ethical insights, MacIntyre argues, is his recognition that "rational argument in the areas of politics and morals will be ineffective with those who lack adequate character formation."[15] Consequently, the central problem for ethical theories is *not* (as many ethicists appear to assume) to decide what actions to perform, to answer ethical questions or to work through ethical dilemmas, but something far more fundamental: namely, the epistemic requirement that we can only engage in an ethical conversation with persons who *already* share at least some of our beliefs, and can only influence their behavior if they already have a commitment to morality. Where do such persons come from? How can they be created? It does no good to tell a murderous tyrant that he should stop butchering his citizens and respect their human rights: his moral landscape already *precludes* appeals to human rights, because, if it didn't, he wouldn't be able to engage in such butchery in the first place. Less dramatically, but equally significantly, at least for the bioethicist, even if we determine that something like the principled approach is, indeed, the appropriate method for resolving the dilemmas bioethicists face, this approach does not tell us how to become those persons who are committed to ethics in the first place.

As we saw in the chapter on virtue ethics, one of the great strengths of virtue ethics is that it takes as central the question of how persons committed to morality are created and provides a compelling answer to it. A contemporary virtue ethicist, then, must answer the question, "What is the relationship between character formation, being able to learn from experience, and being open to political and moral argument?"[16] Recent scholarship on the work on MacIntyre's approach, now labeled "revolutionary Aristotelianism," provides a helpful version of virtue ethics because it takes as central concerns the question of how virtuous selves can be constructed today, and the impediments to this construction imposed by features of the world in which we now live: our tendency to view our lives as a series of episodes, the complex social institutions which comprise much of our shared social life, and the influences of powerful nation-states, wealthy multinational corporations, and technologically-based medicine. MacIntyre's approach, then, completes the model I am proposing because it directly addresses the institutional structures that make the role of trusted advisor for bioethicists simultaneously appealing and seemingly inescapable.

A contemporary virtue ethicist faces a world in which social structures make it difficult to ask Aristotelian questions, or give Aristotelian answers. First, our lives are compartmentalized, divided between "different spheres, each with its own set of norms."[17] We face different expectations at work, at home, when out with our friends, when sitting on an ethics committee, and when encountering a representative of a government agency or playing team sports: "So day after day our lives are compartmentalized into distinct areas to the norms of which we are expected to adapt, so that adaptability itself, social malleability has become an important social characteristic."[18] In such a world, it is difficult to ask what it would mean to flourish as a human being, in the context of a whole life.

Second, an important part of what we need to learn to become adequate moral human beings is how to "distinguish those of our desires that are desires for genuine goods [those that will contribute to our flourishing] from those that are not"[19]: to use Raz's terminology, we often confuse self-interest with well-being because we lack criteria that would allow us to clearly distinguish between the two. However, "we inhabit a social order in which a will to satisfy those desires that will enable the economy to work as effectively as possible has become central to our way of life, a way of life for which it is crucial that human beings desire what the economy needs them to desire."[20] The conflation of what is genuinely good for us with what the economy needs us to want further inhibits our ability to become self-critical about our desires. Moreover, sophisticated manipulative techniques can be employed to make us believe not only that what we *really* want is exactly what corporations want us to buy if they are to make a profit, but also that these things are what we *need*.

Third, our contemporary world is one that tolerates great inequalities of money, power, and social regard, and, indeed, such inequalities are increasing not decreasing. MacIntyre argues that, for Aristotle, a precondition for a rational conversation about the common good requires that social inequalities be reduced. When great inequalities exist, both rich and poor will find it difficult to become virtuous and to flourish: "The poor are driven to defend themselves, in order to meet even their basic needs, and cannot learn how to rule. The rich are concerned with accumulation and self-advancement and cannot learn how to be ruled."[21] In such a social context, then, it becomes nearly impossible to ask questions about what is good for human beings, and what sorts of social arrangements encourage and inhibit human flourishing, let alone provide answers to them. Such questions will not even make much sense, nor find a receptive audience willing to explore them.

Finally, the law and the market are now so well integrated with one another that it is difficult to distinguish between the two. What is lawful is frequently what benefits the workings of the market, and what is unlawful is anything that challenges it. Revolutionary Aristotelianism attempts to transform this social order so that a space can be created in which human beings can become virtuous, can orient themselves with respect to genuine goods, and can flourish, as individuals and as human beings. Revolutionary Aristotelianism, then, is a neo-Aristotelian approach which re-conceptualizes Aristotle's claims in such a way that they not only are capable of being applied to the contemporary world, but also provide a genuine alternative to rival moral approaches. I now want to draw attention to four of the central claims that underpin this approach, and will then apply them to the contemporary state of bioethics.

First, in MacIntyre's view, moral philosophy and social structures are two sides of the same coin: moral philosophies must be capable of becoming embodied in actual social structures, and the social structures they engender, in turn, are concrete actualizations of the moral theories that provide them with intellectual support. Consequently, particular moral theories "are not, as their protagonists often imagine them to be, heuristic or normative ideals existing apart from social actuality. Rather, they are parts of that actuality. They inform belief and motivate action, and therefore they inform and actualize the social relations that are constituted by and reproduced in human action. Theory and actuality are therefore mutually reinforcing."[22]

The fact that moral theories cannot be considered apart from the social activities, relations, institutions, and, ultimately, self-understandings they make possible and actual means that *these* things must also be considered in the evaluation of any moral theory, not simply the theoretical framework it proposes. If a theory, that is to say, legitimates social relationships that are exploitative or alienating, this negates whatever intellectual appeal its protagonists claim for it. The implications for mainstream bioethics, of course, are clear: a moral approach that can justify buying kidneys from impoverished and desperate people, or using homeless alcoholics in drug trials, because it understands the exercise of autonomy and the requirements of informed consent to be distinct from, and unconnected to, the social and economic contexts within which people act is inadequate, both because of what it justifies as well as because of what it fails to consider.

Second, in keeping with its origins in Aristotelian virtue ethics, revolutionary Aristotelianism makes it clear that the activities we engage in and the actions we perform cannot be separated from who we are: if we habitually perform vicious actions, we will become vicious; if we act virtuously today, we are more likely to act virtuously tomorrow. The "moral agent" referred to in many theoretical discussions about the nature of ethics is not some part of us that we need to call on only when we are faced with an ethical dilemma or must make a moral choice, but each of us, all the time. Moreover, following from the claim that moral theories ought not to be considered apart from their actualizations in the social world, what we say and write are not separate from what we do. The ethicist, who works in a comfortable office in the ivory tower writing papers on bioethical issues, or who sits at a table in a corporate boardroom and gets paid to provide an ethical justification for that corporation's policies and actions, cannot consider herself to be unaffected by the moral consequences of the positions she takes on these issues, policies, and activities. They must, that is to say, be considered not merely intellectual exercises but morally significant choices.

MacIntyre argues in a recent paper that moral, political, and economic theories "are not just theories about the social order framed from some external standpoint. They are also theories whose defense functions within the social order to strengthen some conceptions of justice, liberty, and common goods at the expense of others. To achieve them is not just to write about, but to engage in social conflict."[23] It follows from this that MacIntyre, too, is engaging in social conflict, as am I, as I write this; and, indeed, so are all bioethicists. Because the social world is composed, in part, of competing conceptions of the human good, social conflict is impossible to avoid; consequently, each of us must ask which of the contending positions we ought to accept and defend, and simultaneously shaping our own characters. It is, then, not only the case that, as I have argued, we need to think about the virtues that would be demonstrated by a virtuous bioethicist when we think in the moral terms provided by virtue ethics. Even more fundamentally, whether or not particular bioethicists choose to view their activities in this way, their moral characters cannot be detached from the positions they advance, or from the activities their arguments legitimate. In short, because of the phenomenal success of bioethics and the professional recognition of bio-ethicists that has resulted from this success, the arguments presented by bioethicists do not simply provide an objective analysis of activities that are independent of that analysis; rather, through the arguments they present, they legitimate certain activities and, through that legitimation, help create a world in which those activities are not only possible but can be seen as morally acceptable.

Third, while MacIntyre's account (in keeping with Aristotle's position, and like the one presented by Raz) holds that desires must be given an appropriate place within any adequate moral scheme, it asserts, as we have seen, that what we currently desire may be very different from what we *ought* to desire, very different from what is, in fact, genuinely good. What is genu-inely good—something at which we ought to aim—is so because it will genuinely contribute to our flourishing not only as particular individuals but also as human beings. The liberal understanding of autonomy—an under-standing that has been almost entirely embraced in mainstream bioethics and whose central characteristics are embodied in the figure of the Choosing Self—is problematic precisely because it does not give us any way (theoreti-cally or practically) to distinguish between what we desire and what we ought to desire. As Maletta puts it, "Thanks to the often implicit and even unconscious anthropological and psychological assumptions underlying the liberal view of social action, individuals are allowed to use the statement 'I want / desire this' as the major premise of a practical argument, that is, as a valid reason to act independently of any assessment of that will or desire."[24] Like Raz, Maletta connects the worth of autonomy to the value of the things chosen, but he takes Raz's argument one step further by placing it within the framework provided by revolutionary Aristotelianism which seeks to address the social context in which manipulation and exploitation are made possible.

A conception of autonomy that considers the act of choosing to be more important than the things chosen, far from being empowering, becomes al-ienating, and, indeed, its widespread acceptance may be one of the tools by which manipulative and exploitative social arrangements are maintained. Ac-cording to the liberal self-moral-political account, "the subject always rea-sons assuming the viewpoint of a third person, because she avoids assessing the will or the desire that underlies her own practical reasoning and action. She takes them as positive data. We face the case of *an alienation of the subject from her desires and her will*, that is, *from her own self*."[25] An important difference between the liberal self-political-moral account and rev-olutionary Aristotelianism is that while the former makes moral judgments subservient to political arrangements and sees human flourishing as lying in the freedom to choose detached from any substantive judgments about the value of the things chosen, revolutionary Aristotelianism sees this kind of freedom as both alienating and misguided: alienating because it discourages self-reflection on our own desires and leaves us open to having those desires manipulated by others, and misguided because it provides no resources that individuals can use in their deliberations to distinguish between what is genuinely valuable, and what only appears to be so.

There are two significant consequences for bioethics of this kind of alienation. First, because individuals have no standpoint from which to reflect on their own desires, they are vulnerable to manipulation by others who have the means to create desires in them. Consequently, a bioethics that is predicated on respect for autonomy understood as the identification and then the facilitation of an individual's desires needs to ask much deeper questions about the source of those desires and the actual consequences of their realization. Second, Maletta argues, it is precisely this alienation from ourselves that contributes to the rise of the professional expert who can tell us what we ought to do. Professional ethicists, that is to say, are only needed when people no longer trust their own abilities to make moral judgments. But the ethicist who works within a moral framework that provides no clear means of distinguishing what is genuinely valuable from what only appears to be so has no basis for making such judgments about her own choices, let alone making judgments about what might be best for anyone else. We have seen that one paradoxical result of this perspective is that bioethicists end up claiming an expertise in a subject (ethics) in which the very expertise they claim is, given the account of autonomy they employ, impossible. We can now add that because moral philosophies are always actualized in social relations, the "final effect" of the rise of a professional expert like a bioethicist is also "paradoxical: a social order built to defend the value of the individual and her own liberties produces a new form of dependence and alienation."[26]

Finally, MacIntyre asserts that it is only by recognizing that we are historically situated, and that any account of the virtues will itself reflect this, that we can find "grounds for making universal claims both about human nature and about the functioning of the virtues."[27] That is to say, only an historical approach, which allows us to compare our own perspectives, commitments, and beliefs, in light of the way in which they differ from and are similar to those held by persons in other times and places, permits us to see ourselves clearly *and* to see human characteristics that are common to all historical periods—characteristics, in short, of dependent rational animals who enter into relationships with one another, and who create communities together. Any adequate conception of the virtues that we can articulate will be one that takes into account the kind of creature we are, and any adequate conception of what constitutes human flourishing will likewise have to take the implications of our embodiment into account. Of particular importance for bioethics is his insistence on the fact that "physical and mental disability are afflictions of the body and therefore habits of mind that express an attitude of denial towards the facts of disability and dependence presuppose either a failure or a refusal to acknowledge adequately the bodily dimensions of our existence."[28] Any adequate form of bioethics, then, needs to take seriously the moral implications of our embodiment, not simply the physical effects that result from this fact.

MacIntyre, then, needs to answer two questions: first, what account of the virtues and of the nature of human excellence can we give that accurately reflects the kind of creature we are? And, second, what sort of account can be given *today* that reflects our need to see our own commitments, assumptions, and beliefs clearly, given that these very same commitments, assumptions, and beliefs shape what we understand to be meaningful, to be valuable, and to be real? An answer to this second question will require us to employ the Nuerathian procedure: we will have to identify particular beliefs and commitments and then test them by comparing them to other beliefs and commitments, and gradually alter them in light of what we discover as we engage in this process. But the most important way in which we learn to be virtuous is through engagement in practices.

By a "practice," MacIntyre means any "coherent and complex form of socially established human activity through which goods internal to that form of activity are realized in the course of trying to achieve those standards of excellence that are appropriate to, and partially definitive of, that form of human activity with the result that human powers to achieve excellence, and human conceptions of the ends and goods involved are systematically extended."[29] As examples of practices, MacIntyre cites games like chess and football; architecture; farming; the inquiries of physics, chemistry, and biology; and activities like music. Tic tac toe, however, is not a practice, nor is bricklaying, or throwing a football around, even if one does it with skill. We can extrapolate from this list, and come up with other examples: reading Descartes is not a practice, although philosophy is; stargazing is not a practice, but astronomy is. Each of the coherent activities we can recognize as practices aims at some good, and that good is objective; it exists outside of the beliefs and desires of particular participants. Even if I wish to be a good chess player, and believe that I am, whether or not my wish is fulfilled and my belief true depends on whether or not I have actually mastered what chess requires, and those standards are independent of my beliefs and desires. The practice of chess itself, that is to say, determines what it means to be a competent chess player, and what it means to be an excellent one. Practices, then, require us to submit to *their* standards: "To enter a practice is to accept the authority of those standards and the inadequacy of my own performance as judged by them."[30] And, while practices have a history, we cannot adequately participate in them unless we accept their standards as they are at the present time.

A second important feature of practices is that they are cooperative activities which could not exist without the participation of a number of individuals, each of whom is prepared to enter into the practice on the terms that the practice itself sets out; if I manage to invent a wonderful, complex game, but can find no one else who is willing to play it, it can never become a practice. Finally, excellent participants in a particular practice can, over time, extend that practice, take it to previously unreachable and perhaps unimagined places, while remaining faithful to that practice: a chess master may discover a previously unknown set of moves that themselves become part of the practice of chess, a philosopher may develop a theory which pushes philosophical enquiry into new areas of exploration.

Practices, then, contain goods that are internal to them. (In *After Virtue*, MacIntyre calls these goods "internal," but in later works calls them "goods of excellence." I will use both terms interchangeably.) Internal goods are distinguished from what he calls "external goods" (or "goods of efficiency.") To illustrate the difference between the two sorts of goods, MacIntyre asks us to imagine a child who has to be bribed to play chess. We are to imagine, moreover, that this child is also told that if she wins, she will get twice as much candy than if she loses. In such a case, the child has an incentive to cheat, if she can get away with it. But suppose that, over time, this child begins to appreciate the goods specific to chess, such as competitive intensity combined with strategic imagination. At this point, the child will want to excel at chess, and will realize that if she cheats, she is defeating not just her opponents, but also herself. (A similar example can be given when we consider the academic practices engaged in by students: academic dishonesty, even if it goes undetected, cheats the student who engages in it.)

Thus, in the game of chess, the discipline of philosophy, or the activity of playing music, there are some goods that are contingent and external to the game, the discipline, or the activity, such as the candy, a good mark, or fame which can be achieved in alternative ways: by going to the store, by playing the game well, by cheating; by taking an English course instead of one in philosophy, by writing a good paper, by plagiarizing an assignment off the internet; by becoming a popular musical performer, by becoming a notorious criminal, or by winning the Nobel prize. These *external* goods, then, are not specific to a particular practice, and they can be attained in a number of ways, some of which are consistent with the requirements of practices, and some not. *Internal* goods, however, can be attained "*only* by engaging in some particular kind of practice."[31] MacIntyre identifies two ways in which such goods are internal, to which I will add a third.

First, because internal goods can only be achieved through participation in a particular practice, they are internal to that practice. Second, "they can only be identified and recognized by the experience of participating in the practice in question. Those who lack the relevant experience are incompetent thereby as judges of internal goods."[32] They are internal, that is to say, not only to practices, but also only recognizable to those who have internalized them. (The child who never plays chess unless there is an edible reward, or the student who always cheats, will never know what it is that they are missing, nor be capable of recognizing that they are the persons most hurt by their actions.) Finally, in terms of the moral geography set out by MacIntyre, internal goods are internal not only to the individual who engages in practices in the right way, and to practices themselves, but also to a tradition of moral enquiry. This means, as Knight puts it, that practices provide a way of overcoming social alienation by reconciling "the individual to the social constraints [which act] upon her,"[33] because through practices we can exercise rationality and achieve personal excellence, and thereby render ourselves less vulnerable to exploitation and manipulation.

There is another important difference between internal and external goods: "External goods are . . . characteristically objects of competition in which there must be losers as well as winners. Internal goods are indeed the outcome of the competition to excel, but it is characteristic of them that their achievement is a good for the whole community who participate in the practice."[34] For example, only one person may be able to win the chess tournament, but the whole community of chess players benefits by the increased abilities of all the players; while only a few people can receive the scholarship to grad school, everyone who engages in the practice of philosophy for the sake of the internal goods it confers (critical thinking skills, an orientation toward disinterested enquiry) benefits, as does the society in which they live. External goods, then, often come in the form of money, power, or recognition; internal goods, in contrast, make us better, even virtuous people, and in this pursuit of excellence our main competitor is ourselves.

The results of participating in practices, then, manifest themselves not only in activities (playing chess, joining chess clubs, reading philosophy texts and writing essays on them) but in inner transformations as well. As Todd May notes, the conscious self-reflection developed through his participation in the practice of philosophy has become "part of my personal style."[35] Our selves, then, are quite literally constructed out of, and shaped by, the particular practices we engage in, and by the form that engagement takes; it matters, therefore, in which practices we choose to participate, and how we choose to do so. It is because of this internally transforming potential that practices provide the initial training ground for the virtues. This leads MacIntyre to give a definition of a virtue as "*an acquired human quality the possession and exercise of which tends to enable us to achieve those goods which are internal to practices and the lack of which effectively prevents us from achieving any such good.*"[36] (Italics in the original text).

Participation in practices, MacIntyre argues, requires us to recognize the contributions of others and to be prepared to recognize our own inadequacies. This means that necessary components of any practice are the virtues of honesty (which is required for the pursuit of common goods), courage (the willingness to risk personal harm or danger for the sake of those things which we believe to be important), and justice (which requires that "we treat others in respect of merit or desert according to uniform and impersonal standards"[37]). If we are not willing to accept the requirements of these virtues, and to internalize them, practices can never be anything more to us than a way to achieve external goods.

Before discussing the way in which MacIntyre connects practices to institutions, I want to consider an important objection that is sometimes made to MacIntyre's account of practices, namely that this approach is relativistic, and provides no way of distinguishing between evil practices and virtuous ones. Might not this account, for example, suggest that, through practices, one could learn to become an excellent torturer or mercenary? To this objection, a twofold response can be given. First, practices are necessarily teleological: they aim at *something*, and that something is capable of moral assessment. (The skills of an effective torturer, for example, clearly aim at something very different than the internal goods achievable through chess, philosophy, or medicine.) Further, it is not the case that practices *alone* determine what it is to be virtuous; rather, they are the space within which virtues can be developed, that individuals can learn what it means to be excellent practitioners of that practice, responsive to objective standards outside themselves against which their achievements and failures can be measured, and in which vices can be recognized.

Second, any adequate moral approach must take into account what it is to be human, what it means to be frail and embodied, and what is appropriate for a creature of this sort. In other words, whatever human excellence comes to, it is always, and necessarily, tied to inescapable features of our bodies and our lives. This alone gives bioethicists a good reason to treat illness narratives as important sources of ethical insight into the nature and implications of our embodiment. Consequently, we cannot just say anything we want about human excellence; as Knight puts it, for MacIntyre, it is by "locating his own concept of value within the metaphysical scheme of traditional Aristotelianism . . . [that he is] able to find a non-relativistic measure for moral claims."[38]

Practices, MacIntyre argues, should not be confused with a set of technical skills. While practices do require us to exercise technical skills, these "skills are transformed and enriched by these extensions of human powers and by that regard for its own internal goods which are partially definitive of each particular practice, or type of practice."[39] It follows from this that, while someone who engages in a practice only for the sake of the external goods the practice can confer can develop these skills to some degree, he can never develop them to the same extent, or in the same way, as someone who becomes committed to the achievement of internal goods, and is transformed by them, will be. A philosophy student who only takes courses because she wants the credits may do enough work to pass, but self-reflexivity and all that comes with it will never become part of her personal style. A physician who engages in the practice of medicine for the sake of money and prestige, no matter how technically skilled, will never be as good a physician as one who treats patients in a way consistent with the internal goods of medicine, caring for their well-being, and ensuring that they are treated as persons, not as disease conditions. A bioethicist, no matter how clever, who wants to be a trusted advisor because of the professional recognition and personal prestige that result will never become a gadfly or watchdog.

Practices must also be contrasted with institutions. While practices, (such as chess, philosophy, and medicine) are sustained by institutions (such as chess clubs, universities, and hospitals), the latter are concerned with external goods, the goods of efficiency, in a way that the former are not. Institutions, necessarily, "are involved in acquiring money and other material goods; they are structured in terms of power and status, and they distribute money, power, and status as rewards."[40] Institutions and practices, then, require one another, but their relationship is inescapably conflictual. Although practices need institutions, the goods internal to practices are usually oppositional to the external goods the attainment of which institutions understand as their primary purpose: while philosophy professors may challenge the imperatives of global capitalism in their classes, the universities within which they are employed and their classes housed need money from students, governments, and sometimes private donors as well, if they are to continue to exist.

However, institutions need practices, and individuals who engage in them primarily for the sake of the internal goods they confer, if they are not to become corrupt and, ultimately, something other than what they purport to be, and for the sake of which they exist in the first place. A university which limits academic freedom because private donors might be offended by what is said may still grant degrees, but, in an important sense, has ceased to be a university, and a hospital which focuses on lucrative research at the expense of patient care, will eventually, if this trend goes unchecked, be unrecognizable as a hospital.

It is not only that institutions can become corrupt that is important, however, it is also that they can become corrupting: because they have the power to bestow prestige, money, power, and recognition (all external and competitive goods), the goods of efficiency can sometimes, for some people, outweigh the goods of excellence. As Burns observes, "in every social institution there is a conflict or tension between those individuals who identify with the underlying practice (the institution as perhaps it *ought* to be) and these individuals who identify with the institution as it is: a conflict which is paralleled by the different patterns of motivation, namely, duty and virtuous conduct on the part of the practitioners and self-interest (money, status, and power) on the part of the institution's 'managers.'"[41] To which I would add: the conflict between the goods of excellence and the goods of efficiency can lead to internal conflict as well, at least until one has fully internalized internal goods and become shaped by them, particularly in institutions which have already become, or are in the process of becoming, corrupt. In such institutions, for those who are not fully immersed in practices, external goods are likely to appear attractive and compelling.

We are now in a position to begin to evaluate the state of contemporary bioethics, as we have been considering it in this book, and as, most recently, we saw it described by Elliot. Given the framework of practices and the tension between internal and external goods that results from our participation in them, does the desire of bioethicists to become trusted advisors indicate that bioethics has become corrupt? That individual ethicists have been corrupted, led astray by the allure of money and professional recognition, and even a misguided sense of honor? It is clear that bioethics contains many features that are recognizable parts of practices: an extensive body of literature, an educational program, a set of skills practitioners need to master, and institutional spaces in which those skills can be developed and exercised. One way, then, to understand the state of contemporary bioethics is to see it as a corrupted practice, one in which the internal goods have become subordinate to the external goods of money, power, and professional recognition. As a consequence, it has become increasingly unclear what the internal goods of bioethics are, and how we might come to recognize and achieve them.

We are now in a position to consider in more detail what bioethics might look like if we consider it as a practice. What might it mean to *be* a bioethicist, in the sense of being shaped by an internalization of a set of goods internal to a practice? If the creation myth of bioethics tells us that bioethics was developed in order to challenge unethical activities in medicine and medical research in order to protect the interests of the weak and vulnerable, to ask hard questions about the moral assumptions and institutional policies that allowed these activities to take place, and to help persons live better when sick or dying, we can use these goals to identify the *telos*, the particular goods at which bioethical activities should be directed. Given these goals, what moral commitments are required of the virtuous bioethicist, and how might these commitments be reflected in the activities in which he engages?

BIOETHICS AS PRACTICE

Bioethics, as we have seen, was initially developed by outsiders, who were motivated to challenge what they saw as unethical activities in medicine and medical research because of the effects these activities had on those who were weak and vulnerable, and who were, consequently, unable to protect their own interests. When philosophers became bioethicists, they brought with them a knowledge of ethical theories, the ability to identify and critique epistemic and metaphysical beliefs that went largely unnoticed by others working in the field, and they connected moral commitments to larger political, economic, and social structures. As outsiders, their status within the world of medicine was unclear, but their ability to observe what was taking place there was largely uncontaminated by the desire to preserve the professional status that is enjoyed by insiders. Ironically, it is the very success that bioethics has enjoyed and that has allowed bioethicists to take a respected place alongside those whose activities they would once have analyzed rather than participated in that creates a genuine dilemma for bioethicists who wish to critique the practices they have now become an important part of: how can one challenge those who are responsible for allowing one to gain entry into these privileged spaces without being perceived as being so personally difficult that it would be better if someone else took one's place? Conversely, if one refuses to enter into these places for fear of being co-opted, and deliberately remains an outsider, how can one be heard, let alone taken seriously? It is the journey from the ivory tower to the bedside that, paradoxically, transforms the philosopher into someone whose bioethical views should be taken seriously and makes him someone who has very little of ethical significance to say.

Given the place of practices within institutions, the creative tension that exists between internal and external goods, and the way in which internal goods transform those who engage in practices for the sake of those goods, it is through practices, I believe, that bioethicists can find a way to reconstruct bioethics on a virtuous foundation. In this section, I will identify the internal goods that bioethics conceived of as a teleologically-oriented practice would inculcate in its practitioners; the epistemic and moral commitments a bioethicist needs to make to have access to these internal goods, and to further develop and extend them; and the place of courage, justice, and honesty in the exercise of their role. Finally, as an application of this approach, I will consider how a bioethicist who works within the framework provided by virtue ethics might respond to the activities of the pharmaceutical industry detailed in Elliot's account.

While the external goods conferred by participation in practices are largely the same regardless of what practice one is engaged in, and consist of prestige, money, social recognition, and power, the internal goods conveyed by practices are often unique, and only accessible through participation in *this* particular practice rather than *that* one. Usually, when we consider practices, the internal goods can be identified relatively easily. In the case of philosophy, for example, the internal goods include a willingness to question everything, even one's own deepest beliefs, to identify and explore ideas, and to become familiar with the work of others who also call themselves philosophers; in the case of chess, appreciation for the strategic intricacies of the game and the intellectual agility required to master them; and, in the case of medicine, a desire to heal the sick and to relieve the suffering of those facing illness and death.

When it comes to bioethics, however, identifying the internal goods is surprisingly difficult: they must be unique to bioethics, not simply a duplication in a new setting of the internal goods conveyed by the practice of philosophy, or a new application of the internal goods of medicine. The difficulty of identifying these internal goods is related to the fact that bioethics has become procedurally, rather than teleologically, oriented. However, if the purpose of bioethics is conceived, as I have argued it should be, to challenge powerful persons and interests in medicine and medical research for the sake of the weak and vulnerable who cannot make these challenges themselves, and to ask hard questions about ideas and activities that would otherwise go unnoticed, then the internal goods of bioethics must include, at least in part, a willingness to ensure that decisions made in a medical or research context are not merely institutionally efficient or medically effective but also morally sound, and to make the places within which bioethicists exercise their role ethically better than they would otherwise be, even when attempts to achieve these goals come at some personal cost. While these internal goods sound banal, consider, for a moment, how unusual it is for ethicists to have any public role or to receive any social or professional recognition, let alone enjoy the possibility of being perceived as trusted advisors to the powerful. If ethicists fail to make a positive difference to medical and research settings, given the prestige bioethicists currently enjoy, it is unlikely that they will make a difference anywhere.

In addition, while bioethicists should seek to protect autonomy and to facilitate its exercise, the account Elliot provides of the manipulative and deceptive strategies employed by the pharmaceutical industry and endorsed by bioethicists demonstrates why a conception of autonomy that takes articulated choices as givens, as evidence of what individuals genuinely want, is utterly inadequate: we need also to ensure that choices are not the result of such deceptive and manipulative practices, and that they enhance well-being and not merely self-interest.

Finally, the social and economic context within which possibilities are identified and converted into choices is not simply relevant to a consideration of whether or not a choice was autonomously made, but absolutely crucial:

unless homeless alcoholics have an adequate range of morally sound options from which to choose, their decision to participate as paid guinea pigs cannot be conceived of as a fully autonomous choice, even if the appropriate informed consent forms were signed. Likewise, the choice of an impoverished farmer in the Third World to sell his kidney in order to feed his family, while perhaps freely made in the sense that no one else forced him to engage in this transaction, cannot be defended on the ground that it was autonomously chosen. The issue here is not whether or not these individuals were capable, cognitively speaking, of giving such consent or engaging in an economic exchange of this sort; even if they were, if the context within which their consent was given or the transaction was made makes only *this* choice appear reasonable, rational, or even possible, it is disingenuous at best and deceptive at worst to claim that these choices are ethically justified because they were freely chosen.

It follows from this that bioethicists working within the framework provided by virtue ethics must pay a great deal of attention to economic, political, and social structures, in order to identify whether they enhance or inhibit the ability of human beings to flourish. Neo-Aristotelian virtue ethics can be radically revolutionary, not despite its emphasis on human flourishing, but because of it; the concept of flourishing provides a measure against which social, political, economic, and institutional structures can be evaluated because it tells us that structures should be changed (not overnight, perhaps, but over time) so that impediments to human flourishing are removed. We don't need to spell out in elaborate detail all the components of what flourishing consists in to recognize that many of our current structures are falling short; as Hursthouse observes, when we look at the way in which many human beings presently live, it would be absurd to claim that most are flourishing,[42] and it is not difficult to think of practical ways in which their circumstances could be improved.

We refuse to make changes that would create the circumstances in which more people might flourish, not because we cannot agree on what flourishing consists in (no one could plausibly argue, for instance, that it consists in working for very low wages in unsafe garment factories, in struggling to find clean drinking water, or in being a homeless alcoholic), but because we think that measures to address impediments to human flourishing would be too costly or politically unworkable. An important task for bioethicists working within a virtue-based ethical framework, then, is to ensure that the arguments they make contribute to the creation of increased opportunities to flourish, and, conversely, to be self-consciously aware that the arguments they present can be a mechanism through which oppressive, manipulative, and exploitative structures are legitimated and maintained.

In order to function as a virtuous bioethicist, those who take on this role must balance their commitment to the internal goods of bioethics against the temptations offered by the external ones; in order to do this, they must carry with them the epistemic commitments of the gadfly and the moral commitments of the watchdog; and they must be honest when making their moral judgments, courageous when expressing them since their views might make them unpopular, and must work to fight against the deceptions, manipulations, and injustices they encounter in the course of their work. From the perspective of bioethics conceived of as a practice, it is inconceivable that defending the rights of researchers rather than protecting the health and safety of research subjects could be seen as an adequate position for a bioethicist to take, let alone the most convincing one; that a bioethicist would be willing to use his expertise to help a pharmaceutical company market its products; or that he could be so procedurally focused that he could ignore the social and economic circumstances within which individuals make choices, as long as informed consent forms have been signed.

TRADITIONS: SITUATING OURSELVES IN TIME, SPACE, AND HISTORY

While we develop the virtues through our participation in practices, and exercise them as our lives play out, all practices are shaped by the particular stage they have reached, and all lives are lived against a particular historical backdrop that generates certain possibilities and excludes others. As MacIntyre puts it, we are "never able to seek for the good or exercise the virtues only *qua* individuals."[43] Even the same conception of the good life would be lived differently by individuals who possess a similar set of virtues, in different circumstances: "What the good life is for a fifth-century Athenian general will not be the same as it was for a medieval nun or a seventeenth century farmer."[44] All of us, moreover, have different social identities: we are someone's son or daughter, cousin or uncle; we work in particular jobs; we live in particular places; we create obligations to specific people as we make commitments to them; we have spouses and children; and so on. What is good for us, MacIntyre asserts, has to be what is good for someone who inhabits those roles. The givens of my life, the things I cannot avoid and must, therefore, make sense of, include "what I inherit from the past of my family, my city, my tribe, my nation, a variety of debts, inheritances, rightful expectations and obligations,"[45] and it is these things, in part, that "gives my life its own moral particularity."[46]

We should notice that all these things, of course, are things that Rawls asks us to forget as we go behind the veil, and it follows from this that, if the liberal conception of autonomy which follows allows us to achieve a self that remains detached from these sorts of particularities, any conception of autonomy derived from MacIntyre's approach could not be so detached. However, it is important to note that, while these particularities are inescapable (our lives start from somewhere, are enmeshed with the lives of particular others), MacIntyre asserts that we can, in our search for the good, move towards the universal: "the fact that the self has to find its moral identity in and through its membership in communities such as those of the family, the neighborhood, the city, and the tribe does not entail that the self always has to accept the moral *limitations* of the particularity of those forms of community."[47] In other words, we can always rebel against the identity that is placed upon us.

It follows from the claim that no moral perspectives can exist outside time and place, that we need to determine which of the competing and contesting traditions we ought to situate ourselves in. Which tradition offers us the most coherent, comprehensive, and satisfactory perspective from which to articulate and explore ethical questions? Moreover, given that ethical theories also (as I have argued) assume and employ a conception of the self, which tradition offers us the most satisfactory conception of the self, the one that best meets the requirement that our self-understandings contain resources that help us cope with the challenges, temptations, and dangers we face as we move through our lives, as well as allow us to make sense of our embodied nature and the fact that human beings create social spaces, institutions, and political structures together?

It is the epistemic commitments of the gadfly that help us distinguish between rival conceptual schemes, and a comparison between them that helps us determine their relative adequacies and inadequacies. It is through our continual willingness to question our beliefs in light of new evidence that we discover which of our beliefs can be justified; however, these explorations always take place from within the framework provided by some particular tradition. Traditions, like practices, are not static: they progress, they sometimes fail, and they change over time in response to new evidence and shifting social structures. It is against the concept of the requirements of justification, however, that the claims of a particular tradition can be measured: "Progress within a tradition of enquiry must involve progress in that tradition's ability to explain reality, and a tradition always faces the possibility of running into an epistemological crisis in which its protagonists find that their scheme is no longer adequate to explain its objects."[48] Traditions, then, function as a sophisticated version of the Nuerathian procedure identified by Hursthouse as a means of testing elements of our conceptual scheme, even though we can't find a neutral place outside it against which its claims can be measured.

While we can't find a neutral place that is external to any and all traditions of moral inquiry, we can compare traditions to one another, in order to see their strengths and weaknesses more clearly. MacIntyre, of course, argues that the Aristotelian tradition is the most adequate tradition available to us, and I am making a case for his contemporary articulation of the resources it contains. In the moral geography of revolutionary Aristotelianism, then, tradition plays a dual role. It both provides a moral framework within which practices engaged in by selves who see their moral explorations as taking place within the context of a tradition can flourish in an Aristotelian sense—living lives that are oriented towards a teleological conception of the good, and characterized by the exercise of the virtues—*and* it provides the most adequate tradition available to us when compared to its competitors. Traditions, then, mirror practices in the following way: they can be pushed in new directions, they develop over time, draw on the past, and, if successful, will continue into the future, and as simultaneous participants in both practices and traditions, we can learn what it is that they come to, which possibilities they make available and which they exclude, and we are, in this engagement, both shaped by our participation, and, potentially, persons who can further develop the practice or extend the scope of the tradition.

But traditions have boundaries, even if where those boundaries should be drawn can be a topic of discussion and even disagreement. An approach that tries to absorb too many traditions, in an attempt to avoid choosing among them, becomes incoherent. Arguably (and this is the case that I have been making), bioethics is just such an incoherent approach, because it tries to draw on too many incompatible (and, perhaps in some instances, incommensurable) traditions (and traditions which are incompatible and incommensurable because, as I have argued throughout this book, they disagree on something as fundamental as the conception of the self around which they revolve).

The hope of principle-based bioethics, of course, was that it could find a neutral viewpoint outside of particular traditions of moral enquiry by abstracting principles (and sometimes values) from competing perspectives and then asserting that they can be discovered in something called a "common morality." In practice, the result has been a bioethics which is largely focused on procedural questions, and which makes extensive use of a conception of autonomy drawn from the liberal self-moral-political framework that detaches the value of choice from any questions about the value of the things chosen. However, this approach is not neutral, and even its assertion that if we embrace a value-free conception of autonomy and can get our procedures correct, the correct answers will follow (which is, of course, an instantiation of the claim that the right is prior to the good), itself presents a substantive moral position. This emphasis on procedures, that is to say, is itself predicated on a substantive claim about the way in which political and social institutions should be constructed, and what form ethical questions should take, and needs to be defended in the same manner as other substantive moral claims are defended.

This emphasis on procedures helps explain why so many bioethicists are satisfied when, for example, informed consent forms are signed by homeless alcoholics, or when competent persons agree to buy and sell kidneys: if we presume that it is the right procedures that ensure that the good is done, then, indeed, no further questions about exploitation or power, for instance, need to be asked. However, from the perspective of revolutionary Aristotelianism, the liberal self-moral-political framework, supplemented by principles and culminating in the endorsement of the Choosing Self, not only does not provide a neutral perspective from which moral questions can be asked and answered, it is, rather, a perspective which predisposes us to see *only* certain things as morally relevant (and, consequently, to understanding only some activities to be morally problematic), and the activities that it considers to be morally acceptable are those things which are taken for granted within a market-driven society.

Revolutionary Aristotelianism holds that the "rationality of liberalism is institutionalized in capitalism, as is that of bourgeois political economy. Their rationalities are actualized in what they legitimate and the actuality that they legitimate is rationalized by them."[49] Furthermore, these concepts "are not, as their protagonists often imagine them to be, heuristic or normative ideals existing apart from their social actuality. Rather, they are parts of that actuality. They inform and motivate action, and therefore they inform and actualize the social relations that are constituted by and reproduced in human action. Theory and actuality are therefore mutually reinforcing."[50] Consequently, that is to say, for a bioethicist to reach the conclusion that a Phase 1 clinical trial that uses homeless alcoholics as test subjects using the framework of mainstream bioethics for this judgment is not to reach some impartial and simply rational moral conclusion; it is, rather, to help create a world in which such things are possible, and in which moral questions that might be thought both central and essential from another moral perspective become difficult, if not impossible, to ask, let alone take seriously.

The case I am making, then, is that bioethics can *neither* make the case that it somehow taps into a "common morality" that transcends all actual and particular moral traditions, *nor* that it can simply extract the bits of competing moral perspectives that it likes (for example, extract from Kant's ideas the concepts of autonomy and rights, but detach them from his claims about duty, or remove the cost-benefit calculations of the utilitarian from the utilitarian commitment to organizing entire societies on the basis of utilitarian principles); rather, bioethicists need to recognize that they have no choice but to situate themselves inside a tradition of moral enquiry, and that, when they do so, certain trade-offs have to be made. The case that I have made is that a neo-Aristotelian virtue ethics, informed by feminist concerns about gender and power, which understands narratives as important sources of information about the ethical life, and which is oriented around a conception of autonomy that connects the value of autonomy to the value of the things chosen, and which evaluates social practices and institutions on the basis of whether or not they provide the conditions in which we can flourish, can serve this function better than its competitors.

CONCLUSION: THE FUTURE OF BIOETHICS

Unless bioethics shifts its focus, it risks losing credibility, and will end up (in a final paradox) being seen as nothing more than a handmaiden and apologist for all the kinds of activities within medicine and society which it once (proudly) saw itself as fighting against. The move from outsider to insider may have allowed bioethics to gain increased public recognition, and provided a number of individual bioethicists with professional opportunities and recognition, but the more ethicists move "from critic of the machine to loyal servant,"[51] the less reason there is for anyone to listen to or trust what they have to say. The more bioethicists understand themselves to be insiders, and the more they are seen by patients, members of the general public, and health care professionals to be nothing more than individuals who justify rather than challenge the role played in health care by corporations, and who see the role of bioethics as little more than providing ostensibly ethical arguments in support of allowing business considerations to enter every sphere of human social activity, the less respect anyone will have for them. The reason that bioethicists still enjoy a large degree of success, and can find an audience willing to listen to their arguments, results from the importance of the values which led to the creation of bioethics in the first place, and from the belief that bioethicists are still committed to them, and willing to fight for them. As soon as this belief becomes demonstrably false, and is widely recognized as such, the claims made by bioethicists will be seen as having little more merit than those made by advertisers or corporate lobbyists. And if that happens, then the bioethicist's services will no longer be needed because, from the perspective of the powerful, their presence no longer lends legitimacy to the activities they want to engage in, while, from the perspective of the weak and vulnerable, not only do they have little to contribute, but they have also cynically used the language of ethics to justify activities which are ethically unjustifiable.

However, it is only from a perspective external to mainstream bioethics that a case like this can even be made, because, as we have seen, mainstream bioethics often assumes precisely what it ought to question. While feminist approaches offer powerful external critiques, and might reach similar conclusions about the state of contemporary bioethics, I have argued that some form of neo-Aristotelianism, informed by the insights of feminist approaches, is the most powerful external perspective currently available to us. It incorporates narrative insights, is as concerned with the exercise of power as feminist perspectives are, and, because it is built on a framework of virtue ethics, it allows us to address the appropriate place of emotions in ethics, as well as to use the language of virtue, vice, and moral excellence.

Finally, it presents a framework within which individuals can explore what it means to be gendered, embodied, and frail creatures, whose lives often face unexpected and difficult challenges, and who can make sense of the *peripeteia* by placing these challenges within the context of a whole life in which the virtues serve as resources that can be called upon when danger threatens. In short, it is capable of addressing the concerns raised in these other approaches, while encompassing more than they do. For those who care about bioethics, who believe that the problems in medicine and research that prompted its contemporary incarnation were serious and, in many respects, still with us but are no longer being adequately addressed as bioethicists increasingly embrace the role of trusted advisor, neo-Aristotelianism offers a comprehensive scheme from which new questions can be asked, old assumptions challenged, and new conclusions at least provisionally reached. The Situated Self that lies at the heart of this approach, placed as it is within practices, narratives, and tradition, offers both an account of excellence which individuals can employ as they think about their own lives, and a perspective from which social, political, and medical institutions can be examined and evaluated.

NOTES

1. Thomas May, *Bioethics In A Liberal Society: The Political Framework Of Bioethics Decision Making* (Baltimore: Johns Hopkins University Press, 2002), 116.
2. Carl Elliot, *White Coat, Black Hat: Adventures On The Dark Side Of Medicine* (Boston: Beacon Press, 2010), xi.
3. Elliot, *White Coat, Black Hat*, xi.
4. Arthur Caplan and David Magus, quoted in Elliot, *White Coat, Black Hat*, 152.
5. Elliot, *White Coat, Black Hat*, 146.
6. Elliot, *White Coat, Black Hat*, 170.
7. Elliot, *White Coat, Black Hat*, 170.
8. Elliot, *White Coat, Black Hat*, 170.
9. Elliot, *White Coat, Black Hat*, 170.
10. For example, Radcliffe-Richards et al. argues that "In general . . . the poorer a potential vendor, the more likely it is that the sale of a kidney will be worth whatever risk there is. If the rich are free to engage in dangerous sports for pleasure, or dangerous jobs for high pay, it is difficult to see why the poor who take the lesser risk of kidney selling for greater rewards perhaps saving relatives' lives or extricating themselves from poverty and debt should be thought so misguided as to need saving from themselves." Janet Radcliffe-Richards, A.S. Daar, R.D. Guttmann, R. Hoffenberg, I. Kennedy, M. Lock, R.A. Sells, N. Tilney, and the International Forum for Transplant Ethics, "The Case For Allowing Kidney Sales," in *Intervention and Reflection: Basic Issues In Medical Ethics*, ed. Ronald Munson, 8th ed. (Belmont, CA: Thomson-Wadsworth, 2008), 486. To assume that the poor seller and the rich buyer meet as equal parties in this transaction is to ignore, to an astonishing degree, the economic context within which it takes place—an economic context that, indeed, many political philosophers might argue is itself worthy of ethical analysis.
11. John Harris, *Enhancing Evolution: The Ethical Case For Making Better People* (Princeton: Princeton University Press, 2007), 28–29.

12. Harris, *Enhancing Evolution*, 38

13. Harris, *Enhancing Evolution*, 38.

14. Elliot, *White Coat, Black Hat*, 146.

15. Alasdair MacIntyre, "How Aristotelianism Can Become Revolutionary: Ethics, Resistance, and Utopia," in *Virtue and Politics: Alasdair MacIntyre's Revolutionary Aristotelianism*, ed. Paul Blackledge and Kelvin Knight (Notre Dame, Indiana: University of Notre Dame Press, 2011), 11.

16. MacIntyre, "How Aristotelianism Can Become Revolutionary," 11.

17. MacIntyre, "How Aristotelianism Can Become Revolutionary," 12.

18. MacIntyre, "How Aristotelianism Can Become Revolutionary," 12.

19. MacIntyre, "How Aristotelianism Can Become Revolutionary," 13.

20. MacIntyre, "How Aristotelianism Can Become Revolutionary," 13.

21. MacIntyre, "How Aristotelianism Can Become Revolutionary," 13–14.

22. Knight, *Aristotelian Philosophy*, 106–107.

23. Alasdair MacIntyre, "Where We Were, Where we Are, And Where We Need To Be," in *Virtue and Politics: Alasdair MacIntyre's Revolutionary Aristotelianism*, ed. Paul Blackledge and Kelvin Knight (Notre Dame, Indiana: University of Notre Dame Press, 2011), 311.

24. Sante Maletta, "MacIntyre and the Subversion Of Natural Law," in *Virtue and Politics: Alasdair MacIntyre's Revolutionary Aristotelianism*, ed. Paul Blackledge and Kelvin Knight (Notre Dame, Indiana: University of Notre Dame Press, 2011), 183.

25. Maletta, "The Subversion of Natural Law," 183.

26. Maletta, "The Subversion of Natural Law," 187.

27. MacIntyre, "Where We Were," 309.

28. Alasdair MacIntyre, *Dependent Rational Animals: Why Humans Need The Virtues* (Chicago: Open Court, 1999), 4.

29. MacIntyre, *After Virtue*, 187.

30. MacIntyre, *After Virtue*, 190.

31. MacIntyre, *After Virtue*, 188.

32. MacIntyre, *After Virtue*, 188–189.

33. Knight, *Aristotelian Philosophy*, 149.

34. MacIntyre, *After Virtue*, 1901.

35. Todd May, *Our Practices, Our Selves: Or, What It Means To Be Human* (University Park, Pennsylvania: The Pennsylvania State University Press, 2001), 23.

36. MacIntyre, *After Virtue*, 191.

37. MacIntyre, *After Virtue*, 192.

38. Knight, *Aristotelian Philosophy*, 151.

39. MacIntyre, *After Virtue*, 193.

40. MacIntyre, *After Virtue*, 194.

41. Tony Burns, "Revolutionary Aristotelianism? The Political Thought Of Aristotle, Marx, and MacIntyre," in *Virtue and Politics: Alasdair MacIntyre's Revolutionary Aristotelianism*, ed. Paul Blackledge and Kelvin Knight (Notre Dame, Indiana: University of Notre Dame Press, 2011), 47.

42. Rosalind Hursthouse, *On Virtue Ethics* (Oxford: Oxford University Press, 1999), 223.

43. MacIntyre, *After Virtue*, 220.

44. MacIntyre, *After Virtue*, 220.

45. MacIntyre, *After Virtue*, 220.

46. MacIntyre, *After Virtue*, 220.

47. MacIntyre, *After Virtue*, 221.

48. Knight, *Aristotelian Philosophy*, 194.

49. Knight, *Aristotelian Philosophy*, 106.

50. Knight, *Aristotelian Philosophy*, 106–107.

51. Elliot, *White Coat, Black Hat*, 170.

Bibliography

Ackrill, J. L. *Aristotle the Philosopher.* Oxford: Clarendon Press, 1981.

Agar, Nicholas. *Liberal Eugenics: In Defense of Human Enhancement.* Oxford: Blackwell, 2004.

Andolsen, Barbara Hilkert. "Care and Justice as Moral Values For Nurses In An Era Of Managed Care." Pp. 41-68 in *Medicine and the Ethics of Care*, edited by Diana Fritz Cates and Paul Lauritzen. Washington, DC: Georgetown University Press, 2001.

Aristotle. *Aristotle's Nichomachean Ethics.* Trans. Robert C. Bartlett and Susan D. Collins. Chicago: University of Chicago Press, 2011.

Arras, John D. "Nice Story, But So What? Narrative and Justification In Ethics." Pp. 65-88 in *Stories And Their Limits: Narrative Approaches To Bioethics*, edited by Hilde Lindemann Nelson. New York: Routledge, 1997.

Barry, Susan R. *Fixing My Gaze: A Scientist's Journey Into Seeing In Three Dimensions.* New York: Basic Books, 2009.

Bartlett, Robert C., and Susan D. Collins. "Introduction." Pp. vii-xiv. *Aristotle's Nichomachean Ethics.* Trans. Robert C. Bartlett and Susan D. Collins. Chicago: University of Chicago Press, 2011.

Beauchamp, Tom L. "A Defense of the Common Morality." *Kennedy Institute of Ethics Journal* 13, no. 3 (September 2003): 219-230.

Beauchamp, Tom L., and James F. Childress. *Principles of Biomedical Ethics.* 4th ed. New York: Oxford University Press, 1994.

———. *Principles of Biomedical Ethics.* 6th ed. New York: Oxford University Press, 2009.

———. *Principles of Biomedical Ethics.* 7th ed. New York: Oxford University Press, 2012.

Berlin, Isaiah. "Two Concepts of Liberty." Pp. 15-25 in *Liberalism and Its Critics*, edited by Michael Sandel. New York: New York University Press, 1984.

Blatchford, Christie. "Chemo Begins, Public Campaign Continues," *Globe and Mail*, March 15, 2011. 7(A).

Blackburn, Simon. *Being Good.* New York: Oxford University Press, 2001.

Blackledge, Paul, and Kelvin Knight, eds. *Virtue and Politics: Alasdair MacIntyre's Revolutionary Aristotelianism.* Notre Dame, Indiana: University of Notre Dame Press, 2011.

Blackwell, Tom. "Squalling Life After Death," *National Post*, March 9, 2009.

Boetkes, Elisabeth, and Wilfrid J. Waluchow. *Readings in Healthcare Ethics.* Peterborough, Ontario: Broadview Press, 2000.

Booth, Wayne C. *The Company We Keep: An Ethics Of Fiction.* Berkeley: University of California Press, 1998.

Brand-Ballard, Jeffrey. "Consistency, Common Morality, and Reflective Equilibrium." *Kennedy Institute of Ethics Journal* 13, no. 3 (September 2003): 231-258.

Brannigan, Michael C., and Judith A. Boss. *Healthcare Ethics in a Diverse Society.* Mountain View, CA: Mayfield Publishing Company, 2001.

Brock, Dan W. "Voluntary Active Euthanasia." Pp. 391-392 in *Biomedical Ethics,* 4th Ed., edited by Thomas A. Mappes and David DeGrazia. New York: McGraw-Hill, Inc., 1996.

Brody, Howard. "Who Gets To Tell The Story? Narrative In Postmodern Bioethics." Pp. 18-30 in *Stories And Their Limits: Narrative Approaches To Bioethics,* edited by Hilde Lindemann Nelson. New York: Routledge, 1997.

Bruner, Jerome. "Narratives of Human Plight: A Conversation With Jerome Bruner." Pp. 3-9 in *Stories Matter: The Role of Narrative in Medical Ethics,* edited by Rita Charon and Martha Montello. New York: Routledge, 2002.

Buchanan, Allen, Dan W. Brock, Norman Daniels, and Daniel Wikler. *From Chance To Choice: Genetics and Justice.* New York: Cambridge University Press, 2000.

Burns, Tony. "Revolutionary Aristotelianism? The Political Thought Of Aristotle, Marx, and MacIntyre." Pp. 35-53 in *Virtue and Politics: Alasdair MacIntyre's Revolutionary Aristotelianism.* Edited by Paul Blackledge and Kelvin Knight. Notre Dame, Indiana: University of Notre Dame Press, 2011.

Callahan, Daniel. "Universalism & Particularism Fighting To A Draw." *Hastings Center Report* 30, no. 1 (Jan.-Feb. 2000): 37-44.

———. "Individual Good and Common Good: A Communitarian Approach." *Perspectives In Biology and Medicine* 46, no. 4 (Autumn 2003): 496-507.

———. "Bioethics and Ideology. " *Hastings Center Report* 36, no. 1 (Jan-Feb. 2006): 3.

Callahan, Sidney. "The Psychology of Emotion and the Ethics of Care." Pp. 141-161 in *Medicine and the Ethics of Care,* edited by Diana Fritz Cates and Paul Lauritzen. Washington, DC: Georgetown University Press, 2001.

Camenisch, Paul F. "Communities of Care, of Trust, and of Healing." Pp. 234-269 in *Medicine and the Ethics of Care,* edited by Diana Fritz Cates and Paul Lauritzen. Washington, DC: Georgetown University Press, 2001.

Carel, Havi. *Illness: The Cry Of The Flesh.* Stocksfield Hall: Acumen, 2008.

Carrithers, Michael. *Why Humans Have Cultures: Explaining Anthropology and* Social *Diversity.* Oxford: Oxford University Press, 1992.

Cassell, Eric J. *The Nature of Suffering and the Goals of Medicine.* 2nd ed. Oxford: Oxford University Press, 2004.

Cates, Diana Fritz, and Paul Lauritzen, eds. *Medicine and the Ethics Of Care.* Washington, DC: Georgetown University Press, 2001.

Chambers, Tod. "What To Expect From An Ethics Case (And What It Expects Of You)." Pp. 171-184 in *Stories And Their Limits: Narrative Approaches To Bioethics,* edited by Hilde Lindemann Nelson. New York: Routledge, 1997.

———. *The Fiction of Bioethics: Cases As Literary Texts.* New York: Routledge, 1999.

———. "Centering Bioethics." *Hastings Center Report* 30, no. 1 (Jan-Feb 2000): 22-29.

Chambers, Tod, and Kathryn Montgomery. "Plot: Framing Contingency And Choice In Bioethics." Pp. 77-84 in *Stories Matter: The Role Of Narrative In Medical Ethics,* edited by Rita Charon and Martha Montello. New York: Routledge, 2002.

Charon, Rita, and Martha Montello, eds. *Stories Matter: The Role Of Narrative In Medical Ethics.* New York: Routledge, 2002.

Christman, John. *The Inner Citadel: Essays On Individual Autonomy.* New York: Oxford University Press, 1989.

———. *The Politics of Persons: Individual Autonomy and Socio-Historical Selves.* Cambridge: Cambridge University Press, 2009.

Cohen, Richard M. *Blindsided: Lifting a Life Above Illness: A Reluctant Memoir.* New York: Harper Collins Publishers, 2004.

———. *Strong At the Broken Places: Voices of Illness, A Chorus of Hope.*

Coutts, Matthew. "Mother's Age Raises Ethical Concerns," *National Post,* Feb. 11, 2009.

Crimmins, Cathy. *Where Is the Mango Princess? A Journey Back From Brain Injury.* New York: Vintage Books, 2000.

Daniels, Norman. *Just Health Care.* Cambridge: Cambridge University Press, 1985.

————.*Just Health: Meeting Health Needs Fairly.* New York: Cambridge University Press, 2008.

Davis, Dena S. "Genetic Dilemmas and the Child's Right to an Open Future." Pp. 337-346 in *Intervention and Reflection: Basic Issues In Medical Ethics*, 8th Ed., edited by Ronald Munson. Belmont, CA: Thomson-Wadsworth, 2008.

DeGrazia, David. "Common Morality, Coherence, and the Principles of Biomedical Ethics." *Kennedy Institute of Ethics Journal* 13, no. 3 (September 2003): 219-230.

Donchin, Anne, and Laura M. Purdy, eds. *Embodying Bioethics: Recent Feminist Advances.* Lanham, MD: Rowman & Littlefield, 1999.

Drabble, Margaret. *The Witch of Exmoor.* San Diego: Harcourt Brace & Company, 1998.

Duffin, Jackalyn. *History of Medicine.* Toronto: University of Toronto Press, 2004.

Dworkin, Gerald. *The Theory and Practice Of Autonomy.* Cambridge: Cambridge University Press, 1988.

Dworkin, Ronald. "Liberalism." Pp. 113-143 in *Public and Private Morality*, edited by Stuart Hampshire. Cambridge: Cambridge University Press, 1978.

Dworkin, Ronald. *Life's Dominion: An Argument About Abortion, Euthanasia, and Individual Freedom.* New York: Vintage Books, 1994.

Eberl, Jason T. and Kevin S. Decker. *Star Trek and Philosophy: The Wrath of Kant.* Chicago: Open Court, 2008.

Elliot, Carl. *A Philosophical Disease: Bioethics, Culture and Identity.* New York: Routledge, 1999.

————. *Better Than Well: American Medicine Meets the American Dream.*New York: W.W. Norton & Company, 2003.

————. *White Coat, Black Hat: Adventures on the Dark Side of Medicine.* Boston: Beacon Press, 2010.

Fitterer, Robert J. *Love and Objectivity In Virtue Ethics: Aristotle, Lonergan, and Nussbaum on Emotions and Moral Insight.* Toronto: University of Toronto Press, 2008.

Fitzpatrick, Petya, and Jackie Leach Scully. "Introduction To Feminist Bioethics." Pp. 1-22 in *Feminist Bioethics: At The Center, On The Margins*, edited by Jackie Leach Scully, Laurel E. Baldwin-Ragaven, and Petya Fitzpatrick. Baltimore: The Johns Hopkins University Press, 2010.

Frank, Arthur W. *The Wounded Storyteller: Body, Illness, and Ethics.* Chicago: The University of Chicago Press, 1995.

————. *At the Will Of the Body: Reflections On Illness.* Boston: Houghton Mifflin, 2002.

————. *The Renewal Of Generosity: Illness, Medicine, and How To Live.* Chicago: The University Of Chicago Press, 2004.

————. *Letting Stories Breathe: A Socio-Narratology.* Chicago: The University Of Chicago Press, 2010.

Freeman, John M., and Kevin McDonnell. *Tough Decisions: Cases In Medical Ethics.* New York: Oxford University Press, 2001.

Fox, Renee C., and Judith P. Swazey. *Observing Bioethics.* New York: Oxford University Press, 2008.

Gawande, Atul. *Complications: A Surgeon's Notes on an Imperfect Science.* New York: Metropolitan Books, 2002.

Gilligan, Carol. *In A Different Voice.* Cambridge, Massachusetts: Harvard University Press, 1982.

Glannon, Walter. *Contemporary Readings In Biomedical Ethics.* Orlando, FL: Harcourt College Publishers, 2002.

Gudorf, Christine E. "The Need For Integrating Care Ethics Into Hospital Care: A Case Study." Pp. 69-101 in *Medicine and the Ethics of Care*, edited by Diana Fritz Cates and Paul Lauritzen. Washington, DC: Georgetown University Press, 2001.

Gunter, Lorne. "Cheat Nature, But On Your Own Dime," *National Post*, Feb. 11, 2009.

Hardwig, John. "Autobiography, Biography, and Narrative Ethics." Pp. 50-64 in *Stories And Their Limits: Narrative Approaches To Bioethics*, edited by Hilde Lindemann Nelson. New York: Routledge, 1997.

Hare, R. M. "Medical Ethics: Can The Moral Philosopher Help?" Pp. 49-61 in *Philosophical Medical Ethics: Its Nature and Significance,* edited by S. F. Spicker and H. T. Englehardt, Jr. Dordrecht: Kluwer, 1977.

Harris, John. *Enhancing Evolution: The Ethical case For Making Better People.* Princeton: Princeton University Press, 2007.

Held, Jacob M. "'The Rules of Acquisition Can't Help You Now': What Can The Ferengi Teach Us About Business Ethics?" Pp. 117-128 in *Star Trek and Philosophy: The Wrath of Kant,* edited by Jason T. Ebel and Kevin S. Decker. Chicago: Open Court, 2008.

Held, Virginia. *The Ethics Of Care.* Oxford: Oxford University Press, 2006.

Holmes, Helen Bequaert. "Closing The Gap: An Imperative For Feminist Bioethicists." Pp. 45-64 in *Embodying Bioethics: Recent Feminist Advances,* edited by Anne Donchin and Laura M. Purdy. Lanham: Rowman & Littlefield Publishers, 1999.

Hursthouse, Rosalind. *On Virtue Ethics.* Oxford: Oxford University Press, 1999.

Jonsen, Albert R. and Stephen Toulmin. *The Abuse of Casuitry: A History of Moral Reasoning.* Berkeley: University of California Press, 1988.

Kamm, F. M. "A Right To Choose Death?" Pp. 186-190 in *Contemporary Issues In Bioethics,* edited by Tom L. Beauchamp and LeRoy Walters. 6th Edition. Belmont, CA: Thomson-Wadsworth, 2003.

Kant, Immanuel. *Foundations of the Metaphysics of Morals.* Ed. R obert Paul Wolff, Indianapolis: Bobbs-Merrill Educational Publishing, 1969.

———."Our Duties To Animals." Pp. 377-378 in *Contemporary Moral Problems,* edited by James B. White. 8th ed. Belmont, CA: Thomson-Wadsworth, 2006.

Kearney, Richard. *On Stories.* London: Routledge, 2002.

King, Thomas. *The Truth About Stories.* Toronto: House of Anansi Press, 2003.

Kleinman, Arthur. *The Illness Narratives: Suffering, Healing, and the Human Condition.* New York: Basic Books, 1988.

———.*What Really Matters: Living A Moral Life Amidst Uncertainty and Danger.* Oxford: Oxford University Press, 2006.

Knight, Kelvin. *Aristotelian Philosophy: Ethics and Politics From Aristotle To MacIntyre.* Cambridge: Polity Press, 2007.

———. "Revolutionary Aristotelianism." Pp. 20-34 in *Virtue and Politics: Alasdair MacIntyre's Revolutionary Aristotelianism,* edited by Paul Blackledge and Kelvin Knight. Notre Dame, Indiana: University of Notre Dame Press, 2011.

Kymlicka, Will. *Liberalism, Community, and Culture.* Oxford: Clarendon Press, 1989.

Laidlaw, Stuart. "Fund IVF, Experts Urge Governments," *Toronto Star,* Feb. 11, 2009.

Lakoff, George. *The Political Mind.* New York: Viking Penguin, 2008.

Lear, Jonathan. *Happiness, Death, and the Remainder of Life.* Cambridge, Massachusetts: Harvard University Press, 2000.

Lindemann, Hilde. *An Invitation To Feminist Ethics.* New York: McGraw Hill, 2006.

Lloyd, Genevieve. "Individuals, Responsibility, and the Philosophical Imagination." Pp. 112-123 in *Relational Autonomy: Feminist Perspectives On Autonomy, Agency, and the Social Self,* edited by Catriona Mackenzie and Natalie Stoljar. New York: Oxford University Press, 2000.

Macedo, Stephen. *Liberal Virtues.* Oxford: Clarendon Press, 1990.

MacIntyre, Alasdair. *After Virtue.* Notre Dame, Indiana; University of Notre dame Press, 1984.

———. *Whose Justice? Which Rationality?* Notre Dame, Indiana: University of Notre Dame Press, 1988.

———. *Three Rival Versions of Moral Enquiry: Encyclopaedia, Genealogy, and Tradition.* Notre Dame, Indiana: University of Notre Dame Press, 1990.

———. *Dependent Rational Animals: Why Human Beings Need the Virtues.* Chicago: Open Court, 1999.

———. "How Aristotelianism Can Become Revolutionary: Ethics, Resistance, and Utopia." Pp. 11-19 in *Virtue and Politics: Alasdair MacIntyre's Revolutionary Aristotelianism,* edited by Paul Blackledge and Kelvin Knight. Notre Dame, Indiana: University of Notre Dame Press, 2011.

———. "Where We Were, Where We Are, And Where We Need To Be." Pp. 307-334 in *Virtue and Politics: Alasdair MacIntyre's Revolutionary Aristotelianism.* Edited by Paul Blackledge and Kelvin Knight. Notre Dame, Indiana: University of Notre Dame Press, 2011.

Mackenzie, Catriona. "Imagining Oneself Otherwise." Pp. 124-150 in *Relational Autonomy: Feminist Perspectives On Autonomy, Agency, and the Social Self,* edited by Catriona Mackenzie and Natalie Stoljar. New York: Oxford University Press, 2000.

Mackenzie, Catriona, and Natalie Stoljar, eds. *Relational Autonomy: Feminist Perspectives On Autonomy, Agency, and the Social Self.* New York: Oxford University Press, 2000.

———. "Introduction: Autonomy Refigured." Pp. 3-31 in *Relational Autonomy: Feminist Perspectives On Autonomy, Agency, and the Social Self,* edited by Catriona Mackenzie and Natalie Stoljar. New York: Oxford University Press, 2000.

Maletta, Sante. "MacIntyre and the Subversion Of Natural Law." Pp. 177-194 in *Virtue and Politics: Alasdair MacIntyre's Revolutionary Aristotelianism.* Edited by Paul Blackledge and Kelvin Knight. Notre Dame, Indiana: University of Notre Dame Press, 2011.

Mappes, Thomas, and David DeGrazia, eds. *Biomedical Ethics* 4th Ed. New York: McGraw-Hill, 1996.

May, Thomas. *Bioethics In A Liberal Society: The Political Framework of Bioethics Decision Making.* Baltimore: The Johns Hopkins University Press, 2002.

May, Todd. *Our Practices, Our Selves: Or, What It Means To Be Human.* University Park, Pennsylvania: The Pennsylvania University Press, 2001.

McGinn, Colin. *Ethics, Evil, and Fiction.* Oxford: Clarendon Press, 1997.

Mill, J.S. *Utilitarianism, On Liberty, and Considerations on Representative Government.* ed. H.B. Acton. London: Dent, 1972.

———. Mill, J. S. *On Liberty.* London: Dent, 1984.

Misak, Cheryl. "ICU Psychosis and Patient Autonomy: Some Thoughts From the Inside." *Journal of Medicine and Philosophy* 30: (2005): 411-430.

Mullhall, Stephen, and Adam Swift. *Liberals and Communitarians.* Oxford: Blackwell, 1992.

Munson, Ronald, ed. *Intervention and Reflection: Basic Issues In Medical Ethics.* 8th ed. Belmont, CA: Thomson-Wadsworth, 2008.

Murphy, Julien S. "Should Lesbian Couples Count As Infertile Couples? Anti-lesbian Discrimination in Assisted Reproduction." Pp. 103-120 in *Embodying Bioethics: Recent Feminist Advances,* edited by Anne Donchin and Laura M. Purdy. Lanham: Rowman & Littlefield Publishers, 1999.

Murray, Thomas H. *The Worth of a Child.* Berkeley: University of California Press, 1996.

———. "What Do we Mean By 'Narrative Ethics'?" Pp. 3-17 in *Stories And Their Limits: Narrative Approaches To Bioethics,* edited by Hilde Lindemann Nelson. New York: Routledge, 1997.

Naponen, Niko. "Alienation, Practices, and Human Nature: Marxist Critique in MacIntyre's Aristotelian Ethics." Pp. 97-111 in *Virtue and Politics: Alasdair MacIntyre's Revolutionary Aristotelianism,* edited by Paul Blackledge and Kelvin Knight. Notre Dame, Indiana: University of Notre Dame Press, 2011.

Nehamas, Alexander. *The Art Of Living: Socratic Reflections From Plato To Foucault.* Berkeley: University of California Press, 1998.

Neiman, Susan. *Moral Clarity: A Guide For Grown-Up Idealists.* Orlando: Harcourt, 2008.

Nelson, Hilde Lindemann, ed. *Stories and Their Limits.* New York: Routledge, 1997.

———. "Context: Backwards, Sideways, and Forward." Pp. 39-47 in *Stories Matter: The Role Of Narrative In Medical Ethics,* edited by Rita Charon and Martha Montello. New York: Routledge, 2002.

Nicholas, Barbara. "Strategies For Effective Transformation." Pp. 239-252 in *Embodying Bioethics: Recent Feminist Advances,* edited by Anne Donchin and Laura M. Purdy. Lanham: Rowman & Littlefield Publishers, 1999.

Noddings, Nel. *Caring: A Feminine Approach To Ethics and Moral Education.* 2nd ed. Berkeley: University of California Press, 2003.

Nussbaum, Martha C. *Love's Knowledge: Essays on Philosophy and Literature.* New York: Oxford University Press, 1990.

Oberle, Kathleen, and Shelly Raffin Bouchal. *Ethics in Canadian Nursing Practice.* Toronto: Pearson-Prentice Hall, 2009.

O'Neil, Brendan. *Spiked* online, at http://www.spiked-online com/index phn?/site/printable/ 6172/. (Accessed Feb. 12, 2009).

O'Neil, Onora. *Autonomy and Trust in Bioethics.* Cambridge: Cambridge University Press, 2002.

Orenstein, Peggy. *Waiting For Daisy: A Tale of Two Continents, Three Religions, Five Infertility Doctors, An Oscar M , an Atomic Bomb, a Romantic Night, and One Woman's Quest To Become A Mother.* New York: Bloomsbury, 2007.

Pence, Gregory E. *Who's Afraid of Human Cloning?* Lanham, MD: Rowman & Littlefield, 1998.

———. *Classic Cases In Medical Ethics: Accounts Of The Cases And Issues That Define Medical Ethics.* 5th ed. Boston: McGraw-Hill, 2008.

Picard, Andre. "Denying Herceptin Was A Necessary Evil," *Globe and Mail*, March 17, 2011, 1(A).

Plato. *Apology* in *Four Texts On Socrates*, trans. Thomas G. West and Grace Starry West. Ithaca: Cornell University Press, 1984.

Professor, X. *In The Basement Of the Ivory Tower.* New York: Viking Penguin, 2011.

Purdy, Laura M. *Reproducing Persons: Issues In Feminist Bioethics.* Ithaca: Cornell University Press, 1996.

Rachels, James. *The Elements of Moral Philosophy.* 2nd ed. New York: McGraw-Hill, 1993.

Radcliffe-Richards, Janet, A.S. Daar, R.D. Guttmann, R. Hoffenberg, I. Kennedy, M. Lock, R.A. Sells, N. Tilney, and the International Forum for Transplant Ethics. "The Case For Allowing Kidney Sales." Pp. 484-487 in *Intervention and Reflection: Basic Issues In Medical Ethics*, edited by Ronald Munson, 8th ed. Belmont, CA: Thomson-Wadsworth, 2008.

Rawls, John. *A Theory of Justice.* Cambridge, Massachusetts: The Belknap Press of Harvard University Press, 1971.

———. *Political Liberalism.* New York: Columbia University Press, 1993.

Raz, Joseph. *The Morality of Freedom.* Oxford: Clarendon Press, 1986.

Rehmann-Sutter, Christoph. "'It Is Her Problem, Not Ours': Contributions of Feminist Ethics To The Mainstream." Pp. 23-44 in *Feminist Bioethics: At The Center, On The Margins*, edited by Jackie Leach Scully, Laurel E. Baldwin-Ragaven, and Petya Fitzpatrick. Baltimore: The Johns Hopkins University Press, 2010.

Reich, Warren Thomas. "The Word 'Bioethics': The Struggle Over Its Earliest Meanings." *Kennedy Institute of Ethics Journal* 5, no. 1 (1995): 19-34.

Robertson, John A. *Children of Choice: Freedom and the New Reproductive Technologies.* Princeton, New Jersey: Princeton University Press, 1994.

Rorty, Richard. *Consequences of Pragmatism.* Minneapolis: University of Minnesota Press, 1982.

———. *Contingency, Irony, and Solidarity.* Cambridge: Cambridge university Press, 1989.

Rosenstand, Nina. *The Moral of the Story: An Introduction To Ethics.* 5th ed. New York: McGraw-Hill, 2006.

Ross, Lainie Friedman. "The Child as Research Subject." Pp. 149-162 in *Contemporary Readings In Biomedical Ethics*, edited by Walter Glannon. Orlando, FL: Harcourt College Publishers, 2002.

Sandel, Michael J. *Liberalism and the Limits of Justice.* Cambridge: Cambridge University Press, 1982.

Savulescu, Julian. "Procreative Beneficence: Why We Should Have The Best Children." Pp. 320–326 in *Intervention and Reflection: Basic Issues In Medical Ethics*, 8th Ed., edited by Ronald Munson. Belmont, CA: Thomson-Wadsworth, 2008.

Schafer, Arthur. "The Case For Postmenopausal Mothers," *Globe & Mail*, Feb. 9, 2009.

Schneider, Susan, ed. *Science Fiction and Philosophy: From Time Travel To Superintelligence.* Oxford: Wiley-Blackwell, 2009.

Scully, Jackie Leach, Laurel E. Baldwin-Ragaven, and Petya Fitzpatrick, eds. *Feminist Bioethics: At The Center, On The Margins.* Baltimore: The Johns Hopkins University Press, 2010.

Shalof, Tilda. *The Making Of A Nurse.* Toronto: McClelland & Stewart, 2007.

Sherwin, Susan. *No Longer Patient: Feminist Ethics & Health Care.* Philadelphia; Temple University Press, 1992.

Singer, Peter. "All Animals Are Created Equal." Pp. 379-387 in *Contemporary Moral Problems*, edited by James B. White. 8th ed. Belmont, CA: Thomson-Wadsworth, 2006.

———. *AIDS and Its Metaphors.* New York: Picador, 1988.

Spicker, S.F., and H.T. Englehardt, Jr. eds. *Philosophical Medical Ethics: Its Nature and Significance.* Dordrecht: Kluwer, 1977.

Swanton, Christine. *Virtue Ethics: A Pluralistic View.* Oxford: Oxford University Press, 2003.

Talisse, Robert B. *On Rawls: A Liberal Theory of Justice and Justification.* Belmont, CA: Wadsworth, 2001.

Taylor, Charles. *Sources of the Self: The Making of the Modern Identity.* Cambridge, Massachusetts: Harvard University Press, 1989.

Tessman, Lisa. *Burdened Virtues: Virtue Ethics For Liberatory Struggles.* Oxford: Oxford University Press, 2005.

Thiroux, Jacques. *Ethics: Theory and Practice.* 5th ed. Englewood Cliffs, New Jersey: Prentice-Hall, 1995.

Tomlinson, Tom. "Perplexed About Narrative Ethics." Pp. 123-133 in *Stories And Their Limits: Narrative Approaches To Bioethics*, edited by Hilde Lindemann Nelson. New York: Routledge, 1997.

Turner, Leigh. "Zones of Consensus and Zones of Conflict: Questioning the 'Common Morality' Presumption In Bioethics." *Kennedy Institute of Ethics Journal* 13, no. 3 (September 2003): 193-218.

Vacek, Edward Collins, S.J. "The Emotions of Care in Health Care." Pp. 105-140 in *Medicine and the Ethics of Care*, edited by Diana Fritz Cates and Paul Lauritzen. Washington, DC: Georgetown University Press, 2001.

Vaughn, Lewis. *Bioethics: Principles, Issues, and Cases.* Oxford: Oxford University Press, 2010.

Walker, Margaret Urban. *Moral Understandings: A Feminist Study In Ethics.* 2nd ed. Oxford: Oxford University Press, 2007.

Warnock, Mary. *An Intelligent Person's Guide To Ethics.* London: Duckworth Outlook, 1998.

Warren, Mary Ann. "On the Moral and Legal Status of Abortion." Pp. 114-125 in *Contemporary Moral Problems* edited by James E. White. 8th ed. Belmont, CA: Thomson-Wadsworth, 2006.

West, Thomas G., and Grace Starry West, trans. *Four Texts On Socrates.* Ithaca: Cornell University Press, 1984.

White, Becky Cox, and Joel A. Zimbelman. *Moral Dilemmas In Community Health Care: Cases and Commentaries.* New York: Pearson Longman, 2005.

Wolf, Susan M., ed. *Feminism & Bioethics: Beyond Reproduction.* New York: Oxford University Press, 1996.

———. "Erasing Difference: Race, Ethnicity, and Gender in Bioethics." Pp. 65-81 in *Embodying Bioethics: Recent Feminist Advances*, edited by Anne Donchin and Laura M. Purdy. Lanham: Rowman & Littlefield Publishers, 1999.

Index